# LIFESTYLE WELLNESS COACHING

## Second Edition

**James Gavin, PhD**

**Madeleine Mcbrearty, PhD**

CONCORDIA UNIVERSITY

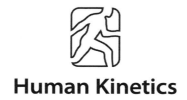

**Human Kinetics**

**Library of Congress Cataloging-in-Publication Data**

Gavin, James, 1942-
  Lifestyle wellness coaching / James Gavin, Madeleine Mcbrearty. -- 2nd ed.
    p. ; cm.
  Includes bibliographical references and index.
  I. Mcbrearty, Madeleine, 1948- II. Title.
  [DNLM: 1. Physical Fitness--psychology. 2. Health Promotion. 3. Teaching--methods. QT 255]

  613.7'1--dc23
                            2012025291

ISBN-10: 1-4504-1484-2 (print)
ISBN-13: 978-1-4504-1484-5 (print)

This book is a revised edition of *Lifestyle Fitness Coaching,* published in 2005 by Human Kinetics, Inc.

The web addresses cited in this text were current as of October 2012, unless otherwise noted.

**Acquisitions Editor:** Amy N. Tocco; **Developmental Editor:** Melissa J. Zavala; **Assistant Editors:** Kali Cox, Casey Gentis, and Amy Akin; **Copyeditor:** Alisha Jeddeloh; **Indexer:** Nan Badgett; **Permissions Manager:** Dalene Reeder; **Graphic Designer:** Fred Starbird; **Graphic Artist:** Dawn Sills; **Cover Designer:** Keith Blomberg; **Photograph (cover):** Ben Blankenburg/iStockphoto; **Art Manager:** Kelly Hendren; **Associate Art Manager:** Alan L. Wilborn; **Illustrations:** ©Human Kinetics; **Printer:** Victor Graphics

Printed in the United States of America    10  9  8  7  6  5  4  3  2  1

The paper in this book is certified under a sustainable forestry program.

**Human Kinetics**
Website: www.HumanKinetics.com

*United States:* Human Kinetics
P.O. Box 5076
Champaign, IL 61825-5076
800-747-4457
e-mail: humank@hkusa.com

*Canada:* Human Kinetics
475 Devonshire Road Unit 100
Windsor, ON N8Y 2L5
800-465-7301 (in Canada only)
e-mail: info@hkcanada.com

*Europe:* Human Kinetics
107 Bradford Road
Stanningley
Leeds LS28 6AT, United Kingdom
+44 (0) 113 255 5665
e-mail: hk@hkeurope.com

*Australia:* Human Kinetics
57A Price Avenue
Lower Mitcham, South Australia 5062
08 8372 0999
e-mail: info@hkaustralia.com

*New Zealand:* Human Kinetics
P.O. Box 80
Torrens Park, South Australia 5062
0800 222 062
e-mail: info@hknewzealand.com

E5536

# CONTENTS

# PREFACE

Anyone affiliated with health, wellness, and fitness professions over the past few decades is not only aware of the exponential growth of career opportunities in these areas but also of the fundamental shifts in the needs and patterns of client populations. Lifestyles have changed dramatically, and along with these changes, profound opportunities and challenges for health, wellness, and fitness professionals have arisen. Clients' work schedules have become increasingly unpredictable with the 24–7 demands characteristic of many careers. Family structures have been affected so much that the concept of the nuclear family is largely anachronistic. Inventions such as smart phones have irreversibly influenced how we communicate and how we live. The ubiquity of Internet access and services has simultaneously simplified and complicated modern life. For instance, it's easier than ever to obtain expert information regarding healthy eating, exercising, or stress reduction, yet the capacity people have for sustaining health-promoting practices appears to be diminishing. A case in point is weight management: Statistical reviews related to obesity and overweight conditions in the Western world are typically prefaced by such terms as *epidemic* and *perilous*.

The adage "Information is power" represents only part of the dynamic influencing human behavior change. In the early 20th century, the reigning paradigm, based in Freudian psychology, was that if people become aware of how they behave and if they begin to appreciate the deleterious consequences of their actions, then they will readily adopt more appropriate behaviors. We now know that this is at best a partial truth. Most Westerners are aware when their weight reaches unhealthy levels. They know when they are insufficiently active, sleeping too little, and eating poorly. They easily identify when they are overly stressed. Moreover, they are also likely to know the steps they need to take to align themselves better with healthy living practices. So, why don't they take action if they know better?

To address this question, social scientists have worked tirelessly to produce practical guides enabling people to move toward healthier and balanced lifestyles. Yet, the portraits drawn by various public health agencies seem to reflect downward trends more than population advances in healthy lifestyle practices. Evidently there is no easy answer, and there doesn't seem to be any single magic bullet.

Within the realm of active living, innumerable initiatives have been implemented with marginal results. Westerners remain stubbornly inactive for the most part. Powerful aids to active living are widely available, and people who take advantage of these tools and services generally note improvements. Take, for instance, the value of personal training. People who hire trainers learn how to exercise properly, and they develop satisfying and effective routines. Nonetheless, it is common to hear trainers lament the fact that their clients exercise only when the trainer is present to babysit them.

Many professionals would argue that modern exercise has been defined too narrowly. As jobs became increasingly sedentary in the second half of the 20th century, the need for programmed physical activity became more apparent. The fitness boom, which began somewhere around 1960, reflected societal concerns about an increasing incidence of heart disease and the positive values of programmed exercise. Yet, in the enthusiasm to get people moving, exercise was most often depicted as running, aerobics classes, and other gym-based activities. Though professionals make clear distinctions among active living, physical exercise, and sport, the popular conception of what it means to exercise may unwittingly exclude millions of people who find gym membership undesirable, unaffordable, or otherwise out of reach.

Similarly, other facets of a healthy lifestyle seem too great a reach for an already overstretched population. Working with a naturopath, consulting a nutritionist, or going to a stress reduction program, among other laudable initiatives, may simply be met with inertia in the face of other life demands.

This isn't a pretty picture, yet it is not overdrawn, either. We seem to be at a tipping point, where the evolving norms for living reveal lowered capacities for health maintenance and disease prevention. Typical are the comments of a seasoned physical educator in an urban high school, reflecting on the adjustments she has had to make in her curriculum: "I used to be able to ask the kids to run around the gym a dozen times as a warm-up. Now, I tell them to walk around a couple times—they just can't do it anymore."

# ALONG COMES THE COACH

It was no accident that in 1995, a new professional field was officially inaugurated through the creation of the International Coach Federation (ICF). Life coaching, in particular, created an immediate media buzz as reports of people transforming their lives through coaching abounded. Unprecedented achievements by ordinary people were attributed to work with coaches. As word spread, increasing numbers of people thought this could, at long last, be the answer to realizing their dreams. Was there a gimmick? What did coaches do that was so different from other helping professionals? And who were the clients who would most benefit from coaching?

In its first decade, the coaching field experienced exponential growth largely fueled by the reported success of clients who hired coaches. Coaching was promoted as a process for people who already had achieved success in their lives and who simply wanted to up their game, grow their life, make a dramatic change, or reach for the stars. It was marketed as a stretch profession—not a rehabilitative, psychotherapeutic, talk-talk-talk process. If you wanted to make dreams come true, you should hire a coach, but be ready to pull out all the stops and get into action. Coaches seemed to have strategies to get beyond your *buts*.

Coaches had a new way of working compared with traditional helpers. They desired proof of change almost as much as their clients did. Each meeting had the quality of facing the music. Clients would codesign challenging tasks to complete between meetings and would be held accountable by their coaches. This was not a soft, empathetic, "Yes, I understand why you couldn't" relationship. Coaches accessed a variety of motivations for client change, including the economic kind. Fees for coaching services tended to be steep. Clients would often take a deep breath before signing their coaching contracts because the bottom line would hit them hard in the pocketbook—and that would be particularly difficult to justify if they were just limping along in their change processes.

Almost 20 years after the official starting point of the coaching profession, some things have changed while others remain much the same. Coaching has broadened its appeal to a variety of populations, with most coaches typically expressing niche specializations. You can find coaches for executives on the rocks or entrepreneurs in training. There are relationship coaches, spiritual coaches, and coaches for people with ADHD. Whatever the specialty, virtually every professional coach subscribes to both the methodologies implicit in the ICF's 11 core competencies and to the ICF's code of ethics. If you walk into an office for coaching and leave without a challenging list of things to do before you meet again, most likely you haven't really been coached. Above all else, the task of forwarding the action remains a hallmark of the coaching field. Coaches may gather historical data and listen to your stories, but their eyes are sharply focused on what actions will best enable you to advance toward your dreams.

# COACHING IN THE WORLD OF HEALTH, WELLNESS, AND FITNESS

When the first edition of this book was published in 2005, boundaries around the coaching profession were not as sharply drawn as they are today. The ICF in particular was just gaining momentum as the worldwide governing body for the practice and evolution of coaching. Anyone could call himself a coach, and although that continues to be the case, one's credibility might readily be challenged if a coach is not certified by the ICF. In addition to certification as a professional coach, there are many niches where high-level specialization in the content matter of coaching is required. A case in point is executive coaching, where a coach's knowledge of business and the dynamics surrounding high-level executives is prerequisite to any coaching conversation. A generic "How can I help you reach your dreams?" simply won't cut it in the executive's world of corporate intrigue, buyouts, and hostile takeovers.

Similarly, the domains of health, wellness, and fitness coaching require extensive professional knowledge and practice-based wisdom. Clients who want to lose weight, improve endurance, regain ambulatory capacities, change eating habits, or balance their lives are likely to require some expert input as they move from desire to action. Knowing the current recommendations of federal agencies regarding dietary composition or exercise requirements isn't enough for professionals to help clients design robust and safe change programs. Unfortunately, many clients may seek out coaches known for their success in promoting change, irrespective of their particular expertise. A coach helps someone finish her long-pursued first novel and a friend thinks, "Maybe this coach can help me run a marathon."

Matters of this sort have ethical implications. How can a coach who has no training in exercise science advise a client on how to run a marathon? An ethical coach wouldn't, but she might forward the action by getting her client to hire a technical specialist in running as part of the overall strategy for goal attainment. The role of coach, then, might be understood as that of a master strategist who coinvestigates and codesigns plans and actions with clients, accessing necessary technical support and advice throughout the process of helping them achieve their desired goals.

## BECOMING A COACH VERSUS ADOPTING A COACHING APPROACH

Because you are reading this book, we will assume that you have strong interests in one of the many health, wellness, and fitness careers. We also imagine that you have established some credentials in one or more of these professional domains. However, we do not presume that you are credentialed in the profession of coaching. Coaching can be understood as one of the approaches you use in your work, or it can be the core of your work, that is, your professional specialization. In many health, wellness, and fitness roles, you are expected to be the expert—to tell people what they should do to reach their goals. In coaching there is a place for expertise, yet the manner of bringing expert information into play in the coaching relationship is rarely the primary focus. As much as expertise is required, we believe that coaching currently exists as a prominent new profession partly because expert advice is considered insufficient to bring about lasting behavior change for many clients who are struggling with health, wellness, and fitness issues.

A distinction we wish to make clearly at the outset concerns the difference between a fully certified coach and a professional using a coaching approach. When we set out to write this book, our deepest desire was to offer useful guidance to those who want to embrace coaching as their primary professional service as well as to those whose principal objective is to integrate a coaching approach into their usual ways of working with clients. Whether you want to occasionally apply a coaching approach or become a professional coach, this book will serve you well.

Virtually anyone with education and training in coaching may apply a coaching approach. They might do so in a particular conversation with a friend, family member, associate, or client. Using the methodology of coaching on an ad hoc basis can have significant benefits for the people concerned. This is quite different than contracting with clients for a coaching relationship. In the latter case, we are talking about becoming a coach and making it public that this is one's métier.

We acknowledge that some of you may not be looking for a major reorientation of what you do or how you work with clients. However, keeping abreast of developments in the exciting field of coaching could add value to your efforts. We believe that reading this book will provide you with the necessary knowledge and skills to advance your current practices.

On the other hand, you may want to become a professionally certified coach. Should this be your choice, the material in this book will foster your development. All of the central concepts and theories presented in our book are embedded in the professional coach certification programs that we have offered over the past decade, with the exception of newer material that has only recently been advanced in the field of coaching. Of course, reading this book represents only a portion of the work that you will need to do in order to gain certification through a professional organization such as the ICF. In the early part of the book, we provide you with some practical guidelines for becoming a certified coach.

## ABOUT THIS SECOND EDITION

*Lifestyle Wellness Coaching, Second Edition,* is not a generic coaching book; rather, it is written specifically for those who currently have or are planning for careers in health, wellness, and fitness. The first author, Jim Gavin, has written in the areas of health promotion, exercise, and sport psychology for over 30 years, and he has conducted workshops, seminars, and training programs for health fitness professionals since the early 1980s. The first edition of this book sprang from his passion for and commitment to promoting the careers of health, wellness, and fitness professionals, particularly because dimensions of their work show parallels with the evolving field of professional coaching. This second edition extends his commitment to the development of health, wellness, and fitness career paths by bringing together the extensive changes in the world of professional coaching since the publication of the first edition with the language, orientation, and concerns of health, wellness, and fitness professionals.

The second author, Madeleine Mcbrearty, also has a passionate interest in the domains encompassed by this book, namely, those concerning the promotion of health and well-being. Her recent and highly acclaimed doctoral dissertation details the experiences of obese women confronting the challenges of owning their bodies and reshaping them accordingly. As a professional coach and researcher, she brings extensive knowledge of the vast literature on coaching to the creation of this book. Both authors have collaborated to offer you the best of their personal and professional wisdom about coaching for your present and future career.

Because the second edition represents a thorough revisioning and rewriting of the original book, we debated long and hard about whether to give this book a new title. Ultimately, we chose to change one word in the title. Thus, *Lifestyle Fitness Coaching* became *Lifestyle Wellness Coaching*. While "fitness" may be understood broadly, there is a possibility of interpreting it solely as it pertains to the domain of exercise, sports, and physical education. Surely, this domain is central to healthy living, but it is not the whole of it. Wellness is a more comprehensive concept that encompasses physical, psychological, social, and spiritual health, among other dimensions. Even when professionals are primarily focused within a specific arena of health and wellness promotion, they are profoundly aware of the interrelationship of all health-related behaviors. A fitness specialist would not ignore a client's dietary habits. A nutritionist would be mindful of a client's social world that influences eating patterns. A wellness practitioner would no doubt explore clients' exercise patterns in a stress management program. The common denominator in the realm of *lifestyle wellness coaching* is that the coach or practitioner comes to her work with professional certifications or degrees that attest to her specialized health-related knowledge and expertise. Unlike generic life coaches, a *lifestyle wellness coach* has a specialized niche in which she has been trained and for which she holds professional credentials. Perhaps more

critically, this niche is an expression of her deep interest, if not passionate concern.

The first edition was strongly geared toward people working in sport and fitness, whereas this edition acknowledges the multiplicity of concerns represented in clients' seemingly simple requests for health-related change. "I just want to get back in shape" soon blossoms into a multipronged change process that incorporates aspects of the client's emotional, interpersonal, somatic, mental, and behavioral patterns. We believe that coaching is about the whole person, and consequently we want our book to be relevant to students and practitioners in a wide range of health-related professions.

The framework for this work, *Lifestyle Wellness Coaching*, is not confined to a narrow interpretation of health. Rather, it extends to the boundaries of what it means for modern men and women to experience full-spectrum wellness in their lives. If your profession is based in nutritional or dietary sciences, you will benefit as much from this book as would other health care specialists. If you are a massage therapist or do another kind of bodywork, you will learn important methodologies for your work through these pages. As a wellness professional or professional nurse dealing with clients' adherence to health regimens, life balance, or quality living, you will find that this book can improve your practice as much as it will if you are a health promotion specialist in a clinic or private practice. Of course, this book remains central to all those professionals and students whose expertise is in physical training, sport, and exercise.

Since the first edition's publication in 2005, the ICF has articulated a cogent framework of competencies required for coaching. None of the competencies was entirely new or unexplored, and there were strong similarities between the ICF's presentations and the material described in the first edition. With considerable excitement, we updated and aligned concepts and methods presented in the first edition with the ICF competency template so that readers who wish to go beyond our book into formal coaching coursework can readily make links between our descriptions and those found in the broader literature on coaching. We want our readers to have the most current and accurate map of the coaching field and its terminology. Even for those who only want to incorporate a coaching approach, our intention is to ensure that all readers are conversant with the wider world of coaching and the language that professional coaches employ.

# PLAN FOR THE BOOK

For those who wish to become lifestyle wellness coaches, this book describes essential skills and processes for competent engagement with clients. To facilitate your learning, we often complement our discussions with case studies and scenarios. We also offer suggestions for engaging the material through guided reflections. We strongly believe that these moments of self-reflection are essential for any practitioner involved in helping others. We invite you to consider these as essential tools to reinforce your learning journey.

Because it is important to describe coaching within the theoretical frameworks that have influenced its development, we present a broad overview of the field in chapter 2. We then identify characteristics that, taken together, might help you distinguish coaching from other models of helping. Given that the fields of psychology and adult learning are integral to coaching, we introduce some markers that link coaching to its root disciplines. We conclude the second chapter with an outline of core ingredients necessary for engaging in effective health, wellness, and fitness coaching.

Knowing what clients may think and do at various stages of a change process enables coaches to decide which types of interventions or conversations would best empower them to identify and reach their desired goals. In chapter 3, we introduce two models that will help you guide clients' progression through significant changes. First, we discuss the popular transtheoretical model (TTM) of health-related behavior change (Prochaska, Norcross, & DiClemente, 1994), which maps the change process through six stages that occur over time. This model suggests that when people want to adopt a new behavior, they move from precontemplation, where they have no intention to change; to contemplation, where they become conscious that modifications to their daily habits are necessary; to preparation, where engagement is imminent; to action; and finally to maintenance of the desired behavior. In some cases, people achieve the sixth stage, termination, where they are no longer tempted to revert to their former ways of living. Following our discussion of the TTM, we present several strategies that are effective in producing movement through the phases of change.

The second model presented in chapter 3 is the learning-through-change model (Taylor, 1986). Although its phases parallel those of the TTM, this framework reveals the deeper layers beneath the surface of change. Clients who are catapulted into change may express goals without identifying critical dynamics that may have initiated this process of transformation. Except for whimsical decisions to try something new, the desire to change health behaviors is typically fraught with important personal meanings that are thoroughly captured in the learning-through-change model.

Of course, we would be remiss if we did not also include concepts that are pivotal to behavior change processes, namely, those of self-efficacy (Bandura, 1997), self-regulation (Vohs & Baumeister, 2010), and relapse prevention (Dimeff & Marlatt, 1998; Marlatt & Gordon, 1985; Marlatt & Donovan, 2008). As an effective coach, you will want to investigate the level to which clients believe that they have what it takes to accomplish what they plan to achieve (self-efficacy). You will also want to find out if they have the inner resources to deal with impulses and conflicting yearnings that could distract them from achieving their goal (self-regulation). And because people rarely make plans for significant change without faltering, you will want to ensure that your clients have strategies to manage momentary lapses or a full-blown relapse so they can stay the course in the long run (relapse prevention).

In chapter 4, we provide a road map for coaching. We introduce our flow model of coaching, which can be used equally well for navigating the entire coaching relationship or a single session. In this chapter, we consider how you will require a clear and mutual understanding of what your client wants to achieve. Once this is in focus, you and your client can collaboratively explore patterns, resources, skills, and other elements pertinent to the creation of a solid action plan. When this has been achieved, you will assist your client in committing to and engaging in action. This model also enables you to appreciate the need for celebration when clients assiduously put forth effort to break through old patterns, develop new competencies, access unacknowledged resources, and experiment with new behaviors.

The ICF has worked diligently to articulate standards for the coaching profession, and its list of core competencies delineates not only what effective coaches need to do well but also the communication strategies they might find useful in empowering clients to reach their goals. In chapters 5 through 11, we move deliberately and carefully through each of the ICF core coaching competencies. This material is intended to give you a thorough appreciation for the methodology of coaching and provide practical tools for your emerging practice.

This book brings together the combined wisdom of the old and the new. It encompasses the broader perspectives of the classic helping professions and their teachings in how we have interpreted the field of coaching. As noted, coaching arises from a long lineage of knowledge and practice in assisting human beings as they cope, manage, and grow. To serve readers' evolving careers, we have extracted the most relevant principles and theories and combined them with the new literature on coaching. We have translated ideas that have been applied in other practices, such as counseling and psychotherapy, so they make more sense for coaching clients and their agendas. We have embraced the optimistic, forward-moving slant of coaching while retaining the capacity to delve sufficiently into clients' histories to extract the energy and dynamism for effective change. And we have also acknowledged that, whatever your past work and experiences, your accumulated learning has great relevance to the practice of coaching. We have written this book so you can readily see yourself taking on the manner and methods of a professional coach, and we offer some final reflections on these matters in chapter 12. In the meantime, we wish you profound learning and good progress as you unveil your own unrealized resources, potentialities, and opportunities throughout the upcoming pages.

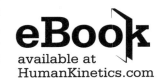

eBook available at HumanKinetics.com

# 1

# INTRODUCTION TO LIFESTYLE WELLNESS COACHING

---

**I**n this chapter, you will learn how...

- health, wellness, and fitness can be optimized through a coaching approach;

- lifestyle wellness coaching, as an action-centered partnership, empowers clients to achieve goals and bring about a desired future; and

- effective coaches accompany their clients as they navigate the uncertainties and emotionality of a change process toward greater health.

---

The living self has one purpose only:
to come into its own fullness of being.

—*D.H. Lawrence*

---

The World Health Organization (WHO) suggests that health is something that can be enjoyed by everyone regardless of physical limitations. Being healthy simply means having the energy to do the things we care about on an everyday basis (Hoeger, Turner, & Hafen, 2007). Health, wellness, and fitness professionals are intimately aware of the interrelationships among health-promoting behaviors such as maintaining a nutritious diet, managing stress, sleeping a sufficient number of hours, and avoiding toxic substances and unsafe practices. They also know that a complete sense of well-being moves along a continuum from optimal wellness to debilitating conditions (see figure 1.1). Wellness presupposes that we endeavor to discover and pursue our life purpose, cultivate fulfilling relationships, engage in meaningful work, seek work–life balance, and care for our environment.

## Health and Wellness

### What Is Health?

In 1946, the WHO defined **health** as "complete physical, mental, and social well-being and not just the absence of disease or infirmity" (p. 1315).

### What Is Wellness?

The WHO definition of health implies that it involves more than physical aspects of well-being. Conse-quently, wellness is often understood as the interaction of seven dimensions: physical, social, emotional, mental, spiritual, occupational, and environmental. To achieve optimal **wellness** and quality of life, a person seeks to move toward the positive side of an illness–wellness continuum on all seven dimensions.

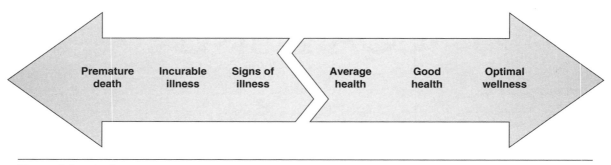

| Premature death | Incurable illness | Signs of illness | Average health | Good health | Optimal wellness |

**Figure 1.1**  The illness–wellness continuum.

## MODERN HEALTH ISSUES

Before we embark on a discussion of how difficult it is to change health-related behaviors, let's look at issues that affect the health and wellness of North Americans:

- Life expectancy at birth is 78.5 years in the United States (Centers for Disease Control and Prevention [CDC], 2012b) and 81.1 years in Canada (Statistics Canada, 2012b).

- Heart disease, cancer, and stroke are the top three causes of death in North America (Murphy, Xu, & Kochanek, 2012; Statistics Canada, 2008). According to the National Center for Health Statistics (NCHS), if all forms of major cardiovascular disease were eliminated, life expectancy could rise by almost 7 years in the United States (CDC, 2009a). Each year, about 250,000 potential years of life are lost in Canada due to cardiovascular disease, including heart attacks and other chronic heart-related conditions (Heart and Stroke Foundation, 2011).

- Eating poorly, being physically inactive, smoking, and drinking too much can prematurely age you by up to 12 years (Lynch, Elmore, & Morgan, 2012).

- In 2011 in the United States, 25.8 million children and adults—8.3% of the population—had diabetes (American Diabetes Association, 2011). In the same year in Canada, 1,793,352 people had diabetes and over 5 million experienced high blood pressure (Statistics Canada, 2012c, 2012e).

- Physical inactivity is a risk factor for developing type 2 diabetes and obesity (CDC, 2011b).

- Three-quarters of American visits to doctors concern stress-related ailments (Mental Health America, 2012). Over 20% of all Americans report extreme stress (American Psychological Association [APA], 2012). The National Institute of Mental Health (NIMH) states that in any given year, approximately one-quarter of American adults (26.2%) are diagnosable for one or more mental disorders (NIMH, 2005).

- In 2009, 10.6% of American men and 3.4% of women were heavy alcohol drinkers (i.e., drinking five or more drinks on the same occasion on each of five or more days in a month). In the same year, 20.1% of all high school seniors used tobacco, 20.6% used marijuana, 1.3% used cocaine, and 2.5% used psychotherapeutic drugs for nonmedical purposes (NCHS, 2011). According to Health

Canada (2010), 10.6% of Canadians aged 15 and over use cannabis, 1.2% use cocaine or crack, 0.9% use ecstasy, 0.6% use psychoactive pharmaceutical drugs to get high, 0.4% use speed, and 0.7% use hallucinogenic drugs. In addition, 5.1% of Canadians surveyed by the organization reported frequent heavy drinking as their usual pattern of alcohol consumption (Health Canada, 2009, 2011).

- At least 2.9% of American adults are either problem gamblers or pathological gamblers in any given year. Studies show that problem drinkers are at increased risk of developing an addiction to gambling (Rehab International, 2012).

Most people know that vegetables make healthier snacks than chocolate bars, that smoking is a leading cause of cancer, that excessive alcohol consumption diminishes health, and that unprotected sex with multiple partners puts them at risk of contracting sexually transmitted infections. Why, then, do people continue to engage in these practices? Why is it that even after consulting with professionals to alter unhealthy habits, people fail to change? And, even when they are successful in their efforts, why is long-term maintenance of change less than guaranteed? We might also wonder why we, as professionals, continually offer people who engage in unhealthy practices more and more information when we typically know they already have the facts?

### REFLECTION 1.1

Pause for a moment and reflect on your own health behaviors. What things do you do that run counter to your accumulated wisdom about actions required for a health-promoting lifestyle? What might be an unwise behavior or practice that you seem to be ignoring? Where might you stretch the limits of accepted standards for healthy living in order to accommodate your current habits?

## PROCESS OF CHANGE

We answer some of the questions just posed through an examination of one component of well-being, namely, participation in **regular physical activity.** Adopting a physically active lifestyle bears strong similarities to other changes that people desire in their pursuit of health and well-being. Such behaviors must be initiated and maintained until one's goals are attained. Then they must be integrated into one's way of life if progress is to be sustained.

Consider for a moment another component of well-being related to healthy weight. If someone resolves to lose weight, he might choose to modify his diet until he reaches a desired weight. During this time, he must initiate new eating habits, self-regulate to stay the course, and use effective strategies to recover from momentary or full-fledged relapses. Once he has reached his target weight, he must continue monitoring food intake to avoid regaining the weight he so painstakingly shed. Unfortunately, as most of us know, our best intentions run an obstacle course in their conversion to desired actions, and they then face other hurdles as we endeavor to make them part of everyday life. Even if the benefits of the positive behaviors are readily apparent, those who have attempted to modify ingrained patterns know that lasting change can be mighty difficult to realize!

## Benefits of an Active Lifestyle

Regular physical activity is a foundational practice that supports a continuing sense of health and wellness. The U.S. Department of Health and Human Services offers recommendations for weekly amounts of physical activity. It recommends that adults between the ages of 18 and 64 accumulate at least 150 minutes of moderate to vigorous physical activity every week in order to be considered physically active. In addition, they should perform muscle-strengthening activities that involve all major muscle groups two or more days per week. It is recommended that children and adolescents (aged 6-17) do at least 60 minutes of physical activity every day (HHS, 2008).

For the vast majority of the population, opportunities to be physically active are both plentiful and potentially exciting. And, on the whole, the benefits of an active lifestyle are commonly understood: Habitual involvement in sport, exercise, and physical activity improves psychological well-being (Miles, 2007); it enhances self-concept (Donaldson & Ronan, 2006) and frequently contributes to better social health (Gümüş, Öz, & Kırımoğlu, 2011). An active lifestyle slows the aging process, increasing longevity (Paffenbarger & Lee, 1998; Walker, Walker, & Adam, 2003) and contributing greatly to quality of life (Bize, Johnson, & Plotnikoff, 2007). In addition, increased physical activity is one of the primary ways to achieve an energy deficit to promote weight loss and curb overweight and obesity (Jakicic, Davis, Garcia, Verba, & Pellegrini, 2010).

**Obesity** is most often defined as excess weight in relation to a person's height (table 1.1). It has been assessed as a risk factor for conditions such as metabolic syndrome (cluster of insulin resistance, dyslipidemia, and hypertension) (Haslam, 2005; Tjepkema, 2004), cardiovascular disease (Field, Barnoya, & Colditz, 2002; Lofgren, Herron, Zern, West, Patalay, Shachter, et al., 2004; Pi-Sunyer, 2002), type 2 diabetes mellitus (Pi-Sunyer, 2004; Rorive, Letiexhe, Scheen, & Ziegler, 2005), and various forms of cancer (Crespo & Arbesman, 2003; Field et al., 2002). The list of potential diseases is even longer, extending as far as premature death (Allison, Fontaine, Manson, Stevens, & VanItallie, 1999; Muennig, Lubetkin, Jia, & Franks, 2006). According to the WHO (1998), "Overweight and obesity are now so common that they are replacing the more traditional public health concerns such as under-nutrition and infectious diseases as some of the most significant contributors to ill health" (p. 17).

In addition to purely physical definitions, obesity is a social construct characterized as body weight beyond the socially accepted norms of attractiveness for specific ethnic and age groups within a given culture (Brownell, 1991; Cooper, 1998). Given the impact of obesity on numerous levels, people who are obese often feel ostracized and discriminated against because of their excess weight (Joanisse & Synnott, 1999; Puhl & Heuer, 2009). They often want to increase their levels of physical activity when they choose to engage in weight-loss efforts.

Worldwide, 1.5 billion adults (20 years and older) were overweight in 2008. Of these, more than 200 million men and nearly 300 million women were obese (WHO, 2012).

In 2009 and 2010, it was estimated that 78 million U.S. adults (35.7%) and 12.5 million adolescents and children (17%) were obese (CDC, 2012a; Ogden, Carroll, Kit, & Flegal, 2012). In Canada, 24% of adults over 18 are obese. Almost 60% of all Canadian adults and 26% of children and adolescents are overweight or obese (Heart and Stroke Foundation, 2011, 2012).

In 2008, the medical costs of obesity in the United States were as high as $147 billion. The average annual medical costs for an obese person were $1,429 more than those of a person of normal weight (CDC, 2012a).

According to the American College of Sports Medicine (ACSM) and the Canadian Medical Association (CMA), between 150 and 250 minutes of moderate-intensity physical activity per week will provide modest weight loss. Greater amounts of physical activity (more than 250 minutes per week) have been associated with clinically significant weight loss. After weight loss, weight maintenance improves with more than 250 minutes per week of physical activity. The CMA also recommends that physical activity and exercise be sustainable and tailored to the individual (Donnelly, Blair, Jakicic, Manore, Rankin, & Smith, 2009; Lau, Douketis, Morrison, Hramiak, Sharma, & Ur, 2007). Less than 20% of obese American adults meet these public health recommendations for physical activity (Young, Jerome, Chen, Laferriere, & Vollmer, 2009).

## Barriers to an Active Lifestyle

As is evident, the benefits of being physically active are numerous. Regardless, fitting exercise into modern lifestyles may be as complex as finding the missing piece in a four-dimensional puzzle when you can only envision three dimensions. While

**Table 1.1 Standard Classification of Body Weight According to Body Mass Index (BMI)**

|  | BMI (kg/m²) |
| --- | --- |
| **Underweight** | <18.5 |
| **Normal** | 18.5-24.9 |
| **Overweight** | 25.0-29.9 |
| **Obesity class I** | 30.0-34.9 |
| **Obesity class II** | 35.0-39.9 |
| **Obesity class III** | ≥40 |

**REFLECTION 1.2**

Based on your experiences with family, friends, or clients, what are some of the reasons you have heard people give for not exercising regularly? Make a list of them and then reflect on this list, exploring the degree to which they make sense to you. As a second step, imagine someone has just offered one of these reasons. What might you say to her as a way of countering her excuse?

some people simply do it, others only want to or perhaps hope they can get by without it. For most of those who don't exercise, something is out of their awareness or beyond their control, resulting in wishes slipping by unfulfilled. As much as they would like to believe their excuses, the reasons why people are inactive are rarely a matter of time, capacity, or comfort. There is something for most every taste, yet for the chronically inactive (see Who Exercises?), regular physical exercise seems forever elusive, unappetizing, or perhaps just the last choice on a long to-do list.

In the final quarter of the 20th century, social scientists talked about the promised land of the **leisure society**; however, this dream state never materialized. We seem to be busier than ever. In meeting the demands of modern life, people appear to be on a grueling flat-out run every day. However, a closer look reveals that many people spend considerable time in pursuits that are optional. This may not always be the case, but it is accurate enough that the relatively stable rate of exercise participation—persistently hovering around 15% to 20% for adults (Smits, Tart, Presnell, Rosenfield, & Otto, 2010) and 25% for adolescents (Katzmarzyk & Ardern, 2004)—might move up a couple deciles if some of that discretionary time got reprioritized. The time excuse is not entirely valid for many reasons: It is the rare Westerner who is working at the extremes of his physical capacities every day. Most people could walk at times when instead they drive. They could trade labor-saving devices for ones that require effort. They could even do sit-ups while watching the evening news. And they might

consider scheduling movement breaks on the hour for standing and stretching. These forms of exercise may seem trivial, but in a world that increasingly structures life as sedentary, small efforts can produce worthwhile benefits.

People offer many reasons other than time for not exercising at levels required for optimal wellness (table 1.2), and these, too, can be deconstructed with relative ease. Reasons such as lack of opportunity, inconvenience, and financial costs, among others, reveal once again a narrow conceptualization of what it means to be physically active. When it comes to transforming a habitual pattern of inactivity, lack of motivation is perhaps an excuse most often viewed as an obstacle. As Prochaska, Norcross, and DiClemente (2002) suggest in their transtheoretical model (TTM), some people have no intention to exercise and seem impervious to the most dramatic inducements to change. Others think about it, try it a few times, and revert to inactivity with an even stronger conviction of their incapacity for or dislike of exercise. **Motivation** (Vallerand, 1997) may well constitute the holy grail for those in health, wellness, and fitness fields (figure 1.2). What can fitness professionals do to help clients discover their internal motivations to pursue enjoyable activities regardless of the benefits they might derive?

In terms of capacity, if someone argues she is physically unable to exercise, you may perceive either a misconception or partial truth. Certainly there are debilitating conditions that preclude much physical exertion, but for most people who have movement restrictions or physically limiting ailments, physiotherapists would strongly argue

## Who Exercises?

In 2009, 49.3% of American adults did not engage in 30 or more minutes of moderate physical activity five or more days per week or vigorous physical activity for 20 or more minutes three or more days per week (CDC, 2009c). Only 19.1% of Americans aged 18 and over met the guidelines for both aerobic activity and muscle strengthening (NCHS, 2011). In recent years, approximately 16% of Americans aged 15 and over participated in sport and exercise activities on any given day (Bureau of Labor Statistics, 2008).

(http://www.apa.org/helpcenter/stress-willpower.pdf)

In Canada, men and women are sedentary for approximately 9.5 of their waking hours. Although 52.1% of Canadians were at least moderately active, 47.8% did not meet the guidelines to be considered moderately active during their leisure time (Statistics Canada, 2010). Men are more likely to be moderately active (54.9%) than women (49.4%). Yet, the number of Canadian men who report that they are moderately active is going down (Statistics Canada, 2010)

Higher levels of education and higher personal income are positively correlated with higher levels of participation in leisure-time physical activity (Statistics Canada, 2009).

## Table 1.2    Incentives and Barriers to Exercise

| Incentives | Barriers |
|---|---|
| Improving or maintaining health and fitness (Carron, Hausenblas, & Estabrooks, 2003) | Internal barriers: Personal beliefs, values, and commitment levels |
| Losing or maintaining weight (Zunker, Cox, Ard, Ivankova, Rutt, & Baskin, 2011) | Interpersonal barriers: Relationships, role conflicts, family demands |
| Enhancing physical appearance (Marquez & McAuley, 2001) | Environmental barriers: Access to facilities, availability of exercise venues, climate (Brinthaupt, Kang, & Anshel, 2010) |
| Developing a fit and athletic social image (Culos-Reed, Brawley, Martin & Leary, 2002; Williams & Cash, 2001) | Other barriers include the following: |
| Experiencing a sense of enjoyment (Henderson & Ainsworth, 2002) and preference (Hill & Hannon, 2008) for a certain sport | Lack of confidence or information regarding proper exercise techniques |
| | Fear that others will see that they are overweight, uncoordinated, or unfit (Culos-Reed et al., 2002) |
| Being with others (Holt, Black, Tamminen, Fox, & Mandigo, 2008) | Misunderstanding of how much they enjoy exercise because of a narrow focus on the unpleasant beginnings of exercise (Ruby, Dunn, Perrino, Gillis, & Viel, 2011) |
| Realizing psychological benefits (Carron et al., 2003; Vallerand & Rousseau, 2001) | Lack of time and interest (Ifedi, 2008, p. 60) |
| | Cost |

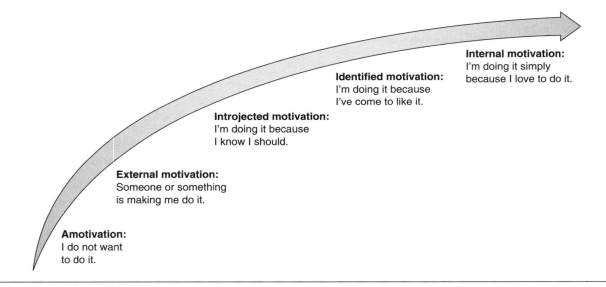

**Figure 1.2**    Motivation continuum.

Adapted from Vallerand 1997.

that they need to do something within a range that is possible for them. Conditions such as **morbid obesity** would seem to pose restrictions on strenuous exertion, but this simply highlights the need to reframe physical activity so that it doesn't always look like an Ironman Triathlon.

Comfort is another matter. After all, physical exercise is by definition stressful; that is, it requires exertion beyond that of sedentary existence. Here,

too, the argument can be seen as a ruse. Movement generally feels good and leaves us psychologically invigorated, though many nonexercisers will argue that their muscles ache when they exercise, or it feels unpleasant to sweat, or they find it emotionally challenging to train in the company of hard bodies at the gym. Their mental model of what exercise is becomes apparent in these arguments. Exercising well beyond one's current capacity will result in sore muscles, moderate- to high-intensity training definitely makes people sweat, and certain gym settings easily lend themselves to unfavorable body comparisons. That said, it's relatively easy to find ways around these objections and even to create joy, if not ecstasy, through physical movement.

To date, the fitness industry has been extraordinarily responsive to the expressed needs of current and potential clients. There are women-only gyms intended to reduce the discomforts women experience when exercising in mixed environments. New techniques, classes, and schedules make access, benefits, and enjoyment more likely. Better instructor training and ever-increasing requirements for fitness professionals enhance client safety and the knowledge base on which clients design their actions. Child care and family programming make regular participation less of a disconnection from the social fabric of clients' lives. Still, there is that fourth dimension referred to earlier—something inactive people cannot quite grasp that interferes with their ability to establish a lifelong connection

to nurturing and sustaining physical activity. To paraphrase Albert Einstein's oft-quoted remark, if people pursue their goals using the same ineffective approaches they have always used, they will continue to reap the same kinds of results—in this context, a failure to sustain an enduring relationship with life-giving patterns and practices.

# COACHING

The premise of this book is that health, wellness, and fitness professionals using a coaching approach can successfully help clients establish resilient bonds to life-promoting practices. Through coaching, they can facilitate clients' access to that fourth dimension, which seems to hold answers to what people need in order to pursue healthy lifestyles.

According to the International Coach Federation (ICF) (2011b), "Coaching is partnering with clients in a thought-provoking and creative process that inspires them to maximize their personal and

## Definitions of *Coach* and *Coaching*

"A coach is a person who facilitates experiential learning that results in future-oriented abilities. . . . [A coach] refers to a person who is a trusted role model, adviser, wise person, friend, mensch, steward, or guide—a person who works with emerging human and organizational forces to tap new energy and purpose, to shape new vision and plans, and to generate desired results. A coach is someone trained in and devoted to guiding others into increased competence, commitment, and confidence." (Hudson, as cited in Stober & Grant, 2006, p. 3)

"Coaching is a catalyzing relationship that accelerates the process of great performance; it's about individuals and/or organizations identifying purpose and living out of that purpose." (Coach U, Inc., 2005, p. 10)

"Masterful coaching is about inspiring, empowering, and enabling people to live deeply in the future while acting boldly in the present." (Hargove, 2008, p. 2)

"[Coaching] is a way of effectively empowering people to find their own answers, encouraging and supporting them on the path as they continue to make important choices." (Kimsey-House, Kimsey-House, & Sandahl, 2011, p. xvi)

"Coaching is unlocking a person's potential to maximize their own performance. It is helping them to learn rather than teaching them." (Whitmore, 1992, p. 8)

Coaching is "that part of a relationship in which one person is primarily dedicated to serving the long-term development of effectiveness and self-generation in the other." (Silsbee, 2010, p. 4)

Coaching is a "collaborative, solution-focused, result-oriented systematic process, used with normal, non-clinical populations, in which the coach facilitates the self-directed learning, personal growth, and goal attainment of the coachee." (Grant, 2003, p. 1)

professional potential." Though there may be as many definitions of coaching as there are authors writing about it (see Definitions of *Coach* and *Coaching*), the ICF's perspective sufficiently captures the essence of this emerging field of human service. Of course, this and other definitions invariably leave you guessing about what has to happen in this partnership so that clients can maximize their potential.

What is it about coaching that holds so much promise for increasing clients' engagement, enjoyment, and lifelong pursuit of healthy lifestyle behaviors? The answer partly lies in how coaching accesses the fourth dimension, or that which is outside our normal perceptions, frameworks, and understanding. Most people have strong self-definitions, which usually include any number of **self-limiting beliefs** such as "I don't have what it takes to succeed," "I always need to be the best," "I must be in control at all times," "I don't deserve to put myself first," "Change is frightening," and so on. These beliefs aren't always wrong or harmful, but they can keep us living within artificial boundaries that block us from appreciating other ways of seeing, doing, and being. In other words, these beliefs can thwart forward movement toward a more desirable or preferred way of living.

Unfortunately, we are not always the best diagnosticians of patterns that keep us stuck, and we do not always choose the most beneficial paths to change. Clients generally hire coaches when their normal success strategies no longer work (Hargrove, 2008) or when they feel trapped in a maze with no evident way out.

Coaches understand the meandering course of change; they appreciate that linear thinking sooner or later leads straight into a wall. No matter how small or how big the client's goal, the whole person is taken into account because even small changes need to be considered in the full context of the client's life. Coaching challenges clients to think outside the box and experiment with manageable steps toward desired outcomes. Skilled coaches, who by definition have mastered critical competencies listed by the ICF (2011c), balance support with challenge. They work collaboratively with clients to make it possible for them to substitute can-do ways for can't-do attitudes. Coaches look beneath the surface; they access unrealized resources for achieving clients' supposedly impossible futures (Hargrove, 2008). They ask unaskable questions. They request that clients dream big and take that longed-for step toward change.

In the early years of the coaching industry, the title *life coach* was prevalent. It had a certain cachet

and paralleled the more traditional helping professions of counseling and psychotherapy, where one hung out a shingle as a psychologist or counselor and waited to see who would walk in the door next and what issues they would present. Coaching has come a long way since its seminal years in the early 1990s. Today, there are innumerable career tracks in the profession. Just as helpers in other professions gravitate to areas where they have accumulated expertise and interest, so have professional coaches increasingly specialized (table 1.3). If you search the websites of professional coaches, you will discover that some prefer to work with women, with business and career issues, with spiritual matters, or with people dealing with major life transitions. It's simply impossible to be an expert in everything.

Clients enter coaching relationships with an agenda to reach certain goals. Even though coaches may apply a generic method or metamodel to their work, clients' topics often require a certain degree of knowledge or expertise beyond coaching. In other words, skill in the process of coaching is a necessary but frequently insufficient condition for effective coaching. For example, when a client is thinking about dramatically altering his eating habits, changing lifestyle patterns, or reorienting physical activities due to injuries or health concerns, knowing what is reasonable, what works best, or how certain health conditions influence the design of action plans becomes highly relevant. These are not matters where coaches can allow clients to formulate goals on their own. Informed guidance is necessary to shape objectives and codesign successful action plans. The fact that a coach has been physically active all of her life does not in itself create the grounds for knowing whether a client's proposed exercise plans are appropriate and likely to produce the desired results. Preferably, a life coach who lacks technical background would team up with a fitness expert and work in tandem with clients who have fitness agendas. However, this life coach would be wise to avoid promoting herself as a lifestyle wellness coach.

Imagine that a woman hires a life coach to help her stick to a rigorous diet that she obtained from a certified nutritionist. The client has never been able to adhere to any sort of program for weight management. The coach's knowledge of the process of change will be invaluable, but ethically speaking, it would be important for the coach to work with the nutritionist and have at least a fundamental appreciation of nutrition and dietary processes. Again, though this coach might be successful in helping clients with weight management and nutrition

**Table 1.3    Sample Coaching Niches**

| Coaching type | Niche |
|---|---|
| Business coaching | Career and career transition coaching<br>Executive and leadership coaching<br>Managerial and supervisory coaching<br>Team coaching<br>Work–life balance coaching<br>Workplace and organizational coaching |
| Personal or life coaching | Transition coaching<br>Conflict resolution coaching<br>Creativity coaching<br>Diversity and culture coaching<br>Emotional intelligence coaching<br>Environmental coaching<br>Family and parenting coaching<br>Financial coaching<br>Lifestyle fitness and personal wellness coaching<br>Mindfulness coaching<br>Relationship coaching<br>Religious coaching<br>Spiritual coaching<br>Student and teacher coaching<br>Youth and at-risk youth coaching<br>ADHD coaching |

changes, unless she pursues content-specific training related to this field, it would not be advisable for her to represent herself as a specialist in weight and nutrition coaching.

# LIFESTYLE WELLNESS COACHING

**Lifestyle wellness coaching** is a coaching specialization that builds on expertise in areas related to health, wellness, and fitness while relying on relevant theories and methods from the coaching field. Lifestyle wellness coaches may work with clients who have specific health, wellness, and fitness goals as well as with clients who have personal or professional goals that can be facilitated through action planning and goal pursuit related to health and wellness.

As described previously, the ICF defines coaching as a partnership that inspires clients to maximize their potential through thought-provoking and creative processes. Lifestyle wellness coaching conforms closely to this definition, adding the requirement that coaches practicing in this area have professional credentials related to the health, wellness, or fitness agendas of their clients. By definition, then, lifestyle wellness coaching is a specialized area within the coaching field. It is an action-centered partnership informed by the coach's expertise in health, wellness, and fitness. Clients are empowered to efficiently realize their goals through inspirational coaching dialogue and creative action planning.

Let's explore this definition further. Lifestyle wellness coaching is a *specialized area within the coaching field* that addresses clients' health, wellness, and fitness as either primary or secondary objectives for the coaching relationship. A client's primary agenda may be to lose weight, or it may be to pursue personal or professional goals that encompass health and lifestyle changes as secondary objectives. An example of a secondary objective can be illustrated by a client who wants to change careers and needs to improve his management of stress, energy levels, and physical presence. Some of the most prevalent client goals in health, wellness, and fitness are as follows:

Achieving and maintaining life balance

Adopting and maintaining an active lifestyle

Decreasing or eliminating unhealthy habits

Dealing effectively with negative addictions

Maintaining healthy eating

Managing stress in all areas of life

Adhering reliably to medically prescribed programs

Incorporating body-centering practices in daily living

Increasing aerobic fitness, muscular fitness, and flexibility

Starting a new exercise routine after a debilitating condition

Training for a sporting event such as a marathon or triathlon

Managing and maintaining appropriate weight

Incorporating mind–body centering practices in daily living

As an *action-centered partnership*, lifestyle wellness coaching moves clients from intention to action and then toward sustainable change. It involves the creation of meaningful goals and the design of viable and robust action plans in areas of health, wellness, and physical fitness. Lifestyle wellness coaching represents a nonhierarchical and collaborative relationship with clear agreements about role relationships and shared responsibilities.

The coach's *expertise* in specific wellness areas informs the coaching dialogue and resultant action planning. A prerequisite to lifestyle wellness coaching is that coaches have professional-level expertise in an area of wellness, health, and physical fitness obtained through academic programs or professional certifications. Lifestyle wellness coaches may have certifications in nutrition counseling or medical backgrounds in nursing, addiction counseling, or other allied health professions. They may have multiple competencies and years of involvement in personal training or specializations within the world of sport and exercise. This is not to say they will act as experts who tell clients what to do. They are coaches, and as the definition indicates, the relationship is a partnership.

The coaching process *empowers clients to efficiently realize their codetermined goals* by creating awareness of inhibiting patterns of behavior and by uncovering strengths, resources, and opportunities thus far unrealized. Effective coaching requires an unwavering commitment by both coach and client to moving forward in action with well-focused, clearly designed, and measurable steps.

*Inspirational coaching dialogue and creative action planning* are at the core of the coaching process. Coaches have an optimistic and appreciative stance toward their clients that fully acknowledges the clients' unrealized capacities and their ability to disengage from self-limiting beliefs and unproductive habits. In addition, coaches work synergistically with clients in a creative process that permits nonlinear and out-of-the-box thinking applied to action planning.

# COMMENTARY

We hope that you now have a better framework for appreciating what lifestyle wellness coaching is and what it is not. If you were to make an appointment with a counselor or therapist for a deeply troubling matter, you would not expect to be told what to do. Rather, you would anticipate a relationship where someone patiently listens, asks good questions, and occasionally interprets the meaning of the experiences you describe. Further, you would probably assume that this relationship would take place over a matter of weeks or months and that you would be required to reliably attend sessions. Finally, you probably would not imagine having to do much in between sessions other than reflect on what you had said and generate thoughts to present in the next session.

Take another scenario. Imagine you are overweight and suffering from fatigue and low energy. You decide to consult a nutritionist. In advance, you are asked to keep a log of your nutritional intake during the week before your appointment. In your first session, the nutritionist reviews your log and asks a wide variety of questions focused on eating patterns and potential causal relations such as the ingestion of certain foods and resultant symptoms. Your nutritionist has a specialization in nutritional supplements and not only gives you a detailed menu to follow but also a number of nutritional supplements to take with your meals. A follow-up meeting is scheduled to take place a couple weeks later. In this second meeting, adherence to the plan is reviewed along with any changes you have noticed. The plan is tweaked and you leave with a follow-up appointment in six weeks.

Finally, let's say that you have been experiencing a lot of work stress and you have completely fallen off the rails in your adherence to any kind of healthy life practices, including exercise, nutrition, stress management, and work–life balance. You decide to consult a lifestyle wellness coach. From what you have read in this chapter, what would you expect to happen? How do you think you would work together? What do you imagine the differences would be in the relationship dynamics with your coach compared with the previous two examples? We leave you with these questions, assuming that you have some beginning responses that will be filled in more completely as you progress through the rest of this book.

The process of coaching involves more than expert advice and compassionate listening. It may contain elements of these approaches yet have a wholly different structure and way of relating to clients. At this early point in the book, it may be hard to fully distinguish all the approaches in coaching from those of other professionals, but by the final page of this book, your understanding of role distinctions will be quite sophisticated. So, please read on.

# 2

# BACKGROUND AND CORE INGREDIENTS OF COACHING

*I*n this chapter, you will learn how...

- the coaching profession came into prominence;

- coaches distinguish themselves from other helping professionals;

- coaching is rooted in the disciplines of psychology and adult education, among others;

- learning styles and human development phases guide effective coaching;

- insight, social support, and a holistic perspective inform coaching relationships; and

- lifestyle wellness coaching differs from other health, wellness, and fitness roles.

> The touch that heals always feels
> and cherishes the other as a unique person.
>
> –*Sam Keen*

The notion of coaching is not entirely new. The word *coach* originally referred to a 16th-century wagon made in Kocs, a Hungarian city between Vienna and Budapest. In the 1800s, *coach* came to mean a tutor or someone who carries a student through a course of study to an exam. Later still, coaching became intricately linked to athletics and sport. Though the term still conjures up images of gymnastics or football coaches, sport coaching is only a small piece of the historical background of coaching (see Historical Landmarks of the Coaching Profession).

Early coaching texts presented the field as something totally new. They used unique terms for techniques, such as *blurting* (Whitworth, Kimsey-House, Kimsey-House, & Sandahl, 2007), and they made little reference to the extant literature of the more traditional helping professions. In our perspective, coaching is strongly rooted in the lineage of the helping professions rather than being an entirely new practice disconnected from the past.

# EVOLUTION OF COACHING

Founders of the coaching field didn't simply armchair-theorize about what people needed; rather, coaching came into prominence because it filled a gap. It embraced the evolution of our modern lifestyles, and it framed ways of helping that fully responded to client needs for forward movement. Present-day coaching is no longer considered devoid of theoretical influences or viewed as simply relying on common sense; its knowledge base includes many arenas of professional endeavor that constitute essential roots of the profession. In addition to studies of psychology and adult learning, these arenas include philosophy, social work, management, motivation, communications, human relations, systems thinking, spirituality, and a myriad of hybrid disciplines (table 2.1).

As the umbrella organization for coaches and coaching schools, the **International Coach Federation (ICF)** came into existence in 1995. Two of the largest coach training organizations at that time, Coach U and the Coaches Training Institute (CTI), were largely responsible for creating the ICF as a community for their graduates and as a regulatory and standards-setting association. Since then, a number of other bodies have appeared on the scene, including the Worldwide Association of Business Coaches in 1997; the Association for Coaching in 2002; the European Mentoring and Coaching Council in 2002; the Association for Supervision, Coaching and Consultancy of Australia and New Zealand in 2002; and the International Association of Coaching in 2003. Even so, the ICF continues to dominate the coaching world. In 1995 there were approximately 200 coaches, whereas currently there are close to 16,000 ICF-certified coaches – one third of the total number of coaches worldwide (ICF, 2012). As well, there is an untold number of unaffiliated coaches, who may or may not have formal training, and who have not been identified in surveys of the field. The coaching profession continues to grow exponentially with a proliferation of innovative methodologies that are disseminated worldwide.

We might question why the coaching field has expanded so significantly. The answer lies partly in the fact that coaching professionals have adapted rapidly to shifts in modern life. Though the frameworks of traditional helping professions often inform coaching, coaches are not hampered by ingrained or hallowed practices and strong traditions. Coaching has taken the best techniques of its root disciplines, coupled them with modern communication strategies and tools, and worked feverishly to prove its mettle. Coaches listened carefully to what people said they needed and then aligned methodologies with the structures of emerg-

## Table 2.1   Major Influences on the Development of Coaching

| Name | Discipline | Decade influence began |
|------|-----------|------------------------|
| Alfred Adler | Psychology | 1920s |
| Martin Heidegger | Philosophy | 1930s |
| Napoleon Hill | Motivation | 1930s |
| Dale Carnegie | Motivation | 1940s |
| Abraham Maslow | Psychology | 1950s |
| Albert Ellis | Psychology | 1950s |
| Carl Jung | Psychology | 1950s |
| Carl Rogers | Psychology | 1950s |
| John Wooden | Sport | 1950s |
| Milton Erickson | Psychology | 1950s |
| Peter Drucker | Business | 1950s |
| Red Auerbach | Sport | 1950s |
| Chris Argyris | Psychology | 1950s |
| Edgar Schein | Business | 1960s |
| Fritz Perls | Psychology | 1960s |
| Ken Blanchard | Business | 1960s |
| Fernando Flores | Philosophy | 1970s |
| John Grinder | Liberal arts | 1970s |
| Peter Block | Business | 1970s |
| Richard Bandler | Psychology | 1970s |
| Werner Erhard | Business | 1970s |
| Zig Ziglar | Motivation | 1970s |
| Wayne Dyer | Motivation | 1970s |
| Robert Dilts | Psychology | 1980s |
| Stephen Covey | Business | 1980s |
| Daniel Goleman | Psychology | 1990s |
| David Cooperrider | Business | 1990s |
| Ken Wilber | Psychology | 1990s |
| Martin Seligman | Psychology | 1990s |
| Mihaly Csikszentmihalyi | Psychology | 1990s |
| Peter Senge | Business | 1990s |

Reprinted, by permission, from V.A. Brock, 2008, *Grounded theory of the roots and emergence of coaching*, 289-290. Available: http://cdn.libraryofprofessionalcoaching.com/wp-app/wp-content/uploads/2011/10/dissertation.pdf

ing lifestyles and work patterns. They realized that the rules were changing—so much so that nothing seemed certain for long. Nine-to-five, lifelong employment with one organization was no longer the norm, nor was the family best characterized by the structure of father, stay-at-home mother, and children. Globalization was the framework and planet Earth our home.

As discussed in the previous chapter, there are likely as many definitions of coaching as there are authors writing about the topic. As a rule, however, coaching distinguishes itself from its root disciplines by its focus on the future rather than on analysis of the past. Coaching is unique in its unwavering commitment to "forwarding the action" (Flaherty, 2010; Whitworth et al., 2007). Coaches work collaboratively with individuals and groups to help them create desired outcomes and set achievable goals so as to improve performance or navigate change in a rewarding manner. Distinguishing characteristics of executive and life coaching models that seem generic to all schools of coaching include the following:

- A fundamental belief in the client's wholeness, resourcefulness, and capacity for growth
- Unbridled optimism concerning the human capacity to learn, change, and thrive

- Trust in clients' abilities to self-reflect and build on life experience and prior knowledge (clients are the experts in their own lives)
- A nonhierarchical and collaborative coach–client relationship
- A clear understanding that the agenda comes from the client
- An emphasis on discovery and reflective practice through powerful questioning
- A focus on solutions rather than on problems
- An appreciative approach that translates into a search for resources and strengths rather than weaknesses and deficits
- A commitment to action in between sessions
- A flexible communication structure that encompasses modern technology (Internet, telecommunications) as well as the more traditional face-to-face meetings

Although not all coaches hold credentials, certified professional coaches have typically received coach-specific training from reputable institutions, they have engaged with mentor coaches to enhance their skills, and they have accumulated a considerable number of hours with clients to obtain certification (table 2.2). In general practice, professional coaches work within specific niches (see table 1.3 in chapter 1, Sample Coaching Niches). They might

**Table 2.2    Current Requirements for ICF Certification (2011)**

| Certification | Requirements |
| --- | --- |
| Associate certified coach (ACC) | 60 hours of coach-specific training<br>100 hours of client experience<br>10 hours of work with a qualified mentor coach<br>2 reference letters from qualified coaches<br>Oral exam administered by the ICF |
| Professional certified coach (PCC) | 125 hours of coach-specific training<br>750 hours of client experience<br>10 hours of work with a qualified mentor coach<br>2 reference letters from qualified coaches<br>Oral exam administered by the ICF |
| Master certified coach (MCC) | 200 hours of coach-specific training<br>2,500 hours of client experience<br>10 hours of work with a qualified mentor coach<br>3 reference letters from qualified coaches<br>Oral exam administered by the ICF |

Adapted from International Coach Federation. Available: www.coachfederation.org/icfcredentials/become-credentialed.

open their doors to whatever business and life issues clients want to address; however, they must then assess whether the issue is appropriate for coaching and whether they see a good fit between their own skill set and the client's goals. Moreover, coaches must determine whether a client is coachable, that is, whether the client has the motivation and commitment to reliably sustain action until the objective is reached.

As mentioned, hallmarks of coaching are goal setting, action planning, and accountability. However, coaching represents far more than these straightforward processes. The best coaches tend to be highly creative, nonlinear thinkers. Helping clients move forward often requires novel thinking, innovative processes, and a unique reframing of the client's issues that unblocks an ocean of energy. Occasionally, the most effective path to a goal will look like retreating, sidestepping, or even doing nothing. Discovering the right thing to do at the right time under the right circumstances represents the genius and creativity of coaching.

At present, coaching clients are largely adults (25+), with the majority (65%) aged 46 and under (ICF, 2012). Clients deal with a wide range of challenges and opportunities. According to the 2012 ICF global coaching study, "The main areas addressed by coaches encompass personal growth (38%), interpersonal relationships (32%), self-esteem (28%), communication skills (26%) and work–life balance (25%)" (ICF, 2012). Coaching clients essentially are people who want to improve their performance and enhance their well-being.

Though coaching might be therapeutic and derived from traditional approaches to helping, it is neither therapy nor counseling. A characteristic often ascribed to coaching clients is that they are relatively free from significant mental health issues that would impede their journey toward goal attainment. As such, an early premise in the coaching field was that clients are typically people who have already achieved considerable success in their lives and careers. With the maturing of the coaching profession, however, more and more applications can be found for coaching people who are struggling or who are engulfed by dilemmas resulting from challenging life circumstances, job promotions, new relationships, or profound awakenings. In many instances, clients may have had far less than stellar histories of goal accomplishments; they may have hit the wall with logical approaches to problem solving or realized that their previous success formulas no longer apply to their current objectives. Coaching has even been used with students who have

had chronic difficulties addressing their academic challenges as well as with professionals, managers, and team members who have fatal flaws in the way they work with people or with job-related matters.

# MODELS OF HELPING AND LEARNING

Though associations such as the ICF have worked hard to draw sharp distinctions between coaching and other helping professions such as counseling and psychotherapy, resultant delineations may be more apparent than real. In truth, as social realities have continually shifted their underlying axes over the past 100 years, virtually every human service profession has had to update its methods of service delivery. Consequently, many helping professions currently incorporate certain aspects of what we might generically refer to as a **coaching approach**. Many clients' agendas may be seen as resembling ones that personal development professionals have addressed for decades, and present-day counselors, psychologists, and human relations professionals may function much the same way that coaches do. Indeed, those of you who have one-to-one practices may well discover that you have been functioning in a manner resembling the ways of professional coaches.

The bottom line is that coaching is multidisciplinary (Williams, 2008) and strongly informed by its root disciplines. Though coaches sometimes claim they have a distinctly different philosophy and methodology than other human service professionals, the lines are never that precise. In the next sections, we discuss recent transformations in two specific fields of study, psychology and adult learning, that have influenced the development of modern-day coaching. The theory and practice of coaching still draw significantly from these disciplines, and coaches' creative and collaborative approaches to clients' agendas are informed by sources within these traditions. As a result, many approaches to coaching parallel the traditions from which they issue.

### Approaches to Coaching

Behavioral coaching

Cognitive behavioral coaching

Existential coaching

Gestalt coaching

Integral coaching

Narrative coaching

NLP (neurolinguistic programming) coaching

Ontological coaching

Psychodynamic and system-psychodynamic coaching

Solution-focused coaching

Systemic coaching

Transpersonal coaching

# Psychology

Early models of helping relationships in psychology and psychiatry relied heavily on a medical view of the client as patient. One needed to be sick to ask for help. The *Diagnostic and Statistical Manual of Mental Disorders (DSM)* was originally published by the American Psychiatric Association (APA) in 1952 and grew considerably over the remainder of the 20th century, representing a trend toward viewing an ever-widening range of human behavior as pathological. With the recent release of the fifth edition of the *DSM*, debate continues to rage about all the new **psychosocial** pathologies that have seemingly cropped up since the fourth edition was published in 2000.

From the early 20th century until now, methods and models of psychological help adapted to the changing conditions of the lives and needs of the populations served. In the early 1900s, psychological treatment would best be described as elitist. For the most part, only the upper echelons of society could afford it. For the masses, the idea of lying on a couch talking endlessly about oneself to someone sitting in a chair probably seemed indulgent and nonsensical. Indeed, not only did the masses raise questions about this manner of help, increasing numbers of helping professionals expressed concerns about the practices as well. The fact that methods of treatment changed so vastly in the 20th century offers vibrant testimony to the commitment of helping professionals to revising methodologies so that they would best benefit clients.

As the fields of psychiatry and psychology developed, an emphasis on growth and the acknowledgment of normative challenges or adjustment issues became increasingly evident in theories and applications, particularly from about 1950 onward. Even the classic Freudian model of psychoanalysis, or the talking cure, morphed dramatically in the works of innovative Neo-Freudian thinkers, among whom were Alfred Adler (1927), Carl Jung (1969), Erik Erikson (1959), and Karen Horney (1939), to name but a few. The much-parodied premises of the Oedipus complex and other archaic interpretations of psychic structures such as the unconscious, id, ego, and superego were transformed into more palpable explanations for why we do what we do as human beings. We weren't all sick; sometimes life was hard and we simply needed a helping hand.

By the mid-20th century, B.F. Skinner's (1938, 1953) model of behaviorism began to take hold in the Western world, supplanting Freudianism as the reigning paradigm from which to view human nature. In this transition, we moved from a perspective where wildly erotic and violent internal forces ruled our lives to one positing that we were little more than stimulus-response machines. In this emerging brave new world (Huxley, 1932), there was little need to be concerned with what people thought. We might simply be manipulated with M&M-like rewards, or we could be controlled in a *Clockwork Orange* (Burgess, 1962) fashion of behavioral conditioning. As happened to the Freudian model, the tide eventually turned against the mindless behavioral premises such that by the early 1970s, human thoughts and feelings were welcomed back into the realm of psychology. Cognitive behavior therapy (CBT) increasingly integrated mindfulness along with the stark manipulations of behavioral psychology.

Other schools concerned with human behavior emerged more distinctly in the second half of the 20th century. Humanistic psychology, existential psychotherapies, and feminist approaches expanded our thinking about human nature and self-actualization. Pioneers in the field of humanistic psychology were pivotal in reorienting psychological thinking toward growth, self-realization, and human potentiality. They believed that not all who sought help were neurotic and not all problems were pathological. Existential therapy advocated a quest for meaning, purpose, and personal responsibility in one's choices and actions. Of particular importance to coaching were feminist approaches, which sought to equalize the power structure between client and helper.

Within the past 20 years, there have been even more profound shifts in psychological theories wherein Eastern and Western philosophies have merged to create a far greater concentration on the present or, as it is more popularly known, *the now* (Hanh, 2007; Kabat-Zinn, 2005; Kornfield, 2008; see Now and Mindfulness). A clear example of this blend is evident in transpersonal psychology, which provided a further thrust toward human potential and realization. Building on the works of Roberto Assagioli (1965), Stanislav Grof (1988), Abraham Maslow (1962), and Viktor Frankl (1969), transpersonal psychology asserted that such practices as spiritual rituals and meditation create strong anchors in the present moment and enable people to move beyond complaint and resistance toward a transcendent consciousness of the normal human issues that they confront (Davis, 2003).

Another instance of mindfulness-based therapy is that of acceptance and commitment therapy, or ACT (Hayes, Strosahl, & Wilson, 2011). As an offshoot of cognitive behavior therapy, ACT, along with other approaches such as brief therapy, solution-focused therapy, and narrative therapy, veers even further away from a pathological perspective of human beings in difficulty. Toward the end of the 20th century, Ken Wilber (2000a, 2000b, 2000c) integrated much previous research and ushered in the integral age with his theory of everything. He and theorists such as Susan Cook-Greuter (2006a, 2006b, 2000) and Don Beck (Beck & Cowan, 1996) merged transpersonal psychology with Eastern

practices to push the envelope of human development and experience. They articulated methodologies to accelerate personal growth and propel the evolution of human consciousness over the course of a lifetime (see Modern Perspectives of Human Behavior).

Coaching has developed strong links to positive psychology as a strength-based approach to human development. Following in the footsteps of such psychologists as Abraham Maslow (1962), Carl Rogers (1961), and Erich Fromm (1962), Martin Seligman championed the cause of positive psychology when he became president of the American Psychological Association in 1998. His classic writings on learned helplessness (1975) and learned optimism (2006) enabled us to realize that we can learn new and more effective ways of being and that we have profound potential for growth. Seligman and Csikszentmihalyi (2000), two essential figures in the field of positive psychology, describe the approach as follows: "Positive psychology at the subjective level is about valued subjective experiences: well-being, contentment, and satisfaction (in the past); hope and optimism (for the future); and flow and happiness (in the present). At the individual level, it is about positive individual traits: the capacity for love and vocation, courage, interpersonal skill, aesthetic sensibility, perseverance, forgiveness, originality, future mindedness, spirituality, high talent, and wisdom. At the group level, it is about the civic virtues and the institutions that move individuals toward better citizenship: responsibility, nurturance, altruism, civility, moderation, tolerance, and work ethic" (p. 5).

A major contribution of positive psychology can also be found in the work of Peterson and Seligman (2004) on character strengths and virtues associated with happiness. The researchers proposed a new

## Now and Mindfulness

A number of traditions focus on cultivating mindfulness. For example, Buddhist mindfulness offers that the goal "is to be mindful of the mind as it takes its own course" (Varela, Thompson, & Rosch, 1992, p. 31). Jack Kornfield, a Western meditation teacher and a cofounder of the Insight Meditation Society, explains mindfulness as "patient, receptive, non-judging awareness" (2008, p. 99). Lama Surya Das (1997) describes it as "relaxed, open, lucid,

moment-to-moment, present awareness" (p. 300), while Thich Nhat Hanh (2007), a Vietnamese Buddhist Zen master and activist, describes mindfulness as "the energy of attention. It is the capacity in each of us to be present one hundred percent to what is happening within and around us" (p. 42). Meditation (e.g., Zen, insight meditation, yogic mediation) is a practice associated with developing awareness and mindfulness.

# Modern Perspectives of Human Behavior

## Acceptance Commitment Therapy (ACT)

ACT is "an empirically based psychological intervention that uses acceptance and mindfulness strategies, together with commitment and behavior change strategies, to increase psychological flexibility" (Hayes, 2009, p. 1). An acronym for ACT could represent the following:

**A**ccepting reactions and being present to current reality

**C**hoosing a valued direction for action

**T**aking action

Further readings on ACT can be found at http://contextualpsychology.org/act and in Hayes, Strosahl, & Wilson (2011).

## Transpersonal Psychology

"Transpersonal psychology is the field of psychology which integrates psychological concepts, theories, and methods with the subject matter and practices of the spiritual disciplines . . . its central concepts are non-duality, self-transcendence, and optimal human development and mental health; and its core practices include meditation and ritual" (Davis, 2003, p. 6).

Further readings on transpersonal psychology can be found at www.johnvdavis.com/tp/index.htm.

## Integral Theory

Ken Wilber, founder of the Integral Institute for teaching and applications of integral theory, offers an interdisciplinary philosophical approach to the study of everything (Wilber, 2000a, 2000b). Through it is a broad survey of Eastern and Western modes of thought and practice, Wilber proposed an integral map (including quadrants, levels, lines, states, and types) of human experience as well as life practices meant to help raise one's levels of consciousness (Wilber, Patten, Leonard, & Morelli, 2008).

The value of Wilber's work lies in its breadth of scope, though he might be perceived as being overly optimistic in generalizing his integral theory to nearly all modes of human inquiry. A recent trend is that thinkers in various fields are incorporating Wilber's integral theory into counseling, coaching, and consulting practices. For example, in the field of coaching, Joanne Hunt (2009) and Laura Divine (2009), founders of Integral Coaching Canada, base their coach training on Wilber's theory. Others, like James Flaherty, founder of New Ventures West and author of *Coaching: Evoking Excellence in Others* (2010), have also been significantly influenced by Ken Wilber's work.

---

classification of character strengths and suggested that positive strengths, if practiced consistently, could result in the good life. These character strengths are as follows (Peterson & Seligman, 2004, pp. 29-30):

Wisdom and knowledge: Cognitive strengths having to do with the acquisition and use of knowledge; these are seen in one's creativity, curiosity, love of learning, and perspective taking.

Courage: Emotional strength relating to the capacity to accomplish goals in the face of opposition; it involves bravery, persistence, integrity, and vitality.

Humanity: Interpersonal strength pertaining to how one cares for and relates to others with social intelligence, kindness, and love.

Justice: Civic strength demonstrated through active citizenship, social responsibility, loyalty, and leadership.

Temperance: Strength referring to self-regulation, prudence, humility, forgiveness, and mercy.

Transcendence: Strength in one's connection to the greater universe; includes a sense of gratitude, hope, playfulness, and faith.

The importance of positive psychology for the field of coaching shows up in its unparalleled focus on the promotion of health and happiness rather than on the treatment of mental illness and pathology. Along with other **postmodern approaches** referred to previously, positive psychology dwells less on what previously happened and more on what people can do now to move their lives forward. It acknowledges the unbounded resourcefulness of human beings with all their unrealized strengths and potentialities. Indeed, this shift toward identifying strengths and resources as a means to promote growth and wellness in individuals, families, workplaces, and communities is foundational to coaching.

As research continued to support the effectiveness of coaching in addressing specific client issues, a new branch of psychology known as coaching psychology grew to prominence in the first decade of the 21st century. Grant (2007) explains coaching psychology as "the systematic application of behavioral science to the enhancement of life experience, work performance and well-being for individuals, groups and organizations who do not have clinically significant mental health issues or abnormal levels of distress. In broad terms, coaching psychology sits at the intersection of sports, counseling, clinical, and organizational and health psychology" (p. 23). Palmer and Whybrow (2007) offer that "coaching psychology is for enhancing well-being and performance in personal life and work domains underpinned by models of coaching grounded in established adult and child learning or psychological approaches" (p. 3). Coaching psychology integrated the considerable shifts in models of psychological treatment with the multidisciplinary contributions of the pioneers of coaching.

## Adult Learning

If we agree with Sir John Whitmore that coaching is helping clients learn rather than teaching them (1992, p. 8), we can then appreciate clients as adult learners. Approaches to helping adults learn are very different than pedagogical principles applied to children or adolescents. To help you better appreciate the influence of adult learning on various approaches to coaching, we offer our reflections on principles of andragogy, experiential learning, and transformative learning.

### Andragogy

Malcolm Knowles (1980) expanded the concept of **andragogy** in North America through his research on adult education. He held the belief that andragogy is not the same as pedagogy because adult learners have a different set of needs than those of children. Knowles proposed that the difference was not between children and adults per se but whether a person approaches learning as an adult or a nonadult (Cyr, 1999). Andragogy has ties to Piaget (1952) and the **constructivist theory of knowing,** which asserts that adults build on previous experi-

ences when faced with new learning opportunities. Knowles further offered that adults are self-directed learners who move toward increasing independence from their teachers over time.

Some key principles of andragogy are as follows: (1) Adult learning is an active process with learners who possess innate curiosity about areas of interest and who are intrinsically motivated to learn, (2) adult learning is greatly influenced by the social environment, and (3) more often than not, adult learning is oriented toward performance rather than cognitive mastery of a topic (Cyr, 1999).

Knowles' assumptions include certain characteristics of adult learners that influence the way they learn. According to Knowles, adults have an inherent need to know. They are self-directed and have a wealth of prior experience with which they approach new learning situations. Furthermore, Knowles tells us that adults are attracted to learn matters that are relevant to them, and they are internally motivated toward problem-solving learning (Bachkirova, Cox, & Clutterbuck, 2010).

Two further assumptions of adult learning theory are crucial for coaching: (1) Rather than being the sole purview of teachers, adult learners and teachers mutually assume responsibility for learning as well as for determining the learner's needs, the objectives of the learning experiences, and the manner in which subject matter is presented (Ratcliff-Daffron, 2003); and (2) evidence of learning must be viewed through learners' behavior change as well as through their cognitive development (Bachkirova et al., 2010). These two assumptions are represented in coaching in the form of nonhierarchical partnerships and an emphasis on action and behavioral engagement of the client. Knowles' assumptions concerning adult learning are foundational to the field of coaching, as is evidenced in the distinguishing characteristics of the coaching models mentioned earlier in this chapter.

### Experiential Learning

David A. Kolb's (1984) four-stage process of **experiential learning** is also of great interest to the coaching field. His efforts follow in the footsteps of the founding fathers of experiential learning, John Dewey (1916), Kurt Lewin (1935), and Jean Piaget (1952). Kolb also acknowledged the influence of Carl Jung (1969), Erik Erikson (1959), Carl Rogers (1961), Abraham Maslow (1962), Paulo Freire (1970), and Ivan Illich (1972) in the development of this concept. His view of experiential learning has strong links to models describing how people continue to develop in their adult years.

According to Kolb, experiential learning emerges through a four-stage process. At the heart of his model is what he describes as concrete experiences (see figure 2.1). Such experiences allow people to reflect and observe, following which they then generalize their learning and sometimes form new theories about how to act in future situations. These new **theories of action** influence new behaviors, which produce another set of concrete experiences. The cycle repeats itself as people observe and reflect upon what they have just done.

Kolb and his colleague, Roger Fry (1975), also defined ways they believed people absorb new information. They created the Learning Style Inventory (LSI) to help learners and educators—or coaches, in our case—understand how to present information so it is more readily processed by people using their preferred **learning style**. According to Kolb and Fry, people navigate along two continua when they are confronted with new information (see figure 2.1): the perception continuum (how we think about things), which ranges from feeling to thinking, and the processing continuum (how we do things), which ranges from observing to doing. Depending on the learner's preferences, new information is absorbed in one of four ways. Kolb and Fry named their four learning styles (see table 2.3) as follows: converging (learn best by thinking and doing), diverging (learn best by feeling and observing), assimilating (learn best by thinking and observing), and accommodating (learn best by feeling and doing). When coaches recognize their

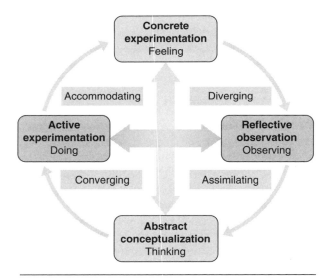

**Figure 2.1**   Kolb's experiential learning cycle.

clients' preferences, they have an edge in helping them navigate the change process more easily.

The concept of experiential learning should become clearer when, in chapters 10 and 11, we discuss the competency development model and the design of intermediate actions in which clients engage subtasks of their agendas. By reflecting on and learning from their experiences, clients acquire new ways of approaching their topics and more effective strategies to reach their goals. Embedded in the philosophy of coaching are Kolb's suggestion that the learner be placed at the center of the learning cycle and his belief that people must assume ownership of their learning and development. Effective coaching serves clients' agendas with a firm belief that people have a choice and that they possess the answer to their issues (Coach U, 2005).

## Transformative Learning

Finally, let's consider yet another constructivist adult learning theory underlying the coaching field. **Transformative learning**, which emerged from the work of Jack Mezirow (1994), is "the social process of construing and appropriating a new or revised interpretation of the meaning of one's experience as a guide to action" (pp. 222-223). In other words, Mezirow thought that learning involves revising our beliefs, principles, and feelings. He identified two dimensions in the meaning structures involved in this reframing. The first was described as *meaning perspectives*, or the lens, most often acquired during childhood and youth, through which sen-

## Table 2.3  Kolb and Fry's Learning Styles

| Learning style | Place on learning continua | Characteristics of learner |
|---|---|---|
| Converging | Abstract conceptualization (AC) + active experimentation (AE) | Greatest strength is the practical application of ideas<br>Performs well when there is a single correct answer<br>Can focus hypothetical-deductive reasoning on specific problems<br>Prefers to deal with things rather than people<br>Has narrow interests and chooses to specialize in the physical sciences |
| Diverging | Concrete experience (CE) + reflective observation (RO) | Greatest strength is imaginative ability<br>Good at generating ideas and seeing things from other perspectives<br>Interested in people<br>Has broad cultural interests<br>Specializes in arts |
| Assimilating | Abstract conceptualization (AC) + reflective observation (RO) | Greatest strength is the ability to create theoretical models<br>Excels in inductive reasoning<br>Concerned with abstract concepts rather than people; not too concerned with the practical use of theories<br>Attracted to basic sciences and mathematics |
| Accommodating | Concrete experience (CE) + active experimentation (AE) | Greatest strength is doing things<br>More of a risk taker<br>Performs well when required to quickly adapt to immediate circumstances<br>Solves problems intuitively<br>Relies on others for information |

Adapted, by permission, from M. Tennant, 2006, *Psychology and adult learning* (New York: Routledge), 89.

sory perceptions, feelings, and thoughts are shaped and consequently limited. The second was called *meaning schemes,* or the set of concepts, beliefs, judgments, and feelings borne out of our meaning perspectives that influence our interpretations. As we mature and become more autonomous thinkers, transformation occurs as our perceptions shift and our worldviews change.

Transformative learning is facilitated by reflection on the rationale for our beliefs: Why do we believe what we believe? Once we make our assumptions about our beliefs explicit, we are then able to challenge them. This critical reflection of our experience is key to transformative learning (Merriam, 2004). Mezirow (1994) tells us that this reflection process usually is awakened when we finally

**REFLECTION 2.3**

Before you continue reading, take a few minutes to reflect on your preferred mode of taking in new information. Which of the following four descriptions best characterizes you?

1. You can usually see right away how new ideas could be applied concretely to solve nagging issues you have been dealing with (converger: thinking and doing).

2. You like to get together with other people and brainstorm creative ideas so as to examine various facets of an issue (diverger: feeling and observing).

3. Most of the time, you create abstract concepts that may not always be recognized as practical by other people (assimilator: thinking and observing).

4. You are a problem solver who likes to do things rather than spend too much time in reflection (accommodator: feeling and doing).

Once you have established your preference, list some of the pros and cons of your learning style. When might it benefit you to make conscious efforts to use another style? When would your style be helpful in a coaching relationship? When might it hinder progress?

our world. *Premise reflection* is where we critique the basis upon which we have defined the problem itself and examine the values, beliefs, and assumptions that gave rise to the issue in the first place. According to Mezirow (1994), the phases of critical premise reflection are as follows.

### Mezirow's Phases of Critical Premise Reflection

- Coming up against a disorienting dilemma
- Self-examining with feelings of guilt or shame, sometimes turning to religion for support
- Critically assessing assumptions
- Recognizing that one's discontent and the process of transformation are shared and that others have negotiated a similar change
- Exploring options for new roles, relationships, and actions
- Planning a course of action
- Acquiring knowledge and skills for implementing one's plan
- Trying out new roles
- Building competence and self-confidence in new roles and relationships
- Reintegrating into one's life on the basis of conditions dictated by one's new perspective

Reprinted from J. Mezirow, 1994, "Understanding transformation theory," *Adult Education Quarterly* 44(4): 222-232.

realize that our old ways of thinking are no longer serving us well. He believes that most reflections of this sort are triggered by a disorienting dilemma in our lives. He identifies three types of reflection that, along with self-reflection, might rise to the surface when we are facing difficult life situations: content reflection, process reflection, and premise reflection. We generally do the first two types of reflection, content and process, on a daily basis as we solve problems or change our minds. We may reflect on the *content* of an actual issue or on the way (or *process*) in which we went about solving a particular problem. For instance, we may reflect on information about nutrition and thereby make changes. Or, we might realize that when we solved a particular problem, we left out of the *process* a consideration of how our new behaviors might affect significant others in our lives.

The last type of reflection Mezirow identified is where the most significant learning takes place; it leads to a self-transformation in how we perceive

Premise reflection is no doubt at the core of most clients' work when they engage coaches to help them with profound personal shifts in their lifestyles. A number of tools and techniques typically described in coaching books (Coach U, 2005; Flaherty, 2010; Stolzfus, 2008) serve the reflective agendas that Mezirow articulated in his work. These include asking powerful questions, challenging limiting beliefs, and brainstorming alternatives.

From this brief overview of historical progressions in the fields of psychology and adult learning over the past 50 years, at least two things have emerged. First, the field of coaching was strongly informed by developments in these areas, and second, coaching needs to be appreciated not as an entirely new field but rather as a creative integration of the invaluable contributions of theorists in adult learning, psychology, and many other related disciplines. It is heartening to see that the present day coaching field has wholeheartedly embraced these frameworks and has built its core around their grounded principles.

# CORE INGREDIENTS IN EFFECTIVE COACHING

Throughout most of the 20th century, needing help or consulting a therapist was thought to indicate an inherent weakness. Today, we are far less likely to stigmatize requests for help for our human condition. It is okay to seek counsel, to not know, to lack expertise, and to acknowledge the wisdom of getting help when we are in over our heads (Kegan, 1995) or when our behavior resembles that of a dog chasing its tail. In the world of health, wellness, and fitness, we often need expert guidance and support to successfully make changes. As professionals, we need to be concerned when out-of-shape clients begin throwing dumbbells around at the gym without guidance or when people who want to lose weight arbitrarily embark on a new diet because a media star advocated it on a late-night infomercial. Likewise, we are likely to appreciate that expecting people to change simply because they know they should is not very realistic. For the most part, professionals acknowledge that there is a process to overcoming old habits, and that the path of change is not always straightforward or best pursued in a solitary fashion.

In the fitness world, a noteworthy contribution to the evolving perspectives of what people need and how professionals can be helpful may be found in the beginnings of one-to-one or personal training. Many psychologists and psychiatrists who were working in private practice in the 1980s are likely to remember stories of clients quitting therapy after experiencing more tangible progress in their relationships with personal trainers. Pioneers in the field of personal training are also likely to remember those heady days when clients who had been stuck for years began to leap forward through their relationships with trainers. A serious dilemma arose when clients began to generalize the trainer's expertise and helpfulness to other domains of their lives, however. Clients not only relied on their trainers to get fit, lose weight, and train regularly, but they also wanted to broaden the conversation to include advice on business, relationships, nutrition, and lifestyle. Journalists at the time enjoyed either lionizing or demonizing the helpfulness of this first wave of personal trainers. No matter the press, the more critical dynamic from the early days of the personal training profession concerns its methodology of action planning and goal setting that closely approximated what we now see in the field of coaching.

Perhaps you are currently a personal trainer or perhaps your métier is in other areas of health, nutrition, bodywork, health care, or stress management. To be an effective coach in today's world means embarking on a steep learning curve whereby you can efficiently sort through your past approaches to helping relationships, extract what is relevant, and then integrate this knowledge with the emerging awareness of what will work now. There are four themes that we want to briefly explore here to create a deeper foundation for lifestyle wellness coaching:

- Balancing action and analysis for forward movement
- Understanding the phases of human development
- Identifying and integrating social support structures
- Recognizing systemic relationships and the holism of clients

## Balancing Action and Analysis for Forward Movement

A caricature of psychotherapeutic models of helping might depict a client lying on a couch while a bearded psychiatrist doodles on a pad. Whatever the client is talking about seems inane and impractical. The impression is that the client interminably analyzes her life, and nothing ever comes of it. In contrast, a caricature of coaching might picture a coach shoving a terrified client in front of her boss to demand a pay raise. The message is one of getting on with it, doing it despite the fear, and certainly not wasting time analyzing the situation. In such images, the risky nature of forwarding the action is laid bare. Imagine this dialogue between a new client and her coach:

**Client:** I need some help figuring out the next steps in my life.

**Coach:** Great. What's your goal?

**Client:** Well, I want to be happier?

**Coach:** What's preventing you from being happier now?

**Client:** I guess one thing is that my husband doesn't really "get" me. He wants things the way they are. I want something new . . . I want more excitement.

**Coach:** What do you want to do about that?

**Client:** Sometimes, I wonder whether we're a good match.

**Coach:** And what do you want to do about that?

**Client:** I did think the other day that maybe we shouldn't be together . . . I even had a flash about getting divorced.

**Coach:** What's the first step you would need to take to make that happen?

**Client:** Well, I guess I could talk to a lawyer.

**Coach:** What would it take for you to get in touch with a lawyer?

Sounds absurd? This is an almost verbatim report of one client's experience meeting her coach for the first time. And yes, she did get divorced. Later on, she regretted it deeply. This example highlights the danger of leaping into action without sufficient analysis. The caricatures referred to earlier highlight the artificial division of skill sets in coaching versus more in-depth processes such as counseling and therapy: Coaches move clients forward through goal setting and action planning, whereas therapists spin their clients in analysis. Such representations do great disservice to all helping professionals. Psychotherapy clients don't just stew in their problematic reflections, and coaching clients don't just leap into action. Just as many therapists might not privilege analysis for the sake of analysis, the best coaches would never advocate action for action's sake; they would want to probe and explore the topic further.

The elegance of coaching is partly represented in how efficiently coaches unveil critical details and relevant parameters to understand client issues. It is also reflected in how they work with clients to formulate robust action plans. Some clients are impatient—they want change *now*. Yet, finding the key to facilitate effective change requires insight into clients' unique histories and dynamics. Analysis is essential to good coaching. It is a distortion to think of analysis as simply delving into a client's childhood experiences. Rather, it is about gaining appreciation of who your client is and what he desires. It involves seeking sufficient knowledge of history relevant to your client's topic rather than excavating a broad range of historical information that may be interesting to know but not essential to moving forward. Coaching is not voyeuristic. Some might argue that asking clients about their past is taboo. After all, you wouldn't want to cross that line into psychotherapy! The fact is that you need to ask about the past; you just don't want to stay there too long. You need to know what clients have tried in the past, what their success formulas have been, who their greatest supports are, what strengths they have demonstrated over their lifetimes, and why this goal is so important to them at this time.

If you are wondering how this is relevant to the type of coaching you might do, consider some of the seemingly clear-cut issues that health, wellness, and fitness clients may bring to you:

I want to lose weight.

I want to eat better.

I want to get fit and build some muscle.

I want to reduce my stress and feel better.

I want to quit smoking.

I want to be healthy.

I want to prepare for a trek up Mount Kilimanjaro.

I need to stick to the plan my doctor gave me.

I want to have more positive energy.

I want to have less back pain.

Could you begin working on any of these objectives without asking at least a few pertinent questions? The critical skill here is knowing which questions to ask and whether those questions are meeting your clients' needs rather than your own. Also, you are probably aware of role boundaries. As a health, wellness, and fitness professional, you may conceive of your role in such a way that precludes you from going too far afield in your questioning. Your notion of relevant knowledge may be limited to questions such as "What's your time frame?" and "What's your target weight?" From a coaching perspective, there are at least two sets of necessary questions for all of these agendas. The first has to do with meaning, for instance, "What does 'losing weight' mean to you?" And the second has to do with importance, that is, "What is it about this goal that so deeply matters to you at this moment in your life?" Beyond these two questions, there are likely many others that effective coaches will need to ask before embarking on the task of action planning.

A number of coaching texts elevate the quality of curiosity (Coach U, 2005; Whitworth et al., 2007) to a high order. A major point regarding the balance of analysis and action is that *appropriate* curiosity is not intrusive and is not psychotherapy; rather, it is essential for cocreating meaningful goals and strategies for action.

## Understanding the Phases of Human Development

When Gail Sheehy (1976) first published her classic work, *Passages*, what many of her readers already knew but may not have had the capacity to articulate was that different things assume primary importance over the years of a person's life. Agendas that were once nonnegotiable surprisingly drop off the list. Sheehy wasn't the first to talk about stages of life; she was simply more successful in popularizing the ideas. In the early 20th century, thinking about

development focused almost exclusively on childhood—to the point of asserting that by our 20s, we are set for life. Erik Erikson was one theorist who definitely had other thoughts about this matter.

Erik Erikson (1902-1994), a developmental psychologist and psychoanalyst, is best known for his theory of psychosocial development, which details eight stages of life (table 2.4). Unlike Freud, Erikson (1959, 1963, 1968) emphasized the social rather than sexual aspects of the life span. He went well beyond the first two decades of life in appreciating the critical themes and issues we need to confront as we age. Erikson believed that at each life stage, we have a pivotal conflict around which our lives revolve. The ways in which these conflicts are eventually resolved inevitably influence our lives and our character. In the successful resolution of stage-specific conflicts, the individual emerges with greater strength and potential for positive development.

You may have encountered Erikson's theory in your previous studies. There are many other frameworks through which we can appreciate clients who come to us at varying points in their lives. None of the theories of life-span development posit that age is the sole determinant of a stage of life, nor is age thought to guarantee that issues akin to those named by Erikson have been resolved. For instance, many 30-year-olds have been known to say, "I'm still trying to figure out what I want to do when

---

**REFLECTION 2.4**

Take a moment to address the following scenario. Imagine that the same words about a desired outcome from coaching are spoken by two people, a 21-year-old woman and a 50-year-old woman:

I want to lose at least 20 pounds, or 9 kilograms, in the next three months.

Jot down the thoughts that come to mind. What questions would you want to ask? What motivations might you assume for each woman? The one variable presented is age. Make a list of all the assumptions you have about age and weight loss.

Our assumptions are that given the aging process and the phases of human development, weight loss might mean different things to these two women. These meanings, along with the personalities these women have built through their life stages, will color the quality and intensity of their work in coaching to achieve this same goal.

---

## Table 2.4 Erikson's Eight Stages of Development

| Age | Stage | Central concern |
|---|---|---|
| Birth to 1 year | Trust vs. mistrust | Sensing that the world is safe and I can trust others |
| 1-3 years | Autonomy vs. shame and doubt | Knowing that I can act on my own and be independent |
| 3-6 years | Initiative vs. guilt | Planning and doing new things and managing my failures |
| 6-12 years | Industry vs. inferiority | Learning basic competencies and comparing myself favorably with others |
| 12-20 years | Identity vs. identity confusion | Integrating my roles into a single, consistent identity |
| 20-40 years | Intimacy vs. isolation | Sharing myself deeply without fear of losing my identity |
| 40-65 years | Generativity vs. stagnation | Contributing to others and society through my offspring and productive work |
| 65+ years | Integrity vs. despair | Appraising my life in a way that allows me to appreciate its significance and meaning |

I grow up," a statement that reflects the identity confusion of adolescence. Nonetheless, knowing someone's age allows us to bring into question concerns that normatively might be awakened at this time. It also permits us to be sensitive to how we can best enter the conversation with clients.

## Identifying and Integrating Social Support Structures

Life is about relationships. It's as simple as that, according to a number of theorists ranging from the Neo-Freudians previously mentioned to modern-day object relations theorists (Cashdan, 1988) and social constructivists (Vygotsky, 1978). How often have you spun in indecision about some important matter and then, through the gift of a friend's listening ears, you achieved clarity and resolution? When we voice our opinions to others, they become more real. Evidence on goal setting continually reminds us that making goals public increases the likelihood that we will achieve them (Donatelle & Thompson, 2011).

So much of what we do in life is for and about others. Reality is a social construction. What words mean to you, what you believe is important, even how you understand your own identity have to do with the social context of your life. There is good evidence that people who have stronger friendship networks live longer and are happier (Friedman & Martin, 2011). As the classic Beatles song reminds us, "I get by with a little help from my friends."

There are group support structures for most of the challenges and difficulties of life. People who want to lose weight find added strength to do so through the social fabric of group meetings. Twelve-step programs have developed for anything that resembles an addiction. Within the world of health, wellness, and fitness, the evolution of the personal training profession and other one-to-one services bears strong testimony to the importance of having social support for our intentions. More currently, the field of coaching has grown partly by virtue of its creative ways of being in relation with clients.

What is it, though, that makes social support so critical? Recently, a 43-year-old friend who has her PhD in education scheduled an appointment with a counselor at a community clinic to discuss some issues she had been having with her 11-year-old daughter. This friend walked into the clinic and was introduced to a 25-year-old graduate student who was single and had no children. An hour later she walked out of the counselor's office feeling relieved and with a clearer sense of direction. She said, "I know the counselor didn't have a lot of personal experience with my problems, but just being able to talk about them—to get them out of my head—allowed me to think more clearly and—hearing myself talk—I could sense that this wasn't such a big deal. I felt I could handle it."

We are strongly influenced by those around us. People we encounter on a daily basis have an impact on us and on our behavior. Politicians, celebrities, and other members of society play a role in shaping our culture, and consequently, in influencing who we are, what we do, what we think, what we value, what we look like, how we take care of our health, and more. For better or worse, we are social creatures! We might seek to emulate our friends, or we may get inspired by our social network to stretch beyond our present limits. Social support is one of the variables that reliably contributes to the ability to change behavior and adopt new and healthier habits (Connor & Norman, 2005).

There is a lot of discussion in professional and private circles about dependency in relationships. In intimate matters, there is talk of codependency. In professional relationships, there is disquiet about dependency on helpers. Some of these concerns are legitimate; however, they might also be traced to our legacy of rugged individualism, particularly in a North American context where we are supposed to be self-reliant. We are expected to just do it. Self-determination and willpower are primary virtues.

From a deeper perspective, however, it would seem that we rarely—if ever—do it alone. We live our lives in a social reality, with people and for people, with the aid of friends, family, and others who figure into our social constructions. Our social character empowers us to reach the unreachable goal—or to believe we can't. Having good role models, being responsible to others for the goals we set for ourselves, seeing others being successful at what we would like to be doing, and expressing our intentions to others all increase the likelihood that we will be successful in bringing about positive changes in our lives (Bandura, 1997a, 1997b; Prochaska, Norcross, & DiClemente, 2002).

## Recognizing Systemic Relationships and the Holism of Clients

We have already established that no man is an island. What is now important to explore is how one alteration in someone changes everything. There is a wonderful concept known as the butterfly effect that posits the question "Does the flap of a butterfly's wings in Brazil set off a tornado in Texas?" (Lorenz, 1972). Everything in our world is connected. Systems theory, which has become the reigning paradigm for appreciating the interrelationships of all things, can be traced to the early works of Ludwig von Bertalanffy (1968). Present-day expressions of systems theory can be found in the works of people such as Gregory Bateson (1979), Fritjof Capra (1997), and Peter Senge (1990).

Let's consider the mind–body connection in light of systems theory. When Hans Selye (1956), a medical doctor, began researching the concept of stress in the 1950s, his colleagues viewed him as eccentric. He argued that mental experiences could affect physical health, a premise that most of us would take for granted today. Though evidence concerning the mind–body connection accumulated at an astonishing rate from the 1950s onward, mind–body medicine struggled to gain a foothold within the medical world throughout the second half of the 20th century. Today, we might say that physical scientists generally accept the relationship of mind and body and have come to describe health as the interaction of several dimensions of our personhood (Engel, 1977; Wilber et al., 2008).

What are the most relevant systemic relationships to consider when addressing coaching topics with clients? Beginning with the fact that our thoughts influence our emotions and vice versa, we also know that our thoughts and feelings influence our physical being—and conversely, the way we relate to our bodies affects our mental and emotional health. Moving out from ourselves, how we are influences others. If we happen to be in a great mood, evidence tells us that this influences the moods of those around us. Thus, our personal realities influence our social realities. In the language of causality, our emotional, physical, mental, social, and behavioral experiences influence one another. Touch one part of us and you influence all other parts to a greater or lesser degree. Touch one person and you touch untold numbers of others in a kind of ripple effect— or, if you will, the butterfly effect.

This theme speaks to an important consideration in effective coaching: working with the whole person. Most helping professions are organized to address specific realms of human existence. Lawyers deal with legal issues, accountants with accounting, and so on. When a client hires a health, wellness, or fitness professional, there are likely to be implicit and explicit boundaries to this relationship. The implicit ones guide both the topics brought forward

and the questions and methods deemed legitimate. The explicit ones pertain to ethics and professional regulations that delimit the delivery of services for which you are trained and licensed.

If we return to the list of possible topics clients might bring to you in your professional role, how do you function as a systems thinker and yet intervene in ways that are within the boundaries of your profession? Take weight loss as a goal your client deeply desires. You may recognize that eating has emotional triggers for this client. You may learn that family and friends have sabotaged weight reduction plans in the past. There might be a history of obesity in the client's family, suggesting genetic factors. The client may also have particular beliefs ("I can't do it") and knowledge ("A book I just read says . . .") that will challenge progress. Can you work with this client by handing him an eating plan or putting him on an exercise program without addressing at least some of these other factors?

A coaching approach is holistic in that it encompasses all that might be relevant and builds strategies for each area where there is likelihood of impact. Not only does this require that coaches be exquisite diagnosticians but also that they be able to codesign and then engage clients in multidimensional action plans that increase the probability of lasting change. Moreover, it necessitates the coach's awareness of potential changes in dimensions of clients' lives that are not part of the specific **coaching agenda**.

# CORE INGREDIENTS IN LIFESTYLE WELLNESS COACHING

Having introduced the broader field of coaching, let's return to how clients with health, wellness, and fitness issues can benefit from coaching. You may already suspect that when client issues are framed holistically, almost all clients would benefit from embracing goals related to their health, wellness, and fitness. Indeed, most coaching clients present multiple interlocking concerns wherein some form of somatic or health-related action planning would be beneficial.

Depending on how coaches represent their areas of expertise, clients will seek to work with them on topics pertinent to these areas. For instance, a business coach will attract clients who want to address business and career matters. Your coaching practice

**REFLECTION 2.5**

Having read the core themes of a coaching approach, reflect on the reasons why health, wellness, and fitness professionals would have a privileged niche within the coaching world. From your experience, what particular knowledge, expertise, insights, strengths, or ways of being would you bring to your coaching relationships? How might these create a unique niche for you?

will probably be targeted to health, wellness, and fitness matters, so clients will seek you out for goals situated within this broad domain. They may show up with histories of marginal eating habits, relative inactivity, adrenaline-fueled lifestyles, and warning signs related to early-stage medical concerns. By general standards, they could be highly successful in life, having realized advanced degrees of education, significant business success, and the creation of well-functioning families. However, in the domain of health, wellness, and fitness, they need your help. Not so long ago, the options available to them in the fitness world would have been limited to club memberships, class instruction, or personal training. In other health and wellness matters, they might have engaged an expert who would have diagnosed them and given them a prescription or program. Now, these potential clients can also hire a coach.

Imagine a coach whose career up to the present has been in nutrition assessment and advisement. She may, in fact, be continuing in these roles while developing a client base where the contract is explicitly for coaching. What might change in her professional behavior? We have identified five elements that highlight some of the more evident differences between the person's behavior as a lifestyle wellness coach versus someone who delivers certain health and wellness services:

1. The context for coaching is likely in an office setting or over the phone.

2. The work is represented in ongoing conversations rather than diagnostic assessments, demonstrations of techniques, or taking the client through a physical program.

3. Though the coach may have accumulated credentials in nutrition counseling, personal training, or some form of massage or bodywork, the coach does not directly engage in any of these practices with her clients. Rather, these practices serve as a backdrop to her coaching efforts, informing her of potential avenues to explore.

4. Although the coach's role is related to an area of expertise, she does not dictate what the client should do; whatever actions derive from the sessions are created in a collaborative manner.

5. The coach has license to explore a wide spectrum of interrelated issues that may extend well beyond matters of health, wellness, and fitness.

Let's take a simple set of presenting issues for someone a coach is considering taking on as a client. George wants to train for a 14-day cycling tour in Europe that is three months away. He lives in the Northeast United States, he is fit, and he has cycled regularly for years but never for great distances. If the coach were to serve in the role of personal trainer, she might map out a program of training, get his buy-in, and start to work. In a coaching role, she would begin by asking a number of questions so that she could situate herself in George's life and understand the dynamics and interacting implications of how he is currently living, what might need to change, and what the ramifications of these changes might be. The resulting action plan would be multipronged wherein one of the strategies might be finding a personal trainer who has great expertise in developing cyclists.

This scenario seems straightforward. George is highly motivated; has a clear, well-defined target; is realistic in his expectations because he is fit and has cycled regularly; and has the wisdom to get some professional guidance in case he has any blind spots in his thinking and planning. Even here, however, important issues for coaching may arise. What if George hasn't accounted for effects on his family? What if the ideal training regimen bumps up against his heavy workload and travel schedule? What if he has a medical condition that may need to be managed throughout this grueling two-week journey? What if his reason for undertaking this venture is to prove something to someone else? Coaching topics may seem simple but do not always prove to be so.

Consider another client, Melanie, who has been obese for most of her adolescent and adult years and has a long, unsuccessful history of weight-loss efforts. She wants to try a combination of dieting and exercising as a way of addressing the issue. No doubt this is a common enough goal. As a personal trainer, you would readily set up a program that is appropriate to her level of fitness, her interests, her schedule, and her intended goals for progression toward a target weight. As a nutritionist, you might assess her dietary intake and provide her with clear guidance about a new eating plan. Putting on your coach's hat, you would begin by asking questions. The result of your work together might include any of the following and even additional options depending on the client's unique profile *and* your level of training as a coach: You might cocreate a process for Melanie to make peace with her body just as it is. She might hire a nutritionist to set up a supportive eating plan while she is increasing her energy expenditures, and you might help her monitor the plan. You might assist her in identifying lifestyle adjustments that increase her activity outside the gym while also aligning her with an inviting fitness center where she feels welcomed; there could also be a particular trainer in that center who would work with her from time to time.

In addition, you might engage Melanie in dialogue to appreciate her social support as well as any relationships that could undermine her intentions; a plan of action would also ensue from these discussions. Indeed, you might help her discover people on a similar path and thereby create new social connections that inspire her to succeed. Further, you might collaboratively generate a list of readings to inform and motivate her at various stages of the change process. All of this would take time, possibly a year or more—not a quick fix, but rather one that is appropriate to the complexity of the goal and respectful of the client's deep desire to succeed in the long term.

George and Melanie illustrate typical client issues as well as differences in working as a coach and as a health and wellness specialist. As noted earlier, most clients who seek the services of professional coaches have either explicit or implicit health and wellness agendas. Explicitly, a client may want to get fit, lose weight, train for an event, or change sports; implicitly, a busy executive may have correlated health, wellness, and fitness issues that have to be encompassed in the coaching process for her to achieve her primary goal of getting a job promotion.

The process of coaching clients with health, wellness, and fitness goals may not be entirely foreign to those who have worked for years with clients in one-to-one relationships around issues of health and wellness. Let us deepen this discussion by understanding what it would mean to specialize in coaching related to wellness. Referring back to George and Melanie, both had health, wellness, and fitness

goals they wanted to achieve. It is quite possible that they might engage a professional coach with no background in health or fitness matters. The public image of coaching is that coaches help organize and motivate clients to achieve their goals, so clients may not always perceive the critical relevance of specialized knowledge. Lifestyle wellness coaches typically bring to their work not only academic and professional expertise but also years of professional practice with clients pursuing similar goals.

Lifestyle wellness coaches may help clients with other kinds of agendas, such as managing stress, being more focused in their work efforts, developing a more disciplined way of living, becoming more attuned to others and their environment, and so on. These types of agendas may be seen as related to lifestyle, yet the ways of developing capacities pertinent to these objectives would likely include somatic practices, health promotion, mindfulness techniques, and even spiritual development. Why would these clients choose a lifestyle wellness coach for these agendas? There are at least two strong arguments: Lifestyle wellness coaches would be well-trained individuals who adhere to professional guidelines for the practice of coaching, and they would presumably have amassed a wealth of knowledge related to the mind–body connection.

To illustrate our second argument, let's examine stress, which was previously presented as a mind–body issue. There is a reciprocal causality in stress whereby mental processes affect physical being and vice versa. Lifestyle wellness coaches should be well versed in the ways in which exercise, eating, meditation, bodywork, and other factors can modulate stress responses. They will also appreciate how engagement in various somatic or health practices can influence personal awareness, sensitivity to others, the ability to be focused or disciplined, and even spiritual evolution.

Having strong somatic awareness, or an appreciation of how the body works and what influences our physical energy, lifestyle wellness coaches may well have an edge on other coaches who have not spent as much time studying health, wellness, and fitness. They know how to develop resilience through healthy living and adherence to character-developing physical training. They know that walking the talk of whatever a client wishes to realize is about the embodiment of one's desired new way of being. Perhaps more critically, they know the boundaries and warning signs when clients want to embark on unrealistic or risky paths of change involving body-centered actions.

## COMMENTARY

It's estimated that people alive today in the Western world will live about 30 years longer on average than their predecessors at the beginning of the 20th century. We also know that change is omnipresent in our lives. Most of us have no clear vision about what the world holds in store for our children. The press of change is so pervasive that most young adults who are currently entering the job market will have to reinvent themselves numerous times before they reach those long-heralded golden years of retirement—if such golden years even continue to exist.

Concerns about health, wellness, and fitness will no doubt become more paramount as the number of centenarians increases and the consequences of poor and even moderate health practices become more pronounced. The role of lifestyle wellness coaches will also evolve in upcoming decades. For now, we know that there is considerable work to be done to motivate and support people to make essential lifestyle changes. We also recognize that there is a powerful literature of theory and practice concerning how professionals can promote change through dialogue and conversation. The upcoming chapters will take you more fully into the core dynamics of change and the methodologies employed by successful coaches. You may be at the beginning of this journey, yet it is exciting to realize that this professional world that you are now considering will blossom in an exponential fashion in the years to come.

# 3

# PATHS OF CHANGE

## *I*n this chapter, you will learn how...

- change is not an isolated event; rather, it is a constant in our lives;

- clients must navigate phases of change before reaching their goal;

- clients' internal worlds will differ significantly in each stage and phase of change;

- coaches' actions must be aligned with client needs in each phase of change; and

- self-efficacy and self-regulation play central roles in the change process.

> As you move forward into your life,
> you will come upon a great chasm.
> Jump. It is not as wide as you think.
>
> —*Advice to a young Zuni warrior*
> *upon initiation into adulthood*

Consider your own life and times when you have wanted to change a particular behavior. How easy was it—or are you still trying to change that behavior? We all have heard stories of people who decided seemingly in a moment to stop smoking or to start exercising, and to this day they have been true to their commitments. If these stories underlie your understanding of change, you may believe that it's all a matter of willpower.

Change is rarely linear. Even in examples of instantaneous conversions of smokers to nonsmokers or nonexercisers to exercisers, the individual's internal story will have more twists and turns than are externally evident. There are, of course, exceptions to the rule. Some people simply make a decision and change. They are rare, yet our rational minds would like us to believe they are the rule rather than the exception. Coaches who have worked in one-to-one relationships for a long time will have success stories as well as tales of defeat and discouragement. You may have found yourself thinking, "If only I had done X, my client would have succeeded." In this scenario you would assume a portion of the blame or responsibility for the client's outcome and no doubt would be investing time figuring out how to be more successful in the future. In this chapter, we offer some perspectives about change that we trust will better inform your practice.

The field of health psychology is replete with theories and models that attempt to explain and predict changes in health behaviors (table 3.1). By far the best-known and most researched model of this sort is the **transtheoretical model (TTM)**, sometimes referenced as the stages of change (SOC) model (Prochaska, Norcross, & DiClemente, 1994). TTM, which is the first model presented in this chapter, is not explicitly a coaching model. It is a theoretical framework that describes how people go through the process of change as they progressively discontinue an unhealthy behavior or adopt a healthy one. The model is nonetheless pertinent to coaching by virtue of identifying where clients might be situated in the stages of change and then suggesting potential actions to propel them forward.

The other framework we discuss in this chapter is Marilyn Taylor's (1986) learning-through-change (LTC) model. Though not as widely researched as TTM, this model provides a powerful inner perspective of clients in change. It likens clients' experiences

## REFLECTION 3.1

Take a moment and ask yourself what your truth is about why people change and why they don't. Think about health behaviors in particular. Why do some people continue unhealthy habits despite all the evidence? What causes someone to yo-yo up and down with a change objective such as losing weight? What about people you know who just do it? What makes them different? Maybe your answers will begin to reflect certain attitudes, such as "For this kind of behavior, people don't have much control (e.g., heroin addiction), but for that behavior (e.g., overeating) they have a lot of control." As a result, your personal map of change might categorize some people as strong willed and others as unfortunate victims or weak willed.

## Table 3.1   Popular Theories of Health-Related Behavior Change

| Theory or model | Factors increasing the chances of change |
|---|---|
| Health action process approach (HAPA) (Lippke, Ziegelmann, & Schwarzer, 2005; Luszczynska, Gutiérrez-Doña, & Schwarzer, 2005; Schwarzer, 1992, 2001, 2006) | Motivational phase: Perception of risks Outcome expectancies Perceived self-efficacy Intention and goal setting Belief in self-efficacy to take action Volitional (preparation and action) phase: Action planning Action control (initiation, recovery from lapses, maintenance) Belief in self-efficacy to maintain engagement |
| Health belief model (HBM) (Rosenstock, Strecher, & Becker, 1988) | Perception of threat: Perceived susceptibility to a condition or disease Severity of the condition or disease Beliefs about positive outcomes of performing the behavior Perceived benefits minus perceived barriers Personal factors (age, sex, ethnicity, personality, socioeconomics, knowledge) Cues to action (internal, external) |
| Social cognitive theory (SCT) (Bandura, 1977, 1986, 1997a, 1997b) | Interaction between personal factors, the person's environment, and the behavior: Self-efficacy beliefs Outcome expectancies |
| Theory of reasoned action and planned behavior (TRA/TPB) (Ajzen & Fishbein, 1980, 2004; Fishbein & Ajzen, 2005) | Behavioral intention as an outcome of the following: Attitudes toward the behavior and its outcomes Influence of significant others (subjective norms) Perceived behavioral control (similar to self-efficacy beliefs) |

to seasonal changes as they move from one way of engaging with the world to another. It reframes change efforts as a cycle of learning and explores interior realities. It further suggests beneficial patterns for navigating the often tumultuous seasons of change. The LTC model bears resemblance to TTM, though it offers more penetrating insights about interior and exterior roadblocks to change. It provides coaches with a compassionate understanding of why some people spin interminably in indecision or insufficient commitment and what coaches can do to help.

As we know, pathways of change rarely form a steady progression toward goals; what helps clients at the outset may be ineffective later on. As clients advance toward their goals, they manifest different needs. Coaches who are unaware of these dynamics may respond inappropriately or be surprised by the kinds of reactions they evoke. In combination, the two models presented in this chapter provide practical maps of clients' likely experiences throughout a coaching experience. As an added feature, we offer brief commentaries about decisional balance, self-efficacy, and self-regulation to further guide your work.

# TRANSTHEORETICAL MODEL (TTM)

How ready is your client to make the changes necessary to achieve her goal? The fact that someone has hired you as her coach affords concrete data that she has moved beyond the starting gate. Even so, your client may not be sufficiently prepared to undertake more than talking about or considering necessary actions. TTM, a model developed by Prochaska, Norcross, and DiClemente (1994), outlines a temporal sequence of stages pertaining to a particular behavior change. It offers practical guidelines for understanding a client's readiness for change.

Take, for example, smoking cessation. Surely you know some people who smoke tobacco and have little intention of changing (precontemplation stage). As well, you are likely to know people who were once smokers but haven't succumbed to temptation even once in years (maintenance and termination stages). In between these extremes are people who are thinking about changing (contemplation and preparation stages) and those who are actively wearing nicotine patches and practicing behavioral techniques to reduce their cravings (action stage).

Though the stages of change represent progressive movement through the process, TTM is dynamic in recognizing that clients sometimes lose their resolve, or relapse, and need to be reenergized in their engagement. Movement toward a desired health goal can be circular rather than linear at times.

Another value offered by TTM for coaching is its inclusion of a **decisional balance** of perceived advantages and disadvantages as a catalyst to change. The model describes a continuum of six stages along which people move as they endeavor to change a current behavior (stop smoking) or adopt a new one (meditate daily). The six stages are summarized as follows.

## Stage 1: Precontemplation

People in this stage have no current intention to change; they are not thinking about doing things differently in regard to a target behavior. They are not swayed by the idea that the negative effects of their behavior outweigh the positive. Perhaps they have tried to change this behavior in the past and failed, maybe they are unaware that they have a problem, or maybe they completely deny that their current patterns could be harmful. Some people who have repeatedly failed in efforts to change a behavior may end up feeling demoralized and as a result give up on the possibility of ever changing.

## Stage 2: Contemplation

Contemplators acknowledge they have a problem, and they are willing to think about their need to change. They may even consider the benefits of a lifestyle change, yet they are not quite ready to embark on concrete actions. Though they have not taken action toward change, they have started to evaluate the pros and cons associated with perpetuating their current problematic behavior. They have, in effect, started filling out a decisional balance sheet (see appendix A for a template and example). A non-exerciser admits that she should exercise to improve her health and well-being. Someone who consumes a lot of junk food will readily concede that he needs to improve his diet. People in this stage are open to information and feedback. Though they speak as if they will take action in the next six months, they can remain in this stage for years. Contemplators realize they have a problem, yet they may be unable to initiate the desired change.

## Stage 3: Preparation

People in this stage are on the verge of action. For them, change is imminent—within the next month! They are setting goals, developing plans, and perhaps even making small changes. They have advanced from a reflective state and are now preparing for engagement. They are establishing priorities and setting themselves in motion toward change. People in the preparation stage are convinced of the benefits of a lifestyle change. A large percentage of new coaching clients are likely to be in this stage. The act of contacting a coach to address a particular issue is a good indication that the client is prepared to change. In this perspective, the process of coaching is well suited to bolstering clients' intentions, reinforcing their self-efficacy belief (see the next section), and enabling them to fully delineate what they want and how best to pursue it.

## Stage 4: Action

People in this stage are actually doing it! They are following an action plan that they have developed to modify their behavior and are keenly involved in the change process. The more they have prepared, the more successful they are likely to be in reaching their desired goals. At this stage, coaches focus on empowering clients to increase their self-regulation and boost their belief that they can successfully remain in action (self-efficacy).

## Stage 5: Maintenance

By definition, one enters the maintenance stage only after consistently engaging in the change processes for at least six months (action stage). However, the maintenance stage itself can last for an indeterminate time or until there is no temptation to revert to the original state. This stage is important to consider for at least two reasons. The first is that it takes at least six months of continuous engagement in a behavior change (action stage) for people to be reasonably solid in their new patterns. A second reason is that being a maintainer in no way implies that people can decrease their vigilance to maintaining action. Although new behaviors or patterns may begin to feel natural in this stage, overconfidence and life stresses can lead to lapses or a full-blown relapse (Marlatt & Donovan, 2008; Marlatt & Gordon, 1985). From this perspective, the duration of a coaching relationship for people addressing changes of significant behavioral patterns is around a year, if not more.

## Stage 6: Termination

In this stage, the new behavior has become such an integral part of daily life that the likelihood of relapse is essentially nonexistent. Some professionals question whether people ever reach this stage, although Prochaska and colleagues (1994) affirm that it is possible for a small percentage of people. Think of people who have successfully given up smoking or who have lost considerable weight through strict adherence to diets.

Years of maintenance may give way to complete relapse in moments of laxity. Consequently, regular follow-ups initiated by coaching clients can be invaluable in ensuring that they remain where they want to be. When clients take on major life changes, it is reasonable to consider check-ins or scheduled sessions every three to six months after the first year.

# CHANGE STRATEGIES

According to the American Psychological Association (2012), adopting effective strategies for change improves the likelihood of success (see What Americans Think of Willpower). Prochaska and colleagues (1994) have recommended 10 intervention strategies or processes of change for stages within TTM. These strategies include methods and techniques that can help people modify thoughts, feelings, and behaviors in the pursuit of desired change (Marshall & Biddle, 2001). Some of these will make sense in a coaching context, while others may not. Moreover, as a coach you are not likely to encounter people seeking your services when they are in the stages of precontemplation, maintenance, or termination. However, you may be interested in creating materials directed toward people in the stages of precontemplation, contemplation, and even preparation. Following are 10 strategies that have been suggested for the various stages of change (Prochaska et al., 1994).

## Strategy 1: Consciousness-Raising

This strategy involves intentional or unintentional exposure to information about oneself or problematic behaviors through such means as lectures, discussion groups, readings, advertisements, films, or even unexpected life events (e.g., a health crisis). Some of what happens here is by-chance encounter or unanticipated life experiences. A lifelong smoker goes to a movie where the main character, who smokes, appears out of control because he is always trying to sneak out for a cigarette. This person had no intention of exposing himself to this message; nonetheless he leaves the movie feeling motivated to explore his own behaviors. Of course, we know

## What Americans Think of Willpower

The most frequently reported goals that people set for 2012 were those aimed at improving health (57 percent reported a goal to lose weight, 50 percent reported a goal to eat a healthier diet, and 41 percent reported a goal to start exercising regularly) or financial status (52 percent reported a goal to save more money, and 37 percent reported a goal to pay off debt). . . . The annual Stress in America survey found that one in four reported that lack of willpower (27 percent) or time (26 percent) prevented them from making the change they were trying to achieve. (p. 5)

Fewer than half of adults who indicate a change was recommended or they decided to make a change when they were interviewed . . . report that they have made or are maintaining the change with the exception of reducing or eliminating alcohol consumption . . . it is likely that utilizing effective strategies to help them achieve their goal will improve the likelihood of success. (p. 6)

Reprinted, by permission, from American Physiological Association, 2012, *What Americans think of willpower* (Washington, DC: APA), 4. Available: www.apa.org/helpcenter/stress-willpower.pdf.

that even with strongly framed messages, such as the warnings on cigarette packages, people can turn a blind eye to the potential hazards they continually invite into their lives.

## Strategy 2: Emotional Arousal

Often accompanying consciousness-raising, emotional arousal targets feelings. Films, books, dramatic media presentations, and fear-arousing experiences including, for example, graphic depictions of diseased lungs or lives ruined through substance abuse can arouse strong emotions. As noted, this type of **intervention** is likely to be a side effect of other kinds of messages that people intentionally or unintentionally experience. There are clear ethical considerations regarding deliberate efforts to upset people about their behaviors or current status (e.g., being obese). A coach may, for instance, know of a particularly dramatic film or novel that pertains to a client's issue and surmise that recommending this film or novel could result in the client's having a strong emotional reaction. Such suggestions need to be carefully considered and offered with an unambiguous advisory about the nature of the content and its possible impact.

## Strategy 3: Social or Environmental Control

External social or environmental forces may exert control over a person's behavior with or without consent. Examples include nonsmoking areas, alcohol-free parties, broken elevators that force people to take the stairs, and sanctions such as social ostracism for behaving in certain ways. Increasingly, the Western world has become intolerant of public smoking so much so that smokers need to inconvenience themselves to continue their habit. Taxation or, to the contrary, insurance rate reductions pertaining to certain habits can also influence behavior. Companies may have policies and programs that reinforce certain behaviors, such as exercising regularly or managing one's weight. People may have no expressed desire to address these matters; the situation simply conspires against them. Coaches are not likely to direct their professional efforts toward these kinds of interventions, though as private citizens they may support their application.

## Strategy 4: Environmental Assessment

This strategy involves appraising the negative impacts of the behavior on the person's environment. For example, smokers may realize that smoking is harmful to the environment, or they may become aware of the effects of secondhand smoke on people around them (e.g., their children). Better yet, they may want to act as a model to be emulated by their children and those whom they regularly see.

## Strategy 5: Personal Revisioning

This strategy involves looking toward the future by imagining life after changing problematic behaviors.

Revisioning, or self-reevaluation, enables people to appreciate how their behaviors may conflict with core personal values and thereby generate motivation to change. This type of intervention is well represented in the toolkits of professional coaches. There are a number of ways coaches encourage their clients to create a compelling vision of their desired future in order to drive current actions in that direction. People who are willing to imagine a more gratifying future open themselves more readily to considering new behavior patterns.

## Strategy 6: Commitment

Choosing to change, accepting responsibility for change, and then publicly announcing one's commitment are core features of this strategy. It typically includes clear delineation of the intended change through a contract or other means of making the commitment explicit. This strategy constitutes a core element in the coaching process. Even at the level of small actions planned in individual coaching sessions, clients are typically asked how committed they are to engaging in the designed actions. Making overt commitments to their coaches is a form of public expression for which clients then become accountable.

## Strategy 7: Rewarding

This strategy relies on praise and other rewards to reinforce positive behavior change. Many of the changes that clients undertake in coaching relationships represent a significant challenge. Though many sources of motivation for change are accessed in effective coaching, building in tangible rewards for attaining particular levels of achievement or adhering to commitments can help reinforce the emerging changes. Of course, if clients continue to rely on reward strategies after six or more months of sustained action, coaches might have legitimate concerns about the degree to which the new behavior patterns are being internalized.

## Strategy 8: Countering

In this strategy, people substitute healthy behaviors for unhealthy ones, such as doing tai chi for five minutes instead of having a late-night snack or picking up a compelling book instead of turning on the television. This approach relies on identifying and controlling internal reactions, such as being aware when an urge arises and then substituting a preplanned healthy behavior.

## Strategy 9: Environmental Management or Stimulus Control

Similar to countering, environmental management involves controlling one's world, but the focus is on the external environment. Environmental management involves deliberately manipulating one's surroundings to support change. For instance, the act of engaging in exercise is strongly supported by reconfiguring the nonexerciser's environment so that the probability of exercising on a regular basis is greatly increased. Examples might include signing up for a gym membership with an organization that has multiple locations, packing an exercise bag the night before a morning workout, booking a hotel with a fitness spa on a business trip, having some home workout equipment for days when going to the gym isn't practical, and creating workout stations for one-minute exercises at home, among others. Planning for these kinds of strategic interventions is part of the normal dialogue in coaching relationships.

## Strategy 10: Social Support

Involving friends, families, colleagues, and professionals can definitely help people advance through the stages of change. Of course, coaching relationships in themselves offer understanding, acceptance, and guidance for clients as they progress through the challenges of change. However, a coaching relationship is by definition temporary. In understanding clients' issues and the actions they pursue, ongoing and appropriate **social support** from others is typically considered. Coaches not only explore the nature of current relationships with others implicated in clients' change initiatives, they also investigate untapped resources and the creation of new social networks that can support commitments to action.

# APPLYING TTM STRATEGIES IN COACHING

Throughout the previous section, we indicated that certain strategies might be more appropriate or effective at certain stages of change. In your role as a coach or as a professional working to promote health and wellness, you might want to avoid some interventions for clients who are in the early stages of change because they are likely to backfire. For example, encouraging someone to commit to action during the precontemplation or contemplation stage will most likely fail. The client has not sufficiently worked through his internal connections to the problematic behaviors or developed an adequate plan to deal with the side effects of self-change. Once you have worked with the client for some time and have witnessed his progress toward action, other strategies may prove more effective (see table 3.2 for a list of suggested interventions applied to each TTM stage of change).

Two intervention strategies, environmental assessment and consciousness-raising, may be especially helpful for people in the stages of precontemplation

**Table 3.2    Interventions at Each TTM Stage of Change**

| Stage of TTM | Suggested TTM interventions | Suggested coaching intervention |
|---|---|---|
| Precontemplation | Environmental assessment<br>Consciousness-raising<br>Social and environmental control<br>Emotional arousal | Identify the behavior and clarify its impacts on self and others.<br>Get information about negative consequences of performing or not performing a behavior.<br>Recognize the influences of the social environment related to the behavior.<br>Awaken emotions through the coach's empathetic feedback or through books, films, and such that arouse emotions. |
| Contemplation | Self-revisioning<br>Interpersonal (social) support<br>Decisional balance and force field analysis<br>Self-efficacy | Create positive vision of the future self.<br>Identify people who could provide support for change.<br>Weigh the pros and cons of change.<br>Increase self-efficacy by seeing others implement the desired change. |
| Preparation | Self-revisioning<br>Commitment<br>Interpersonal (social) support<br>Self-efficacy | Set clear goals to achieve vision of future self.<br>Make concrete action plans, make public commitment to change, take small steps toward change.<br>Review social circle to identify those who detract change efforts, enlist others' help for change (including coach's support).<br>Increase self-efficacy by experiencing small successes toward change and getting positive feedback from coach. |
| Action | Countering<br>Environmental control<br>Rewards<br>Commitment<br>Interpersonal (social) support<br>Self-efficacy | Brainstorm alternatives for undesired behavior and adopt new behaviors to replace unwanted one.<br>Design environment to support change.<br>Link rewards and celebrations of success.<br>Self-monitor and tweak action plans, contract for persistent action, design self-regulation strategies, continue public affirmation of goal pursuit.<br>Find new sources of social support.<br>Increase self-efficacy by reframing negative internal feelings toward change. |
| Maintenance | Commitment<br>Self-efficacy | Review action, evaluate progress, determine frequency of lapses (if any), review self-regulation strategies, appreciate pros of change, celebrate success.<br>Increase self-efficacy by reviewing success and getting positive feedback from coach. |
| Termination | Self-efficacy<br>Embark on new change process | Increase self-efficacy by celebrating maintenance of the desired change.<br>Make plans to contemplate future change if desired. |

and contemplation. To facilitate environmental assessment, you might work with your client to help her discover the negative effects of her behaviors on others around her. Consciousness-raising might take the form of giving a sedentary person a pamphlet on the health risks of inactivity or suggesting that the person have an in-depth discussion about inactivity with her doctor. Sometimes unexpected events in a person's life, such as learning that a friend who smokes was diagnosed with lung cancer, can serve as a wake-up call. This kind of intervention, of course, would be unplanned.

Another intervention that is helpful in the early stages of change (precontemplation and contemplation) involves social or environmental control. Surrounding conditions in the social or physical world influence our behavior. Increasingly, the wisdom of having candy dispensers or pop machines in public venues is being questioned; instead, having healthy snacks available in these locations could have a significant positive impact on behavior. At a social level, work and community groups may exert pressure to reinforce positive behavioral norms, such as work–life balance.

Although coaches may not be able to control social or environmental factors, they can use other interventions, namely, emotional arousal and self-revisioning. A client may experience emotional arousal as a result of his coach's expression of concern for his well-being. Let us assume that you are involved with a client concerning a nonhealth-related issue such as career transition and you notice the impact of certain unhealthy habits—poor diet, smoking, or other harmful behaviors—on the client's coaching topic or general wellness. Your empathic feedback in these moments can heighten clients' emotional concern for their own state of health.

As noted previously, emotional arousal may occur when a client views a film or reads a book related to the changes that she is contemplating. In working with people who are searching for motivation to change life-threatening behaviors, you might respond to that cry for help by recommending books, films, or discussion groups that can arouse emotions that direct energy toward commitment. Of course, it is essential to be clear about the content of the recommended material and its potential impact.

Another strategy, self-revisioning, builds on the effects of emotional arousal. Here, you may focus clients toward a positive image of future life after a change has occurred. You can encourage them to imagine themselves after the change process has been successfully completed.

Interpersonal support is a strategy that applies to all stages of change, and simple actions represent it exquisitely. Listening to clients with compassion and warmth enables them to open themselves to their inner wisdom and self-caring. Hearing them without judgment and with concern and empathy allows them to find the strength to change. Beyond the coaching relationship, clients may be encouraged to surround themselves with those who will facilitate their change rather than derail them in the process.

Because many clients are already on the path of change, they will likely have reached the stage of preparation or even action in relation to some aspects of their goals. In these latter stages of change, the most helpful strategies include rewards, environmental control, and enhanced commitment through contracts.

People need feedback to grow, and positive feedback (reward) has the most beneficial effect on behavior (Johnson, 2009). Although some clients may be so dedicated to their programs that you take their commitment for granted, it continues to be important to regularly praise and reward their efforts without necessarily acting as a cheerleader. According to TTM principles, you may want to strategically celebrate clients for specific results they achieve. You may also work with them to collaboratively design rewards that are contingent on achieving intermediate successes on their way to attaining their ultimate goal. A caveat applies here: It is important that the reward be realistic, be commensurate with the achievement, and not detract from the overall goal. For example, buying an expensive exercise outfit for every two weeks that one trains may not be economically sustainable, and getting a chocolate caramel latte and a piece of cheesecake for every five-pound weight loss is not a highly congruent reward strategy.

Another way to help clients in the more advanced stages of action and maintenance is to periodically review their goals and programs. In doing so, you reinforce awareness of their commitment to change and to themselves. Because making public commitments increases adherence, you can also encourage clients to tell others about their goals and plans.

A third strategy for the advanced stages of change is countering. This is where you can exercise your creativity. You might, for instance, engage clients in a brainstorming process where both of you generate as many positive substitutes for problematic behaviors as possible and then evaluate which ones are likely to work best. One of the many values of a coaching relationship is tailoring a practice to clients' unique situations and personal styles. In this way, countering behaviors will have good alignment with clients' shifts in commitment, motivation, and energy to engage action. Although some people may be entirely reliable in meeting their commitments when they are on their normal schedules, holidays, vacations, and travel can create trouble spots for adherence. Dialogues with clients to manage their environments in support of change agendas can promote reliable adherence. As a coach, you can encourage them to plan for situations that previously led to relapse. Especially as people move toward the end of the coaching relationship, it will be important to embed perspectives of how they can continually orient themselves to their worlds so as to capitalize on opportunities that enhance commitment.

In setting goals and ensuring the robustness of an action plan, it is essential to explore obstacles to engagement and incorporate actions that support clients' commitment to change. One of the many gifts of a coaching relationship is how sensitively coaches work to raise clients' awareness of their internal reactions, sensations, or other experiences that signal potential capitulation to an old habit. Coaches collaborate with clients in developing practices to increase self-knowledge that alerts them to potential slippage. As well, they cocreate alternative actions that clients can enact when tempted by deeply ingrained behavioral patterns.

---

**REFLECTION 3.2**

Once upon a time, you may have been inactive, a smoker, in an unsatisfying relationship, in a university degree program that didn't fit you, or in some other unworkable situation. Pick a clear example where you responded successfully to the call for change. Recall the sequence of events from beginning to end. Recollect when you first began thinking about changing and when you realized that you had successfully completed the process of change. Bring to mind as much of your history in this change experience as possible. Remember whether the change was sudden or whether a gradual awakening occurred.

Can you identify the phases of change as described by TTM? If so, what change strategies helped you move from precontemplation to maintenance or perhaps termination?

---

# SELF-EFFICACY, SELF-REGULATION, AND RELAPSE PREVENTION

Of all the variables influencing the change process, perceived self-efficacy (Bandura, 1997a, 1997b) is by far the most widely used in theories and models of change. And though self-efficacy and self-regulation are not explicitly listed among TTM strategies for change, they are core constructs of the model. The influence of self-efficacy on the adoption, performance, and maintenance of health-related behaviors has been researched and validated in numerous contexts (Allison & Keller, 2004; Bandura, 1992, 1995, 1997a, 1997b, 2000; Dallow & Anderson, 2003; Schwarzer, 1992).

**Self-efficacy** and **self-regulation** involve the degree to which people are confident that they can perform the behavior they want, that they can exercise control over challenging situations, and that they can regulate themselves (e.g., thoughts, feelings, motivation) to effectively pursue changes they want (Bandura, 1997a, 1997b). Self-efficacy beliefs naturally differ from person to person. According to Bandura, people with higher levels of self-efficacy set more challenging goals for themselves, consistently visualize successful outcomes, expend more effort, and persevere longer to achieve their goals. They are also more resilient in the face of setbacks compared with those who have low confidence in their abilities, and they cope better with stress in difficult situations. Bandura (1998) offers four sources through which self-efficacy beliefs can be developed:

1. Mastery experiences or learning by successfully doing—"I can jog for six minutes! I think I will be able to jog for eight."

2. Vicarious experiences or learning by observing similar others succeed through persistent effort—"If my friend Jack can do it, then I can do it too."

3. Social persuasion—"Others tell me I can succeed; now I believe I can."

4. Reframing psychophysiological states—"Just because I feel stress and fatigue right now doesn't mean that I can't succeed in the long run."

An important consideration when working with TTM and perceived self-efficacy is that clients' beliefs in their abilities are stage specific. Typically, confidence is low or nonexistent at the precontemplation stage and increases throughout the remaining stages of change. Although some people might have general levels of self-efficacy at the beginning, believing that they are competent to tackle novel tasks and cope with adversity in a wide range of challenging situations (Luszczynska et al., 2005), they may nonetheless need to work with a coach to set realistic goals or to make robust action plans that will ensure success (preparation stage). Furthermore, they may need coaching to devise coping and recovery strategies so that they can generate a grounded belief in their capacity to maintain newly acquired behaviors (action and maintenance stages).

Self-regulation implies that people have the ability and determination to control their thoughts, emotions, impulses, or appetites in service of reaching a desired goal (Vohs & Baumeister, 2010). Baumeister, Heatherton, and Tice (1994) suggest that without self-regulation, past experiences, learning, habits, inclinations, or even innate tendencies might detract from reliable goal attainment. According to these researchers, self-regulation acts include countering, whereby a person substitutes a normal or habitual response to a situation (e.g., eating a calorie-laden snack) with a response more aligned with the outcomes she wants to achieve (e.g., having a piece of fruit as a snack). Without strategies to self-regulate, clients' achievements may be strongly compromised.

People fail to control their actions for a wide variety of reasons. As mentioned in our discussion of TTM, change does not invariably progress from contemplation to action. It may represent a cyclical process whereby people revert to contemplation from the action stage. Sometimes, clients will experience failures when positive or negative triggers distract them from pursuing their goals (Larimer, Palmer, & Marlatt, 1999; Marlatt & Donovan, 2008; Marlatt & Gordon, 1985). A positive trigger might be a big family celebration that calls for a few drinks and, as a result, the client abandons his change agenda. A negative trigger could be emotional states such as anger, boredom, or depression that overshadow the determination to move forward. At other times, people might experience peer pressure to revert to habits they want to break. Similarly, they might let other priorities (e.g., work and family demands)

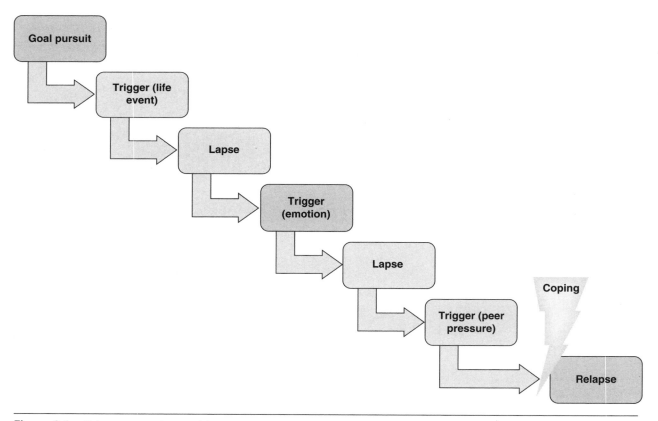

**Figure 3.1**  Relapse prevention model.
Based on Marlatt 1999.

interfere with desires to modify behaviors. Or, they may get discouraged when they don't achieve the results they want as quickly as expected. Without doubt, you can add a few reasons of your own regarding why people experience setbacks.

These setbacks can range from momentary lapses (the smoker who wants to quit smokes a few cigarettes on a particularly stressful day) to a full-blown **relapse** (even though the smoker still wants to quit, she gives up the effort altogether when she experiences too many lapses) (see figure 3.1). It is imperative for coaches to ensure that clients have coping skills and strategies for **relapse prevention** so that they consistently maintain progress without getting distracted along the way.

Strategies to bolster self-regulation include some of the TTM processes of change. Others that have been identified include the following (Vohs & Baumeister, 2010):

- Self-monitoring whereby performance is consistently measured against the desired goals—measuring the current reality against what the client seeks (e.g., weekly weigh-ins to determine progress in weight management, food diaries)
- Setting concrete goals and keeping awareness on the target behaviors so that distractions are minimized
- Expanding realistic effort, that is, acknowledging and doing the work required to predictably bring about positive results

A prerequisite for self-regulation is a strong sense of self-efficacy to ensure that effort is exerted for successful goal attainment. According to theory and research, self-efficacious people—those who develop strong intentions to stay the course, set clear goals, and consistently and effectively monitor their behavior—reliably exert the necessary effort to reach their objectives.

# LEARNING-THROUGH-CHANGE (LTC) MODEL

Changing long-term lifestyle patterns is likely to involve deep restructuring of thoughts, feelings, and behaviors (Gollwitzer, 1999; Gollwitzer & Brandstätter, 1997; Mcbrearty, 2010). As an observer, you may witness the results of long-term deliberations about change in a single moment when a person smokes his last cigarette or steps on a treadmill for the first time. By contrast, you can observe anew

a commitment to positive actions such as exercise each time a person shows up to train. When clients commit to new behaviors or cease old ones, the change process is likely to unfold over time. In this respect, modifying behaviors or shifting patterns can be conceived of according to various phases or seasons of change.

To better understand the personal face of change, Taylor (1986) formulated the **learning-through-change (LTC) model** that illuminates the internal world of those confronting change. As in TTM, LTC tracks the change process over time. Taylor takes the perspective that people in a change process face challenges to learn different things at different times as they cope with and adapt to disconfirming events in their lives. In this respect, she describes change as a potential learning experience. Moreover, she likens the cyclical process of change to the four seasons and seasonal adaptations. Coincidentally, framing change in the language of the four seasons implicitly acknowledges the length of time it may take to effectively work through significant behavioral adaptations, that is, one year.

Appreciating the inner processes of clients who have embarked on a journey toward a healthier life will certainly benefit the coach who has been hired to facilitate change. Moreover, the LTC model offers guidance about the types of interventions or styles of coaching that would be most supportive for clients in specific seasons of change.

If you imagine an area of the world where there are four distinct seasons, you will realize that there are parts of the year that seem to be in between seasons. The LTC model not only describes four distinct phases but also four phase transitions that serve to shift the person from one distinct climate to another. The model (see figure 3.2) relies on the fact that we commonly live in a state where elements of our existence feel more or less in balance. Motivation for change may arise from an accumulation of experiences or from a single event. Someone may grow weary of waking up every morning with a hacking cough resulting from a two-pack-a-day cigarette habit, while someone else may be shocked into awareness when a friend dies of lung cancer.

The roots of change are not always predictable; however, it is clear that people don't randomly decide that today would be a good day to change. It is as if discontent about *what is* and dreams about *what could be* reach a critical mass, causing people to come tumbling out of their comfortable worlds to enter a cycle of events (or phases) that eventually return them to a new equilibrium. This new state of equilibrium may or may not represent an

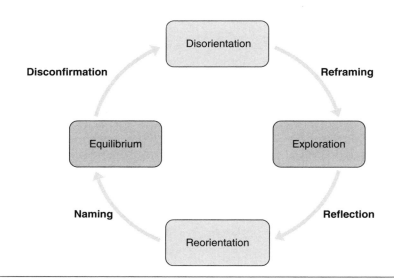

**Figure 3.2** Taylor's LTC model.

Reprinted from M.M. Taylor, 1986, "Learning for self-direction in the classroom: The pattern of a transition process," *Studies in Higher Education* 11(1). By permission of Marilyn M. Taylor, PhD.

improvement over their old way of being, depending on how the change process is managed.

The LTC model describes a cycle of events and experiences. It considers typical thoughts, feelings, and actions of clients as they move through the phases. As orderly as this cyclical flow might appear, any change process can be easily derailed if certain conditions prevail. Human beings gravitate toward balance and a state of equilibrium (Sheldon, Cummins, & Kamble, 2010), whatever shape that may take for each of us personally. We don't often choose to roll the dice with our lives unless something has provoked us to pursue change. Even though there is a sense that modern life is akin to a permanent white-water state (Cabana, Emery, & Emery, 1995) where change is omnipresent, we seem to be capable of finding a balanced path even while shooting the rapids. Change of the kind we are addressing throughout this book is different from the day-to-day pacing of our lives. It represents a need or perhaps a demand for us to be different—to show up in our lives with new perspectives, actions, values, styles, and other aspects of self-presentation.

Whether we choose to engage in change or are thrust into it involuntarily, we are in for a ride. The journey is one that moves us out of a state of equilibrium into a sometimes chaotic world that we must confront and eventually manage in order to regain a new and hopefully more evolved sense of balance. Here's how the cycle unfolds according to the LTC model (see table 3.3 for a list of suggested interventions applied to each phase of the LTC model.

# Transition 1: Disconfirmation

Clients who voluntarily commit themselves to a coaching process do so with reason. Sometimes a big push comes from something such as a medical report. At other times a gradual accumulation of dissatisfactions tips the scale and topples the person out of balance. This first transition is called *disconfirmation* because some aspect of the person's old world no longer works or makes sense. There is inherent discomfort in disconfirmation. It may be like wearing pants that are a size too small—or even worse. Feelings have broken through the surface and can't be pushed back down. The mind is drawn like a magnet to the emerging issue. Things don't seem right and trying to meditate or medicate the issues so they go away just doesn't work.

The idea that life crises open up possibilities for growth or decline is well documented (Ogden & Hills, 2008). This first transition is pivotal. There is real risk that another kind of transitional shift will occur, one that closes down the client's potential and narrows his perspective of self, others, and the world. Think of people who have encountered traumatic injuries or losses. The risk exists for them to spiral downward into a despairing view of themselves and the world. They may nurture the persona of a victim over time. We believe that no matter what the loss, there is a possibility for learning. The path of growth may require extraordinary effort, but in the end is there really a better alternative?

**Table 3.3     Interventions for Coaches According to Transition/Phase of LTC Model**

| Transition/phase | Internal states | Suggested coaching intervention |
|---|---|---|
| Disconfirmation/ disorientation | Dissatisfied with current state<br>Experiencing negative emotions<br>Self-rejecting<br>Blaming self and others | Obtain emotional support.<br>Review past influences on current state with focus on forward movement. |
| Reframing/ exploration | Acknowledging current state without blaming self or others<br>Self-accepting<br>Yearning for new knowledge<br>Keen for human connections<br>Experiencing glimmers of hope | Engage in self-affirmation.<br>Discover unhelpful patterns (beliefs, thoughts, behaviors).<br>Identify resources (people and things) to obtain information.<br>Brainstorm and evaluate new avenues, new ways of being, new beliefs.<br>Discover new motivations.<br>Make decisions to move forward. |
| Reflection/ reorientation | Self-reflecting<br>Introspective<br>Contemplating new identity formation | Find ways to promote self-reflection.<br>Formulate action plans and engage in action.<br>Increase self-efficacy.<br>Self-monitor and self-regulate. |
| Naming/ equilibrium | Self-affirming<br>Accepting of new identity<br>Excited<br>Understanding of self-change process<br>Eager to advocate change for others<br>Self-efficacious | Reflect on new reality.<br>Celebrate success.<br>Reflect on the change process and derive learning for future change.<br>End the coaching relationship in relation to the current agenda. |

# Phase 1: Disorientation

When excuses seem lame, when emerging realities trump rationalizations, and when old solutions no longer work, people in a process of change may feel defenseless. They can no longer justify their behaviors. They cannot maintain their previous way of living. This first phase can be a highly emotional time. People may spin in confusion, anger, blame, sadness, frustration, or guilt. Taking a hard, cold look at themselves in the mirror, they may be saddened or repulsed to see what they have created over years of inactivity or personal neglect. They may seek someone to blame, or they may simply wallow in self-pity. When clients drop the mask behind which they have hidden the truth, they may feel extremely vulnerable. Although they may try to make light of this new awareness, there is an inner voice that continually reminds them of the way it really is. The first phase, disorientation, may last for days, weeks, or even months, depending on the nature and extent of the disconfirmation that people have experienced. It is unlikely they will stay here too long, however, because it is just too uncomfortable. The critical question is whether they will address this emergence in a way that is constructive or destructive.

The disorientation phase generally corresponds to the stage of contemplation in TTM. However, the label *contemplation* has a distinctly different feel than that of *disorientation*. The LTC model provides insights about the client's inner world and how unsettled it is.

Though someone might grow accustomed to wearing pants that are a size too small, it is more likely that over time this person will either buy larger pants or address her weight. From the perspective of TTM, the person who buys new pants retreats to precontemplation or hovers on the boundary between precontemplation and contemplation.

The LTC model clearly identifies the risks that clients run throughout this phase. If the model describes a cycle of change, a downward spiral toward a new equilibrium could be achieved by adopting a more negative self-identity. For instance, the client whose pants no longer fit might redefine herself as a fat person, a couch potato, or simply a lazy and unmotivated person.

Through a coaching relationship, clients in disorientation will have strong support for forward or upwardly spiraling movement. Coaches must remain attentive to where the pain lies and in what direction—inward or outward—it is pointed. They need to create ample space for emotional expression without allowing emotional relief to become the sole purpose of the sessions. The inner terrain of the client's world needs to be explored and historical contributors to his current state identified. However, emotional support and the generation of first steps on a path forward would normally characterize the coach's emphasis at this time.

## Transition 2: Reframing

Imagine someone who finally confronts the fact that she is out of shape and 50 pounds (23 kg) overweight. Perhaps she went to her 20th high school reunion and felt shame when comparing herself to some of her former classmates. The experience of disconfirmation (transition 1) may have pulled her out of equilibrium and thrust her into disorientation (phase 1). This phase normally lasts until the person is able to reframe what is upsetting her without blaming herself or others. As long as she spins in self-rejection or fails to get to the root of what bothers her, she will continue to ride the tumultuous waves of disorientation.

Forward movement requires perspective about core issues. We can describe this as a state of acceptance, which is not to be mistaken for resignation. Though it may be accurate enough to say that the out-of-shape, overweight client bears some responsibility for creating whatever conditions she is now trying to address, the perspective that she needs to develop in this second transition is one of acknowledgment of her present state—without blaming herself or projecting responsibility on others. She begins to understand that she has a choice about a new path forward and that it will be far easier to opt for positive alternatives when self-judging and critical emotions are put aside through compassionate self-acceptance.

There is no doubt that many people are motivated to act based on the emotional charge of anger, resentment, blame, and even hatred. However, the direction of change formed from these emotions is not likely to be generative and uplifting. We need to be ever watchful in appreciating the energy sources that clients rely on for change. Positive motivations must replace negative ones. Life-giving perspectives need to be discovered to prevent a shriveling view of self and others. Effective coaching is not just about getting clients to do things differently; it involves grounding action in affirmations of self and others that breathe new life into their potential.

## Phase 2: Exploration

As the spinning slows and the fog begins to lift, the path forward peeks out in the strangest ways. It is as if signposts appear everywhere. The challenge in this phase is to remain open-minded and in an exploratory mode long enough to appreciate the value of all the potential avenues before choosing one particular path. Consider someone who has recently broken up with her long-term partner. With some help, she has moved beyond blame and out of an emotional spin. Is this the right time for her to enter a new relationship? You will probably think that it's not, and recommendations based on the LTC model support this belief. People in this kind of life change are encouraged to take time to explore what they need, what did not work in their previous ways of being in a relationship, and what changes they want to incorporate in the future.

Imagine that, due to an injury, a client has been forced to give up a sport that he has practiced for over 20 years (transition 1). After he has identified issues without blame (transition 2) and has entered the phase of exploration, he can then consider his options and sample the possibilities in a process of experimentation. This phase is typically an intensely social time. People who are trying to figure out new habits and ways of functioning in a changed personal reality need other people, especially those who are in a similar phase of change or perhaps a step ahead. In this social context, they can openly examine their ideas, plans, and proposals. They also welcome knowledge and information from books or other sources. Clients signal to their coaches that they have entered this phase by their keen interest in facts and information, their need to talk about what they are doing, and their efforts to socialize with others who are walking a similar path. Having resources readily at hand and perhaps scheduling extra time to talk with clients is helpful for them to efficiently move through this phase.

The exploration phase generally coincides with the preparation stage in TTM. What the LTC model adds are an appreciation of the need to experiment, the relevance of like-minded others, and the importance of gathering relevant information. Clients need to sample the options and discover the fit between possibilities they are discovering and their emerging new selves. If we go back to the example of the recently separated woman, we can readily predict that without sufficient experimentation and reflection, she is likely to end up in another relationship with at best a slightly improved version of her old partner. The core work of coaching takes place in this stage. The client needs to progressively develop a new way of orienting herself to the world, and this requires significant alterations in her processes of thinking, feeling, and behaving. This phase is highly active, yet without a commitment to a single path. Of course, depending on the nature of the issue, sorting through the options may be relatively quick or quite protracted.

## Transition 3: Reflection

Deep and sometimes extended reflection marks the transition to the next phase in the cycle. The person may begin to withdraw into himself to consolidate thoughts and feelings and to generate a coherent strategy for action. From the outside, the person may appear more introspective. He may reduce his requests for feedback and no longer ask for readings or other sources of information. We need to be sensitive to this shift by allowing clients space for reflection rather than continuing to offer ideas, suggestions, and encouragement for further experimentation.

Reflection does not come naturally to some people. As important and helpful as it can be, clients may want to short-circuit this transitional time. From the coach's perspective, when clients go inward, there needs to be a keen awareness of the action-packed potential of this interior journey. In support of their clients' work, coaches may recommend such strategies as journaling, meditating, taking long walks, or recording one's thoughts to be listened to at a later point.

When clients don't allow this time, what is at risk? They may conclude their deliberations and explorations with a somewhat nebulous foundation if they don't take enough time to contemplate and solidify their understandings. Coaching relationships often follow a biweekly meeting schedule, so there should be ample material for review if clients commit to contemplative assignments between sessions. It is unlikely that they will stall here for long, but coaches need to be mindful of how long the transition is taking as clients move from active experimentation to the next phase of systematically engaging action.

## Phase 3: Reorientation

Clients generally enter the reorientation phase with a plan. The plan may be rudimentary, but they are usually committed to testing it out and determining how well it works. Maybe the plan is a particular training schedule coupled with a variable routine for other activities. Perhaps it is a healthy eating program that the person has derived from explorations of how to lose weight sensibly and promote wellness. As a health, wellness, or fitness professional, your role in the reorientation phase may take on dimensions of expert feedback and advice so that clients can fine-tune their programs. Your interventions could represent a more technical level of input during this phase. Rather than facilitating the decision-making process as you did during the exploration phase, you are now engaged in setting goals and managing progress and accountability. A kind of shakedown occurs in this phase in which clients make final adjustments to plans before consolidating them into ongoing processes.

The reorientation phase parallels aspects of the action stage in TTM. What the LTC model adds to our understanding are the multidimensional shifts that clients need to internalize during this phase. Consider a person who has committed to a healthy eating plan, which is resulting in gradual but consistent weight loss toward a target goal. If this client was obese for a long time, the shifts that are occurring are not restricted to behavioral eating patterns. Emotionally, this client will feel as if he is living in a new skin. Cognitively, he will begin to know himself in the world differently. Coaches are attentive to this layered change process and guide their clients not only on the technical side of health behavior change but also along the lines of their evolving self-image, emotional realities, relationships, and mental models.

## Transition 4: Naming

You have undoubtedly met people who have recently succeeded in a smoking-cessation program or who have become regular exercisers. Usually, these people enjoy broadcasting their successes wherever they can. They want to help others who have struggled with the same challenges they have overcome. Clients who have made it to this point are excited about their accomplishments and want others to feel as good as they do. Beyond the obvious satisfaction they experience with their achievements, they are able to articulate exactly what has changed for them and how they managed to generate their successes.

This transition represents a self-affirmation of who the person has become through her journey. There is no doubt or vacillation in these announcements. The cycle is almost complete and clients realize their transformative work is nearing an end. At this point, coaches typically validate clients' successes by acknowledging their achievements and by making space for them to talk openly about their journeys. Creating opportunities for them to name publicly what they have learned and accomplished makes it more real for them and provides them with abundant opportunities to celebrate.

## Phase 4: Equilibrium

The LTC model depicts a cycle that begins and ends in equilibrium, although the new equilibrium hopefully represents a healthier and happier way of being. It is characterized by the display of new patterns and orientations that have been tested and refined. It can be seen in the demeanor that the client presents as a result of successfully challenging out-

moded or unproductive ways of living. It shows up in transformed ways of thinking, feeling, and acting. At this point in the change process, the coach's role may be close to ending, at least until the next challenge knocks at the client's door.

The equilibrium phase corresponds to the TTM maintenance stage. However, it provides a broader perspective of the person at this point in time. It allows us to see the various facets of change that are represented in how the person orients herself to the world. For instance, it isn't simply that the person now exercises regularly; rather, she has changed her outlook on life, her self-perception, and no doubt her relationships and emotional interior. The value added by the LTC model lies in understanding that life-affirming health and wellness changes reposition people in their lives such that they are on an upward spiral of growth and evolution.

If this seems over the top, consider the contrary experience. A person initiates a self-change process to finally lose weight, and this commitment to change has been a long time coming. He engages fully, going to great lengths to stick to the plan, but somehow he hasn't embraced the essential ingredients for success, such as controlling his stress and the impact it has on his eating. Sadly, he fails. Is this story simply about nonadherence to a program? We can imagine that this person will feel somewhat demoralized. He may rationalize and make an uneasy peace with his unhealthy eating habits. It is unlikely, though, that this experience will boost his self-esteem or increase his self-efficacy about changing other things in his life. He has potentially entered a downward spiral of self-limiting beliefs and critical self-perceptions.

## APPLYING PRINCIPLES OF THE LTC MODEL

Understanding why clients decide to address a particular change agenda at this precise point in time helps coaches discover the wide-ranging ramifications of these choices. If the decision arose in reaction to certain life events (e.g., marriage or divorce, change in jobs, illness or injury), the coach will need to remain sensitive to the client's inner turmoil. If the decision to change represents a last-ditch effort on the heels of innumerable failures, the weightiness of this work needs to be acknowledged.

As clients progress through phases and transitions, certain cognitive, emotional, interpersonal, and behavioral patterns prevail (Taylor, 1986). In

---

**REFLECTION 3.3**

If you have been working with clients for a while, you may be able to identify a particular person you know well who successfully changed a certain behavior, such as moving from a sedentary lifestyle to an active one. On the other hand, you may not currently be working with clients, in which case you might think about someone you know well who went through a significant life change. Reflect and explore your knowledge of this person's experience. Estimate wherever possible this person's thoughts, feelings, and actions that might shed light on the phases and transitions suggested in the LTC model. Give special attention to the transitional moments in the change process. For instance, can you point to the moment when this person shifted out of a state of blame (of self or others)? Was there a time when this person seemed to broadcast her change at every opportunity and advocate that others follow a similar path?

particular, the required support differs markedly in each phase: Clients in disorientation seek emotional support, those in exploration require guidance and encouragement, and those in reorientation need expert input and affirmation. Cognitively, clients in disorientation have difficulty thinking clearly, those in exploration need to work at remaining open-minded, and those in reorientation need to be more analytical. Throughout the disorientation phase, clients are often unable to effectively address tasks that require strong shifts in perspective and action. Small steps oriented toward self-acceptance are likely to be helpful. In the exploration phase, clients will hopefully display a kind of playfulness as they experiment with new approaches and patterns. During the reorientation phase, clients need to be task focused and exhibit high levels of commitment to action.

The ways in which clients relate to their coaches also vary over the cycle of change, from a sense of dependency to one of codirection and independence. The varying needs of clients and the styles that they prefer in their coaching relationships are intimately related to their phases of learning and development. For example, as the exploration phase is ending, clients need to reflect more privately to create internal order of their thoughts, feelings, and actions. A person who has formerly been open and talkative may become more solitary and self-sufficient. Having a map for clients' internal worlds during change demystifies so many of the alterations in the patterns that coaches witness in their work.

# COMMENTARY

Each client you meet has a unique constellation of precipitating reasons for initiating change as well as a richly textured history that needs to be explored in order to help you enter conversations that maximize opportunities for connection and forward movement. The two models we have presented are general frameworks for what clients are likely to go through as they step forward. The fact that there is overlap between TTM and the LTC model is encouraging; it speaks to the validity of the processes described by both models. Yet, utmost attention needs to be focused on your clients' actual experiences without forcing them to fit into any model. In your private moments of reflection on clients' progress, you may want to examine how they seem to be following these generic models and where they might be carving their own roads toward the future. If there is an overarching message that derives from these models, it is that people behave differently at various points in their change processes. Sometimes they will be more emotionally sensitive, while at others they will crave action and evidence of change. We invite you to consider the models while nurturing your own flexibility of styles in working with your clients.

# 4

# FLOW MODEL OF COACHING

## *I*n this chapter, you will learn how...

- the flow model of coaching metaphorically represents the movement of change facilitated by coaching;

- the model characterizes what happens in a single coaching session as well as representing the entire coaching relationship;

- the model helps clients clarify intentions, generate insights, identify patterns, and discover unimagined resources for change;

- the process of collaborative action planning is a core component in effective goal pursuit; and

- the coaching journey pivots on clients' commitment levels and their capacity to address emergent challenges to change.

---

Beyond living and dreaming there is
something more important: waking up.

—*Antonio Machado*

---

Flow is a way of being. For most of us it is elusive and not easily sustained, but it is an aspiration for how we want to experience ourselves in daily life. Our intention in this chapter is to describe a model of coaching built on a number of theories and perspectives about how people shape their visions and energize themselves to undertake the demanding journey toward creating new and more satisfying realities. As witnessed in the previous chapter, intentional change is often more complex than typically imagined. Twists and turns along the way, blockages, or even relapses may result in discouragement and a loss of resolve. The **flow model of coaching** demonstrates the elements necessary for you and your clients to cocreate an experience of continuous flow toward their desired future. We rely on two case studies to illustrate the model and bring it alive.

# CLIENT DREAMS

Clients come to you with dreams, big and small. Something is missing from their present world. They want change. For as long as they can remember, they may have dreamed of a different life. Or perhaps they have this seemingly simple thing that they can't manage to do. Many of the issues they present may appear straightforward. These may have arisen sharply in the recent past or they could have been long-lingering concerns. Whatever the case, one thing is clear—clients need help, and for whatever reasons, they have identified coaching as the approach they prefer for meeting their needs. So, they contact you. Let's meet your clients: Bob and Amy.

## Bob: The Nostalgic Boomer

Bob is 65 years old. He is semiretired and has created a comfortable balance of work and personal pursuits. As happy as he is, he is searching for something more. Before retirement, he pushed the envelope in all fronts of his life. He was a senior executive in a large biotech company. He served on multiple committees within his community. He raised a family of four boys with his lifelong partner. Somehow he found time to be involved in a number of recreational sport activities; in his youth, he had been an accomplished athlete.

When Bob first calls to set up a meeting, he apologizes, saying that his issue really isn't that big. He thinks it will take just a few sessions to get the forward momentum he needs. In the first session with you, he describes his issue as follows: He is in good physical condition; he has maintained his weight and aerobic capacity over the past few years even though his activity patterns have changed significantly. He completely dropped out of all the recreational pursuits he used to love around the time that he retired from his job and began his part-time consulting practice. He tells you that he wants at least two things from his work with you: first, to understand why he is feeling so reluctant to do some of the things he thinks he should be doing, and second, to develop a strategy to get moving differently than he is at the moment.

Bob describes his home-based routine of calisthenics and weight training but remarks that this program gives him little satisfaction. He thinks it is necessary for his health, and he adheres to it religiously. However, his eyes light up when he discusses the old days of playing basketball regularly, of skiing in winter and cycling with friends in the summer. He is puzzled about why he doesn't just get back to doing these things since he can't find any good reason not to. Bob has lots of extra time compared with when he was working full time, and he remembers distinctly how good he felt when he was active.

## Amy: The Stressed Marketing Executive

Amy wants to reduce her stress. She's 48 years old, recently divorced, and feeling lonely. Her two children are away at college, and she is working harder than ever at her marketing job. The divorce left her feeling a bit wobbly and she admits that she still has a fair amount of anger and resentment toward her ex. She believes her stress is largely related to the ever-increasing demands of her job and the need to keep up her earning power so her children can complete their schooling.

When you meet Amy for the first time, she seems fearful and anxious. Her work requires a lot of travel, and this translates into little exercise and poor eating habits. She knows better, of course, but finds herself running off madly in all directions. She seems at a loss about what to do, though she is on top of doing things her children need and managing all the agendas previously handled by her husband. She thinks that with your expertise in coaching people in issues of health, wellness, and fitness, you can help her set up a plan that will enable her to feel more grounded, less stressed, and more energetic.

Amy says her mind is sometimes like a runaway train. She starts worrying about things and then begins imagining worst-case scenarios. For instance, although she considers herself to be relatively young, she knows there are a number of eager beavers in her company who would love to have her job. On the other hand, she realizes the extent of her skill set and her glowing reputation in the industry. She has always been a bit of a worrier, but her ex-husband helped reassure her throughout the years of their marriage. She imagines that he simply got tired of it and that's why he left. As she continues talking to you, she brings the topic back to what she most wants help with: first, developing a way of relaxing with some kind of program that

Both of the clients described in this chapter present different issues. Before reading further, take a moment to reflect on the dreams and needs that Bob and Amy are bringing forward as they enter the coaching relationship. What do you know about each of these clients? What are the changes they want in their lives? What exactly is their coaching topic? Bob and Amy are clearly in the preparation stage of the TTM. Are there TTM processes of change that could help them move into action? How much self-efficacy do you detect in each client?

she can do regularly, and second, getting serious about exercise.

Implicit in each client's description is the question of whether you have the requisite background and expertise to help as their coach. Additionally, you will need to assess whether the topics they present are appropriate for coaching. For now, we will assume that both these topics can be dealt with in a coaching relationship. What we have to discover are the elements of the paths forward.

# METAPHOR FOR COACHING

Clients initiate coaching with an intention to change or to create a new way of being and doing things. When thinking about this pivotal moment in the coaching relationship, our first question was "What gives rise to this new sense of purpose?" Our assumption was that clients enter coaching with a need to get out of their habitual mind-sets, especially when old patterns continually drive them up against insurmountable walls. It was also apparent to us that clients rarely realize all the resources they have within themselves and in their extended networks. The more we reflected on clients who deliberately pursued a course of change, the more we gravitated toward a particular metaphor for the process of coaching. Before examining the central elements of the flow model of coaching, we will introduce it as metaphor.

Imagine a mountaintop lake sitting at a high altitude in a pristine wilderness area. This lake is so high that it feeds innumerable rivers and streams coursing down to the sea. As seasons come and go, the rivers and streams fluctuate in the force and volume of their flow. Heavy rain may overfill this lake, giving rise to new streams that chart their unique paths toward the sea. So, too, times of drought may cause some of the streams to dry up—at least until the next heavy rainfall.

Each new stream has to make its way down the mountainside. Sometimes there isn't enough flow to sustain a stream's coursing path, so it diminishes, its waters absorbed into the earth; it never makes it to the sea. Other times, a stream may encounter barriers that block its flow. It may become a pond and once again never make it to the sea. And with heavy rainfalls, new streams may burst forth over steep cliffs, giving rise to spectacular waterfalls. With such volume and power, these streams rush relentlessly toward the sea.

How many rivers and streams can this one lake feed? Which ones will continue to flow even in the dry seasons? What is the landscape that allows a new stream to carve its bed down the mountainside toward the sea?

How do we coach people so they can experience a sustaining flow of energy to reach their destinations? Clients vary in the energy they present for change. The same person may show fluctuations over time in how easily his energy flows for change projects. As clients' intentions become clarified and small actions are initiated, their flow may become stronger, or there could be disruptions and obstacles that diminish their intentionality. No matter how well intended clients are, other events may arise that demand their immediate attention. How much energy remains to sustain momentum?

No doubt there are some paths down a mountainside that are steeper and more direct to the sea, while others meander along flatlands and through thickly wooded areas. When a person charts a course of change, is it the most direct path? Or perhaps progress needs to be slow and wandering, giving rise to rich growth along the way. What helps the flow when source waters are low or when a meandering path turns uphill for a short while? Water seeks the lowest ground. Even so, occasionally a deliberate intervention is needed to ensure that obstacles preventing this natural gravitation can be managed.

Coaching relationships represent a partnership that increases the client's resources for change. Though support systems are derived from elements of the client's personal ecosystem, ultimately the flow of energy required to sustain commitments must come from within. Coaches are temporary members of the client's personal environment, cocreating novel routes around seemingly insurmountable obstacles. They help clients discover new resources, and they can also lend a hand in burrowing through blockages in the clients' flow to their desired destinations.

# FLOW MODEL OF COACHING

The flow model of coaching characterizes the client's journey as one of flowing toward the sea from a high source above the clouds. When someone announces her intentions for a coaching relationship, it is essential to appreciate the source of her wishes. It is not that a coach is so interested in why the client has these desires; rather, he needs to understand whether initiating motivations will sustain the journey over time. What if the client has many wishes and dreams that she aspires toward? What if a particular aspiration comes amid the dry season?

In the previous chapter, we reasoned that the initiation of a change process is not a random or whimsical event. It derives from deep places of desire and intentionality that may have been more or less evident for long periods. Clients in coaching, unlike those in counseling and psychotherapy, arrive with an objective in mind; they rarely show up with a wish as vague as the desire to do better or be happier. Before the first conversation occurs, it is likely that the client has identified his desired direction and potential outcomes. These initial intentions are often transformed through the process of coaching to even clearer articulations of the dream, of the desired state of being that has manifest and measurable properties.

In the broad realm of coaching relationships, client dreams may be as concrete as buying a new house, getting a new job, or finishing a doctoral degree. Equally so, client wishes may be represented in an ongoing commitment to a course of action, such as eating more appropriately, managing stress effectively, or exercising in a way that gives joy and vitality to life. In all cases, the interior world of the client will change significantly throughout the coaching process.

The flow model is divided into two major phases: engagement and goal pursuit (see figure 4.1). Within each phase are three critical areas of focus. In the engagement phase, the areas are insight, patterns,

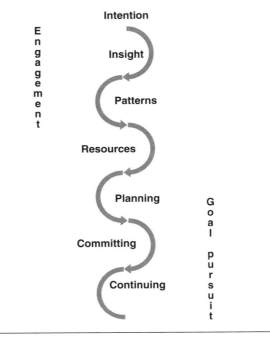

**Figure 4.1**    Flow model of coaching.

and resources. In the goal-pursuit phase, the areas are planning, committing, and continuing. In the engagement phase, the areas of focus may occur more or less simultaneously, whereas in the goal-pursuit phase, the areas tend to be more sequential. Let us begin to explore the model to understand how coaches cocreate with their clients an experience of flow toward dreams and visions.

## Engagement Phase

The waters spill over in a new direction today! What has happened to create this shift? What is it about today that is different from yesterday? A client may have had your name for weeks or just found it today. A call is made; a connection begins.

Coaching is still an emerging profession, and it is therefore important to ask what the client knows about coaching. What are her expectations? Are her desires appropriate for a coaching relationship? Are the two of you a good match? Because the success of coaching often hinges on the strength of the relationship between coach and client, a good fit between the two partners is essential. Honestly answering questions such as "Can I see myself working with this particular client?" and "Is there good chemistry between us?" will increase the chances for successful outcomes.

There are preliminary details to address in order to begin on a professional footing. In the first meeting with prospective clients, you need to ensure that they understand what coaching is and what it is not. In particular, they need to know that it is action oriented rather than a protracted analysis of their issues. You then want to determine whether the client's topic is appropriate for coaching and whether you are the right coach to work with this specific client. Following this, terms and conditions are carefully reviewed until an agreement is reached (see appendix B). Among other elements, the introductory session includes discussions of fees, meeting structures, time frames, and mutual expectations. Assuming all these aspects of business contracting and role clarifications are agreed upon, you will now enter the first area of focus.

Throughout the early work of the relationship, the coach's task is to open up the conversation to gain as much understanding of the client as possible. Correspondingly, through the engagement phase, with its focus on creating insight, uncovering patterns, and discovering resources, the client will likely gain new appreciations of himself in relation to his aspirations. Unique solutions may spontaneously emerge. The goal itself may evolve so that it is both more easily achieved and more fulfilling.

## Focus on Insight

What is the client's larger story? Who is this client in the context of her life? How does the wish that she presents mesh with her other dreams, visions, needs, and realities? What else is her life energy feeding? How well does she understand herself at this juncture in life?

Each client begins with a wish or intention. It may be broad or circumscribed, short or long term, concrete or abstract. This intention cannot be separated from the rest of the client's existence, and as a coach, your role will be to understand this desire in context. The great advantage of this phase of the flow model is that as the coach expresses genuine curiosity in deepening his understanding of the client, awareness is also created within the client. In the safe space of the coaching relationship, the client begins to put together the pieces of her own puzzle.

Let's turn to our two coaching clients as they begin their journeys in coaching.

**Creating Insight With Bob**   Bob says that he is puzzled about why he just doesn't take action. He knows that recreational sports have been a source of joy and excitement in the past, yet he let them

---

### Focus on Insight in the Engagement Phase

For clients, a focus on insight might include the following:

- Understanding the self in context
- Seeing the self clearly
- Comprehending "all of me" in the world
- Identifying the interaction of all the forces at play
- Appreciating the larger picture of other visions, dreams, needs, and realities
- Exploring with a long-term view of intended and unintended changes
- Identifying the deeper wants and needs that will be met by this pursuit

---

go shortly after he retired from his demanding executive position. He says he now has more time than ever, though his days are still quite full. He notes that his routines have changed considerably. He doesn't go to an external office for work but rather consults from his home office. When asked about his network of friends with whom he played basketball, skied, and cycled, he looks downcast and says that many of them have moved away to sunnier climes. He sighs as he adds that some of them have just gotten old.

He mentions nothing about his own age, 65, as an impediment to playing the sports of his past. To the contrary, he reasserts that he is in great shape and could get back into the game without a lot of additional training. You notice some extra weight around his waist and explore his training regimen in greater detail. It amounts to 20 to 30 minutes on three or four days a week. Sometimes he walks fast on his treadmill or outdoors; at other times he engages in a limited weight training program.

Then, you ask Bob an essential question: "Has anything happened that has made this topic more important today than it was over the past couple years when you were doing the same thing?" He muses about how his world seems to be getting smaller. He pinches his gut, pulling at a couple inches of skin and fat trapped between his fingers as he reminisces about being on the basketball court in his glory days. Then he mentions his recent birthday celebration that left him feeling somewhat depressed.

It would be easy to skip this step or speed through it, but that might not allow Bob to fully access his deeper motivations and the degree to which his intention may represent a mix of agendas, including ones for companionship, intensity, and reliving the past. Though he has framed the issue as one of getting back into his favorite sports, might there be other avenues for revitalization? Further, the questioning in this stage would allow him to learn what the core ingredients for success need to be and how to make them all work in his present state of physical being. We can also witness Bob's growing awareness when, in spite of his assertion of being fit, he nonverbally acknowledges the extra weight around his waist. Are there other things happening in his life that are pushing this agenda? Is this the only change he is contemplating right now, or is his lake spilling over into other streams, so to speak? What other insights might you want to generate at this point in the relationship?

**Creating Insight With Amy** Amy presents a potentially more complex portrait than Bob. She wants to find a way to relax, and she wants to get serious about exercising. She drifts back and forth between reflections about her job and her family, notably her ex-husband. You learn that the divorce was just finalized, though they separated a little over a year ago. She tells you that she did see a therapist for a while when first separated, and she has that person's phone number in case she needs it. You also deem it important to learn about her medical history, so you sensitively inquire. The good news is that she had a physical recently and is generally fine. Her weight is a bit high, but more critically she notes that she has little muscle tone.

When asked why she chose coaching, she tells you that she lacks knowledge about exercise and also about how best to relax. She further notes that work takes priority over everything these days, so she believes she needs someone to monitor her and hold her accountable to do what she says she will do in terms of increasing her physical activity. She volunteers that her ex was the family motivator, always organizing her and the children to do things like going on trips and embarking on new nutritional plans. He also did most of the cooking.

Her response to that essential question, why now, brings in another piece. Amy feels lonely, and she believes she will have to get rid of the extra 15 pounds (7 kg) she's been carrying around for a decade before she can start dating again. Also, she thinks the wolves in the office can smell fear, so she figures cultivating a Zen attitude toward life is her best defense against someone taking her job.

Questioning Amy could be tricky. You don't want to be invasive, yet you need to know about some potentially sensitive matters. Amy volunteers that she has seen a therapist, and she provides a broad picture of her life at the moment. It is reassuring that her medical markers are within the normal range. If someone hasn't had recent medical workups, making an appointment for medical assessments may be an early action step in the coaching process. There might be other things you would want to find out from Amy as well, such as what a typical workweek looks like. Examining her schedule more closely might help you codesign ways she could begin creating practices for stress reduction and exercise.

Of course, Amy opened up another agenda by talking about dating. This might lead to a line of exploration about relationships and family support. You might also wonder how much you need to know about the threats at work. Given that her goals would be positive additions to most people's

---

**REFLECTION 4.2**

What insights do you now have about Bob? Before you read on, take a few minutes to articulate insights that you believe have been brought to Bob's awareness. As his coach, what have you discovered that can provide direction to help him move forward? How has his coaching topic evolved at this point? What questions would you ask Bob in order to generate more insight?

---

**REFLECTION 4.3**

What did you learn about Amy through this area of focus? Before you read on, take a few minutes to articulate insights that have been brought to her awareness. As her coach, what have you discovered that can provide direction to help her move forward? How has her coaching topic evolved at this point? What questions would you ask Amy to generate more insight?

lives, there is a question about the degree to which you get into her story as opposed to moving directly toward action. What other avenues of inquiry might you want to explore with her before proceeding?

A focus on insight is about generating awareness. It is meant to provide strength and clarity for the journey. However, it is not an end in itself. This stage is intended to ground clients' dreams in the practical realities they will likely face. As is discussed in chapters 10 and 11, when the distance to the goal seems far, it is helpful to create intermediate goals that can signify progress along the path. Helping clients appreciate their intentions within the broader frame of their lives facilitates action planning that accounts for all relevant elements. For instance, Bob knows how to exercise but realizes that his current fitness plan may not have kept him in as fine shape as he had originally asserted. Through artful and sensitive questioning from her coach, Amy seems to have uncovered an important source of motivation, her budding desire to explore new relationships.

Creating insight does not imply finding out all the little ways in which clients may be lying to themselves; rather, it is about standing on firm ground beside clients as they launch into the future. To do so, it is important to fully comprehend the terrain.

### Focus on Patterns

> We all flow differently. What are clients' patterns of engaging their worlds and getting things done? What styles do they prefer? What are their habits of mind, body, and spirit? What makes them tick? What are their needs, inclinations, and sources of motivation? How do they go about pursuing their dreams and their daily lives?

Take something as common as your waking rituals. What do you do first? When do you eat? What's your preferred way of starting your day? All these patterns are uniquely yours, and that's simply the way it is. You have developed your ways of doing things over many years. They are habitual for you—so much so that when some of the steps are out of sequence, you feel slightly off.

One of the gifts of a coaching relationship is how it enables people to appreciate their current patterns so as to approach things in novel ways. Our patterns show up in how we address new projects, and they are accentuated when we are under stress. Coaches need to appreciate how their clients go about change and what happens when things don't work as planned. Some aspects of clients' patterns may have

---

> ## Focus on Patterns in the Engagement Phase
>
> For clients, a focus on patterns might include the following:
> - Patterns of daily life
>   - Preferred ways of scheduling life events
>   - Ways in which clients prioritize life agendas
> - Habits of mind, body, and spirit
> - Go-to places or defaults when they are stuck
> - Patterns of reaction when they are under stress
> - What makes them tick, what their inclinations are, and what turns them on or off
> - What drives them; what they are passionate about

---

fostered success. Some aspects may have resulted in unsuccessful outcomes when applied in certain situations. For instance, a client may have a pattern of making jokes when life gets too serious. This can be helpful in reducing stress, but he may need to be more serious in a work situation. The implication is not that he has to become completely stern and somber, but rather that he needs to discriminate between times when it's okay to be funny and when a more focused attitude is required.

When exploring clients' patterns, coaches try to uncover ways in which they make decisions, move forward with their plans, get things done, or create joy in their lives. Sometimes they discover useful patterns that can be readily transferred to the coaching agenda. More likely, they find aspects that don't fit and that something elusive is keeping them from achieving the outcomes they desire.

**Uncovering Bob's Patterns**   Bob had been the chief financial officer in a biotech firm until he retired. He had a strong command and control style in work relationships. At play, he was the leader of the pack. Everyone relied on him to get things rolling, and he did this well. He was always reliable and liked to stick to the routine in whatever he did. He tells you that adjustment to semiretirement was a challenge at first, but now he has it down. He gets up early and, on the days he exercises, he has it taken care of before he jumps in the shower. Then it's breakfast and right down to his home office. He's not big on surprises or trying new things. In fact, he expresses pride in how he keeps his clothes forever and dresses pretty much the same way he always did.

You ask him to tell you how he was so successful in managing all the things he did while keeping up a highly active sport life. He happily tells you that it was all about scheduling. He considers himself a master at making time work for and not against him. On his busiest days, he had arranged his sports so they rarely conflicted with his work and family responsibilities. He notes, "Usually, this meant the boys and I would have a 10 p.m. basketball game on Tuesday and Friday nights." You are aware from other things Bob has said that he now heads for bed by about 10 p.m. each night. You also know that many of "the boys" aren't around anymore. When you inquire into his excitement about his earlier athletic days, he offers examples of all the postgame socializing ("Having a few beers after a good game!") he took part in and the magical moments when everyone was playing, skiing, or cycling in sync.

Bob seems to be a creature of habit, enjoying routines and rituals. He also likes to be in charge of things: He's the boss, the go-to guy, the one who makes things happen. You also appreciate that some of his excitement about sport is linked to social connection and teamwork.

Bob certainly is capable of change, but he's not big on experimentation. The challenge will be working with him to shift his patterns without undermining his need for control and predictability. Although he never stated this, you might also be aware of his pattern of being the decision maker. How do you think he feels spending time with a coach, who in certain interpretations of the role is the one who calls the shots?

**Uncovering Amy's Patterns**    You ask, "Amy, you've no doubt had to make changes before. How did you go about making them happen?" She responds by first talking about her ex and how he was always the one to take the initiative. She then tells you that in other instances, friends or experts told her what to do and she pretty much followed instructions. You inquire about how well this worked for her, and she shrugs, saying, "Sometimes fine . . . but then, what may have been

> ### REFLECTION 4.4
>
> What have you learned about Bob's patterns? Before you continue reading, jot down new discoveries you have made about this client. What are some of the patterns, styles, and habits that could describe him and his ways of being in the world? What other patterns do you detect? As a coach, how would you generate information about them? What questions would you ask?

good for someone else wasn't always my thing. After giving it my best, if it didn't fit for me, I just dropped it—or if for some reason I had to do it, I probably felt resentful."

You are aware of Amy's job anxiety and want to probe more around her motivations for change. She has trouble going beneath the surface, even though she offers you lots of information about her life. Without being fully aware of her own words, Amy lets you know that fear is a strong motivator. You hear that she is afraid of losing her job, afraid of being alone for the rest of her life, and afraid that her children are going to be mad at her if their economic situation changes so that they have to switch to a local university and come back home. What you surmise is that fear works for her—it gets her out of her comfortable ruts and into action, such as hiring you as her coach.

You explore other motivations with Amy. In answering, she surprises herself in discovering that her success at work has been largely driven by the fact that she has fun doing what she does. She also realizes that her sons keep telling her that she's the one who creates fun in the family. Her ex may have gotten things going, but then her fun-loving inner child kicked in. As you explore fun with her, Amy provides another insight to how she functions: She says that fun is an attitude and that once she starts something, no matter how hard it is, she always tries to find the places where joy can be created. She notes this is particularly true at work.

You remember her remark about her mind resembling a runaway train in regard to her job and ask her about her patterns under stress or when things aren't going her way. She admits that she can spin in states of worry, but talking to certain people helps her gain perspective. She says she has a short but reliable list of go-to people in her life when she needs to stop the train. Here, she refers again to missing her husband.

REFLECTION 4.5

Consider what you just learned about Amy. Before you continue reading, jot down new discoveries you have made about her. What are some of the patterns, styles, and habits that could describe this client and her ways of being in the world? What other patterns do you sense in her? As a coach, how would you inquire about these patterns? What questions would you ask?

Up until now, you may have wondered whether Amy was going to be someone who becomes dependent on you for creating the programs she will follow. You may have also been concerned about her basing a positive life change solely on the motivation of fear. What comes through in this segment of your session is that Amy seems to rely on fear to kick-start her into action, but once in action she appears to have a clear capacity for generating fun. And there's another pattern you notice: She isn't afraid to ask for help. Moreover, she willingly accepts input from others and makes a sincere effort to use their advice. Implicit in her comments is the sense that she also knows what works for her. This inner knowing as a basis for action may be well ingrained.

In line with her ability to ask for help, Amy gives evidence of her pattern of talking out her issues in order to stop herself from spinning. What you don't know yet is whether what makes her stop spinning is simply talking or having someone tell her not to worry so much.

A focus on patterns is not necessarily distinct from the previous focus on insights. All along, you are trying to understand who your client is—how she functions, what she values, how she knows, what helps her start, and what stops her. After learning about these things, coaches will have a sense of where the client will leap forward and what might stop her cold in her tracks.

Patterns are usually ingrained ways of being or habitual manners of thinking, feeling, and acting. There is a sequencing that is represented in patterns of behaviors, feelings, or thought processes. One thing leads to another, and then a certain, perhaps predictable, outcome occurs. It is likely that when people hire coaches, one of their dominant patterns for creating success in their lives is no longer working. They may have experienced a number of disappointments in relying on their tried-and-true ways. If that's not the case, it may simply be that they don't yet foresee how their old patterns are ill suited to their new intentions. That road hasn't been taken yet.

## Focus on Resources

Invariably there are challenges, opportunities, and a need for resources. What are your clients' resources and capacities? What are their supports? Who is there for them? What opportunities are opening for them? What skills will they need for their journey?

Clients have previously traveled the roads of change, and they have likely learned that other people offer critical support along the path. Resources may emerge miraculously. Help pops up in the strangest places. Beyond social support, clients may need certain skills and capacities to achieve their desired goals. Do they already have these skills and capacities, or will they need to be developed? Similarly, the practicalities of concrete resources, such as locations of services, weather conditions, finances, and access to facilities, must be factored into the client's emerging plans for change.

A focus on resources does not necessarily occur separately from ones on insight and patterns. Coaches elicit information and listen carefully; they

## Focus on Resources in the Engagement Phase

For clients, a focus on resources might include the following:

- What are their skills and abilities?
- What resources are present, and what can they create?
- Where are their social support networks? Which ones have they not yet tapped?
- What opportunities are opening up for them in their worlds? Which ones seem to be closing down?
- What obstacles might appear, and who or what can help the client with them?
- Who will oppose or resist clients' efforts to change? What capacities and resources will be needed to address them?

then sort what they have sensed into various lenses for viewing their clients. In focusing on resources, they want to bring forth clients' awareness about the social fabric of their lives. Our networks are often more extensive than we realize. Clients may not have intimate contact with key people who can help them in their quest, yet friends of friends of friends might be invaluable.

Just as there are likely to be strong supporters of clients' intentions, there may be others who are less enthusiastic or even obstructive. Mapping strategies to address how clients can deal with unsupportive people may make the difference between success and yet another failed attempt. For instance, family members may be ambivalent about intended changes because these changes will affect them personally; they may conclude that they will have to look at their own lifestyles or act differently because someone in their midst will have altered her ways of being.

In addition to social support, a focus on resources encompasses more concrete matters such as finances, facilities where plans can be engaged, and times when actions can be completed. The robustness of action planning relies on the depth of consideration given to all the elements that can foster or disrupt flow. Coaches encourage clients to explore the obvious, the possible, and the yet-undiscovered resources that will enable them to successfully move toward goal realization.

**Exploring Bob's Resources**   Bob has ample time to commit to his plan, and he lives in a community where there is an abundance of sport facilities. He tells you about all the great networks of people who played sports with him in the past. Though the sport centers are close by, his network of friends has shrunk considerably. He describes his wife as supportive and easygoing. You wonder whether Bob is holding onto his nostalgic memories so fiercely that anything different from what he once had simply won't do. You ask him about joining up with some of the local cycling groups or masters swim teams. His response is that it would take effort—it would feel like starting all over again.

You explore Bob's social habits—how he makes friends, what groups he belongs to, and how at ease he is with casual connections. The picture he draws is one of a person with great social skills. He is charming and friendly. It doesn't take much for him to strike up conversations with strangers. You make note of this as a significant resource he can rely on to activate his plans.

Basketball was one of Bob's passions in the past. You inquire about what it might be like for him to go to some of the centers and join a few pickup games. Age comes into focus for the first time. He tells you he would probably be the oldest guy on the court. When asked how that would feel, he remarks that age itself isn't an obstacle, but his current physical condition might be. As he reflects on this, he comments, "Well, that's easily solved."

You want to know if he has thought about doing any other sports beyond the ones he mentioned. He pauses. "You know, I'm a creature of habit . . . but I have been thinking about some of these fitness classes friends have told me about." The more he talks about this, the more animated he becomes. You ask him where he heard about the classes, and he tells you that friends who belong to a sprawling new fitness center in town have been raving about the class choices available to them.

There appear to be ample opportunities for Bob to engage in various forms of physical activity in his area, and certain elements of his social support system are clearly in place. His spouse supports him and he has strong social skills to build new connections. There are no apparent time or financial restrictions that would affect his intentions, and he has ample skill in the athletic arena. He is aware that he may need to regain a higher level of physical conditioning before he plays full-court basketball in a pickup game, but he seems to understand what will be required for him to achieve this level of fitness. Of course, you would want to explore this further with him.

You sense that Bob not only has a nostalgic connection to the way things were but also discomfort around starting over again with new people. Strategically, you check out how he might feel doing other activities. At first, he hesitates, but then his enthusi-

---

**REFLECTION 4.6**

What have you learned about Bob's resources? Take a moment before you read on and make a list of all the resources that could help him attain his two objectives: uncovering the reasons why he is so resistant to adopting new ways of doing things and embracing new avenues to being physically active. Are there other resources you would like to examine in order to coach Bob effectively? What questions might you ask to enable him to discover additional resources?

asm builds. You might guess that he is beginning to realize that there is a ready-made social structure in these fitness classes, so he doesn't have to find his niche within a new group, especially as the oldest guy in the class.

Overall, Bob's path forward does not appear to have significant obstacles. You have likely brought forth awareness of one of his biggest causes of resistance—the loss of his old gang. He may have imagined himself trying to replace this rich social network and the required effort dampened his enthusiasm. The resource of great fitness classes that he can join at will seems to inspire new energy for engagement.

**Exploring Amy's Resources**  "Time is a big concern for me," says Amy. "I'm very busy both at work and at home." You inquire about her ideal schedule for exercising and engaging in a process that would help her feel calm and relaxed. She says, "If I had a 9-to-5 job, that would be an easy question to answer, but I can be out of town three or four days a week for stretches of time." She acknowledges that to accomplish what she wants, she will have to exercise most days of the week, and you concur.

At present, finances are likely to have little impact on her planning. Though she worries about keeping her job, her current income is substantial. She also tells you, "I have a buffer put away for rainy days."

Her knowledge level is low regarding both aspects of her intention, that is, exercise and relaxation. In regard to the relaxation agenda, she tells you, "I don't have time to go away to a monastery for a few months." In terms of physical activity, she acknowledges that she hasn't exercised much over her lifetime and has no idea how to design a reasonable training program. Her home seems to have space for a well-equipped workout room, and she tells you she is open to spending money on setting this up.

You wonder about her capacity to stick with demanding schedules and things that don't come naturally at first. In a sense this is about her patterns, but it also pertains to her capacity to adhere to a rigorous program on her own. You certainly don't want her to invest in training equipment and not use it. When you inquire, she tells you a few important things. First, though she likes being with people, the nature of her marketing job sometimes makes her want to retreat to a quiet room somewhere, and the idea of having a private training center has appeal. She also believes the private time would help her deal with the stress she experiences at work. A

> ### REFLECTION 4.7
>
> What have you learned about Amy's resources? Before you continue reading, list all the resources you have discovered that could help her reach her two goals: establishing a regular relaxation program and getting serious about exercise. Aside from exploring the kinds of social supports she might desire versus what is currently available to her, what other resources would you want to look into with Amy? What questions might help her explore these other resources?

second element has to do with her body image. She says, "I don't look like the models in fitness ads and would probably feel more comfortable with no one watching me." A third piece is potential injuries: "I don't know much about all this stuff, so what if I do things the wrong way and hurt myself?" Finally, she notes that her whole life seems to have been about doing hard things. "That's a no-brainer," she says. "If I need to do it, I'll do it—I just want to do it right."

Amy has financial stability that will allow her to create the conditions for training and relaxation programs, but her knowledge base is low. She has the capacity to go it alone and stick with a challenging agenda. You don't know much about her social supports, although you remember she has her list of go-to people. You recognize that she will need solid guidance in both exercise and relaxation. There may or may not be support for her plans from colleagues, but with her work schedule and the competitive job climate, you doubt whether having training buddies at work is much of an option. Nonetheless, this merits exploration.

Time is a major concern for her, and it needs to be addressed in all elements of the design of whatever she agrees to do. Of course, there are workout resources in most business hotels these days, but does her schedule take her into evening social events when she is on the road?

Amy doesn't seem fatigued, and she doesn't seem to be entering this process of change with a large deficit of energy. Perhaps she has more flexibility than she is aware of regarding how she structures her time outside work, and this can allow her to engage in her exercise and relaxation programs when time becomes available. All this leads you to believe that she has more than adequate resources to make things happen.

It's not always clear how resources differ from patterns; in fact, they may overlap. Resources pertain to what a client can bring forward to support and sustain action toward goal fulfillment. Areas you might want to investigate include the following: What do they know about their topic? What would pursuing this topic and achieving their goal require of them? Whom do they know who can help, and who might try to block their progress? What skills will they need in order to do what they wish, and do they have them? If skills are lacking, what will it take to acquire them? What kinds of opportunities are currently available for their agendas? What else may be happening soon that could influence their plans? Are there any obstacles that need to be acknowledged and addressed? In comparison, patterns have more to do with ingrained ways of thinking, feeling, or acting. They refer to our habits. Someone can be a habitually easygoing person, and that might serve certain goals but not others. When viewed from a resource perspective, habits like this one might be considered as a capacity to get along well with others.

## Goal-Pursuit Phase

Has the flow of energy grown or diminished through the engagement phase? Did the client retreat into doubt, or did she find new sources of strength and motivation? It may take one session or many to move through the various explorations encompassed in the engagement phase, yet the process is anything but static. If there have been multiple sessions, the client will have left each session with a plan of action—to gather information, investigate possibilities, talk to particular people, or accomplish tasks that create foundation and momentum. Just as a new stream must make its way around boulders and through flatlands or even create underground passageways, so too the client needs to find creative ways to address factors that will propel his journey.

A coaching relationship has been formed through work in the engagement phase of the flow model. The client will have learned firsthand what coaching is about and the requirements for progress. Moreover, she will have developed trust in the coach as a reliable sounding board and guide for the journey. A way of partnering in discovery and action will have evolved through the sessions. Coaches will know how clients like to work and where they need to be challenged. Clients will understand what the coach's tasks are and what they can expect in their work together.

Although action has been occurring throughout their time with each other, a clearer emphasis on tasks directly pertinent to the goal now emerges. In some cases, this phase is about taking one big step into the dream and experiencing it fully. In other cases, the dream is a complex construction that requires a sequence of big steps, each of which brings the client closer to a complete realization of her desires.

In the engagement phase, we saw an almost simultaneous process of exploration across the three main areas of focus. In the goal-pursuit phase, the areas of focus have more of a consecutive flow. Clients must first plan, then commit, and finally take action on a continuing basis.

### Focus on Planning

Wishing alone won't make things happen. How will clients reach their goals? What's their plan? Does the plan address all the elements of who, what, when, where, and how? What's the overall strategy? How robust is it? Do clients understand what will be required

## Focus on Planning for the Goal-Pursuit Phase

For clients, a focus on planning might include the following:

- Determining the overall strategy or master plan
- Understanding the sequencing of actions as building blocks
- Identifying who, what, when, where, and how for each action plan
- Using SuPeRSMART action goals and action plans:
  - Self-controllable
  - Public
  - Reward determined
  - Specific
  - Measurable
  - Adjustable
  - Realistic
  - Time detailed

each step of the way? Is the plan fixed, or will it evolve based on what happens at various points on the forward journey?

Planning happens in each session, and gradually a master plan emerges. In the early sessions, clients may be gathering data and experimenting. Plans for these actions are articulated in the coaching sessions. In some cases, there is only one path of action, and even here, the client may not be ready to take it. She may need to build competencies (see chapters 10 and 11), obtain further resources, develop support structures, and so on. Planning for these preparatory actions represents a significant part of the coaching dialogue. In time, the groundwork will be laid and planning will become more squarely situated in actions that more clearly reflect the client's dream.

As we know from the earlier discussion of the TTM and the LTC model, when clients are moving through a change process, adaptation to a new way of being is not complete—it has yet to be integrated into their lifestyle. Planning in the latter stages of a coaching relationship represents a kind of fine-tuning or adjustment process wherein the client explores how well he is sitting in this new life that he has chosen.

Let's see how a focus on planning plays out in coaching sessions with our two clients. In their scenarios, we want to consider planning for action as it evolves through a series of sessions. In order to depict this, we will illustrate both clients' paths of action.

**Designing Bob's Plan**   From previous discussions, you and Bob have come up with some likely avenues that can be tested. First, it seems that Bob will need to improve his current level of fitness in order to achieve that adrenaline rush from full engagement in physical activity. He says, "I keep assuming I'm in good shape, but it wouldn't hurt to find out what the facts are." Together, you plan for him to undergo an evaluation at the new fitness center he wanted to check out. In order to do this, he agrees to take out a trial membership. As he discusses this option, he comes up with a novel thought. "You know, I've always gone off with my buddies to do my sports, but things are different now. My wife isn't working and my time is flexible. I wonder whether she'd be interested in joining me."

Another agreement he makes is to observe some of the fitness classes that match the times when he would like to exercise. In a later session, you realize that Bob has made good progress on his agreements, including involving his life partner in his fitness

plans. He notes, "This is a real bonus. She wanted to do more exercise and I feel as if I'm helping her get motivated. And now I've established a baseline for how fit I am and I know exactly what I want to achieve."

Bob feels a bit intimidated by some of the fitness classes he observed: "I've always been athletic, but some of the moves in those classes would make me feel like I have two left feet." You strategize with him to sample two of the beginner classes, one cardio cycling class and one circuit training class. He reports back with glowing results: "Wow! Had I known about these classes years ago, I would have jumped right in." He is on track and actively pursuing his goal.

A couple of months go by and Bob feels ready to get back on the court. He is definitely more fit than when he started, and he is having a great time with his newfound exercise partner. He has checked out the options and has happily found a seniors' league, where he coyly mentions that he could probably attain star status after a while.

All the elements for robust action planning were fully in place as you got down to discussions about engagement. Bob was ready, and he was also aware of the steps he needed to take in preparation. He discovered novel aspects of his plan as he put himself into play. He realized that bringing his wife into his plans would have unexpected benefits all around: He would have a buddy to accompany him to the gym, and he could share his passion with her. An unanticipated benefit was that Bob's partner got to achieve one of her goals—getting more exercise. He also discovered that doing new things wasn't so bad after all. He began to enjoy the fitness classes and predicted that he could challenge himself with more advanced classes once he had mastered the basics.

Nonetheless, Bob had a yearning to get back on the court. This aspect of his plan remained integral. A little research revealed the existence of a seniors'

---

### REFLECTION 4.8

Planning for Bob is relatively straightforward. Take a moment and detail the action plan he developed in working toward his ultimate goal. What exactly did he do? How was the plan designed? What else did Bob discover to help him along the path? What do you think would have happened if you sent Bob directly to the court? What else might you consider for him at this time?

league in his area, and that satisfied a number of agendas: He liked being the star, and he imagined that among his peers, he would be able to shine. He also missed the friendships that developed around the games he once enjoyed. Playing with younger athletes might not have worked as well for him due to their lifestyle differences, including the times when games were scheduled.

As we will see in the sections on committing and continuing, Bob readily made plans, committed to them, and engaged without hesitation. Although at this point in his story his path seems obvious, it wasn't always this way. He arrived in a fog. He didn't understand his resistance. He needed to talk it out and gain clarity. Through careful questioning, he was able to identify the key elements to a viable plan. Once these were in view, he seemed to be in flow.

**Designing Amy's Plan**    You have a number of the ingredients for effective planning, but not enough to pin things down. You ask, "Amy, what interests you when you think about exercising?" Her answer surprises you. "Interests me? I never thought exercising would be all that interesting. It just seemed like a necessary evil. I've never really enjoyed the time I've spent at the gym."

You inquire about her second agenda, "What has worked for you in the past as a way of relaxing?" Again, you hit a wall: "Well, vacations are great and, as I mentioned, talking to my husband when we were married or to friends would help calm me down. But I think I'm looking for a do-it-myself kit." You explore some of the options for practicing body and mind relaxation, and Amy seems intrigued by them all.

Ensuring success for Amy will take careful planning and a fair amount of experimentation. However, you don't want her to be trying so many things that she fails to experience some of the benefits she desires. You go back to the home gym idea. She likes the thought of having a trainer who brings his own equipment, and she proposes that she would like to train twice a week. The first step, however, is clearing out one of the rooms in her home. She agrees to do this and reports success in the next session. She also commits to calling a couple of reputable trainers in her area. She will do a trial class with each one before you meet next.

So far, so good! You ask her to read about some of the relaxation and meditation techniques that you have discussed. She does this thoroughly and comes back with lots of questions. You both agree that she will choose one of the relaxation CDs she

**REFLECTION 4.9**

Planning for Amy is a multilayered process. It's not just doing one thing and sticking to it. Take a moment and detail the layers of the plan Amy followed to engage in full-fledged action toward her ultimate goals. What exactly did she do? How was the plan designed? What did she discover to help her along the path?

has researched, and she will structure some time to practice.

Meanwhile, weeks have passed without her actually practicing relaxation. Happily, though, Amy reports that exercising is having some unexpected benefits. "I'm surprised," she says. "It's been fun. Caroline [the instructor she chose] makes it interesting, and I feel so relaxed after a session. I've even been going to the hotel gyms when I'm on the road, and I find that just 15 minutes on the treadmill makes me sleep better."

The challenge with Amy is getting her engaged quickly enough for her to reap some clear benefits without putting her at risk of quitting. She needs to experiment, but not so much that she can't point to tangible results. If Amy is as time challenged as she describes, it will continue to be an evolving program with minor to major adaptations until it becomes fully integrated into her lifestyle. That will probably take about a year, if not more.

Bear in mind that Amy has both a primary and a secondary goal. She wants to exercise for health reasons, but she is also aware of her new status as a single woman who might want to begin dating in the future. Exercising for health may be different than body shaping through rigorous training.

When she begins a relaxation program in earnest and its results sink in, Amy may begin to move forward in other areas of her life. Rather than worrying about losing her job, she may aspire to the next level—and why not? If she is as good as she says she is, it may be time for her to get off the road by moving into more of a corporate position.

We don't know how all this will unfold for her, but we do know that she is currently addressing some fundamental needs that will create greater solidity in her life. Planning for change becomes a creative process that is fed by the results of previous actions successfully undertaken. So far, we find that tailoring the change steps to her unique profile is working. The steps aren't too big, and they fit well into her life patterns. Moreover, as planning is translated into action, positive results generate further motivation for engagement.

Planning is about the big and the small, the immediate and the long range, the preparatory and the final steps. It is an integral part of each coaching session, though early planning is often exploratory or directed toward building the foundation. Planning hopefully results in clear actions, which then produce new data and insights about clients' intentions and possibilities. Just as a new stream may branch out in many directions until it finds the one pathway that allows it to continue flowing, so too clients may investigate a variety of options in the beginning of their coaching relationships. In this respect, planning does not always result in forward movement, but it needs to generate a sense of momentum that motivates clients through the understandings they derive and the concrete samples of their dreams.

## Focus on Committing

When the plan has been fully detailed, there remains the doing. How strong is the client's resolve to do it now? What's the level of her determination? How can she commit herself without traces of hesitancy? What's required to ensure that her commitment doesn't dissolve between coaching sessions?

Determining commitment often means listening for the hesitancy in clients' resolutions or the qualifications they make about committing. "I'll try" is a classic red flag for commitment. The coach responds, "What would it take to move that 'I'll try' to an "I'll do'?"

### Focus on Committing in the Goal-Pursuit Phase

For clients, a focus on committing might include the following:

- Distinguishing between the ways in which clients express commitments
- Evaluating their commitment to their action plan on a scale of 1 to 10
- Finding where they might be holding out and what they can do to let go or transform resistance into a positive resource
- Recognizing hesitancies and fine-tuning plans for higher levels of commitment

Coaching is often about stretching a client from a comfortable action objective to one that is likely to require greater engagement and hopefully clearer payoff. There are times when someone takes on a project for which he has little initial enthusiasm. The hope is that in engaging the process, excitement will grow. However, sometimes clients don't engage, or when they do, their resistance builds. Coaches don't always know in advance how things are going to go; experimenting with new behaviors is part of the client's work in a coaching relationship.

When clients look for loopholes in the details of planning, a way out, or an opportunity for adhering to the letter of the agreement but not its spirit, effective coaches don't revert to cheerleading or badgering. Coaching involves a genuine inquiry into aspects of the plan that haven't fully landed in the client's resolve to move forward. In this respect, it's not just about changing "I'll try" to "I'll do." When you explore the hesitancy, you may find that somehow in the creation of the plan, a particular aspect was more your idea than your client's. Clients have to own the plan, and that may take some redesign. If you opt for always stretching your clients to do more than they are ready to take on, they may build resistance or they may not follow through.

We can illustrate this delicate negotiation with Bob and Amy as they move into some difficult terrain in their journeys. As coaches we need to always bear in mind the clients' intentions and dreams and not what we think would be best for them.

**Determining Bob's Commitment**    Initially, Bob wanted clarity about why he wasn't doing what he loved, and perhaps more critically he wanted to get back into action. From your perspective he has made significant progress on both agendas. "I told you this wouldn't take a lot of time," he says. "I just needed to figure things out and get moving." You have noticed that although he and his partner go to the gym regularly, Bob's mostly running on the treadmill and weight training. The group fitness classes have dropped off. He acknowledges his diminished participation in the classes, but he doesn't even mention the seniors' league. When you inquire, he admits that he did not join.

In discussing this turn of events, Bob confesses, "I thought I'd get good at these classes fairly quickly, but they're harder than I thought. Also, I watched a few practices at the court and I realized that the guys in the seniors' league looked like a sorry bunch of amateurs." As he explores this, he fully admits that he doesn't like the feeling of being a novice in the fitness classes. With some reluctance, he suggests trying the classes again and proposes a plan of taking two different types of classes each week for four weeks. He says that he will wait until next month to take another look at the seniors' league.

You move to commitment: "Bob, how committed are you to this plan?" He replies, "I'm going to do my damnedest." You ask, "Does that mean you're going to do eight classes without fail over the next four weeks in addition to other types of training you do while at the gym?" He says, "Well, why not? I said I would and it'll be good for me." You hear a big *should* in his commitment. "Bob, I'm getting a feeling that you think you should do this, but you're not 100% confident that you will. Is this possible?" He pauses. "You know, I like to be in control, and these classes are a bit different from other things I've done. I like the people in the class, but there's something that feels foreign to me." You acknowledge his observations and ask him how he thinks he wants to deal with that other than by forcing himself to do it.

Bob thinks out loud. "If I could look at this as part of a learning curve, it might make more sense to me. I thought it would have been more straightforward, but I guess most real learning always has a few twists in it. This may just be one of those twists." He continues examining this theme, and then concludes, "You were right to stop me. I wasn't ready to commit, but I think I am now."

Clients' resistance to following through on an action plan is not necessarily about their motivation so much as it may be a reflection of the way in which the plan has been construed. Coaches need to be attentive to the verbal and nonverbal signals of clients' connections to a plan. When clients intend to make changes, they often have to travel through uncharted areas. The unfamiliar creates excitement at times and discomfort at others. The coach didn't push the agenda of novel fitness classes on Bob; rather, he showed genuine curiosity and interest in the beginning. Maybe in this scenario the coach has a hunch that Bob is going to get himself into a rut going to the gym and doing the same things he was previously doing at home. So, he inquires about the classes and Bob rapidly orients the discussion to his need to recommit to action.

It is in the discussion around commitment that the hesitancy and forced nature of the agreement become more evident. The coach has to be aware of how the client describes his commitment, and he must ensure that he does not clinch the deal just for the sake of ending with an action plan. Deep commitment derives from an internalized sense of ownership of the agenda. When the plan comes from a feeling of obligation or perhaps even inadequacy, it is likely to be sabotaged.

Bob is insightful when pressed by his coach to examine his motivations. Left to his own style of doing things, he might have charged ahead and built up increasing resistance with each class he took. However, with a changed perspective about the experience and his own preferences for action (i.e., being in control), he now has a way of framing his discomfort (i.e., a learning curve) that will allow him to experience it more constructively.

**Determining Amy's Commitment**  Amy shows up at this session like a changed person. She looks different and has dressed in clothes that flatter her transformed body. She seems justifiably proud of herself. "I'm going to run a half marathon," she announces. "Wow. Tell me more about this. I'm eager to hear," you reply. She goes into a detailed story of her progress with Caroline, her trainer, and then says that Caroline is putting together a running group for "people just like me." In six months, they will all run in a local half marathon. "I'm committed, but it will require some real adjustments in my schedule," Amy adds.

"How do you think that will play out for you, Amy?" you ask. Amy answers, "The marathon thing wasn't on my radar, but it seems like such a good idea." You also inquire about how the half-marathon goal fits in with other goals she has for herself. She replies through a request for you to work with her in putting together a big-picture map of how this can all happen.

As you work with her on elements of her schedule and other plans that now include meditation and reaching a challenging sales goal that "will guarantee another promotion," you notice that Amy's energy keeps dropping. You have identified a number of ingredients for effective planning, but not enough to pin things down. More importantly, you notice she even begins to raise objections to many of the ideas she comes up with herself!

---

**REFLECTION 4.10**

What clues did Bob give to indicate that he was not committed to his plan? How would you restructure the plan to incorporate all the necessary elements to support his engagement? As a coach, are you satisfied with his commitment level at the end of the session? How would you pursue this further?

**REFLECTION 4.11**

In reviewing Amy's commitment to run a half marathon, what prompted further discussion about this newfound goal? What would be a clear indication that Amy was not intrinsically motivated to pursue this goal? What might have been the danger for her if you simply agreed to her request of putting together the big picture of how she would incorporate training with her other goals? What else do you think is going on with Amy in this brief segment?

Midway through the session, you decide to check in with Amy: "How committed are you to this new goal that you've chosen for yourself?" She answers, "Well, Caroline says I can do it. She thinks I've got such great determination." Of course, you acknowledge her fabulous progress in training and her strong determination in all areas of her life. Then you inquire, "Amy, from all I know about you and the great progress you've made, I also believe that you can do it. My question has more to do with whether this goal comes from inside of you." Amy looks doubtful. She describes her weight loss, the new clothes she's able to wear, and the compliments she's been receiving. Again, you acknowledge her, and add, "Let's take a few minutes to figure out together whether training to run the half marathon is on the path you want to take." She looks relieved.

Motivation has many roots, some within the client and others from outside sources. People may want to make changes to please someone else, and though this can sustain progress for a while, unless the motivation becomes internalized it is likely to diminish. Amy has taken on a number of important changes throughout her coaching relationship. She is exercising, meditating, and working hard. Within the goal-pursuit phase of the flow model, we need to ask how much energy Amy has to direct toward change and whether there is a risk of burnout from all the personal development she is undertaking.

As discussed in chapter 2, coaching represents a holistic approach. Coaches don't simply consider a goal in isolation from the client's broader realities and commitments. Sure, Amy could probably train for a half marathon and run it successfully. However, she needs to be clear about balancing this goal with all the other elements of her world that she is trying to advance. The coach raises the question not to create doubt but for Amy to put this new purpose into perspective.

This coaching session also offers another angle on commitment. Amy enters the session with an explicit commitment to train for a half marathon. Because this constitutes a new element in her agenda, the coach needs to inquire about the robustness of her plan. As the inquiry proceeds, she seems to become more hesitant and her energy declines. In essence, she has made a quasi-commitment in the absence of self-analysis and the specifics of engagement. Often enough in daily life, we hear people making statements of this sort: I am going to lose a certain number of pounds, go to Europe, climb Kilimanjaro, quit my job and open my own business. In truth, these aren't commitments as much as they are wishes or nascent intentions. The bottom line is that Amy entered the session with an emerging intention rather than the robust commitment that we would seek in coaching.

When focusing on commitment, coaches don't ask in a rhetorical manner whether clients are committed to what they have been discussing for a good part of the session, nor do they inquire with an expectation of compliance. They genuinely want to know whether clients can imagine themselves fully engaging in the activities they are cocreating. When they hear reservations, they work to fine-tune the plan so that it has greater resonance with the client.

There are countless examples of people who encourage others to do things with a rhetorical question, such as "You're really going to do this, aren't you?" Relationships between coaches and their clients are intentionally egalitarian; the coach doesn't have special powers over clients to make them comply. Yet, as social beings, there may often be a people-pleasing element to requests from others: "The coach wants only the best for me, so who am I to deny her simple requests?" Indeed, this dynamic may be stronger than we would hope in coaching relationships. It is for this reason that we need to be extra sensitive to the qualifying commitments that clients offer: "I'm going to do my best." "You can count on me." "I'll do it [for you] for sure!"

Many times clients will try their best, and that may be good enough. Each coaching session ends with a commitment to action, and sometimes the client may simply not get as far as anticipated during the interval between sessions. Life happens. What a coach looks for are patterns of behavior related to commitments that clients make. A once-in-a-while lapse in follow-through is different from a string of excuses over several weeks or months.

Committing is a process, not a single action. It represents a discussion rather than a yes-or-no answer. It needs to open up discussion as easily as

## Focus on Continuity in the Goal-Pursuit Phase

For clients, a focus on continuity might include the following:

- Identifying the standards for actions and goals
- Detailing exactly what clients have to do to achieve these standards today, tomorrow, and next month
- Choosing or creating ways for clients to monitor their actions
- Knowing how to make adjustments and develop contingency plans
- Having reliable ways of getting back on track should lapses occur
- Developing self-efficacy related to relapse prevention

it leads to closure. A coach's question about commitment has to be presented on an open hand, to be accepted or refused without judgment. It needs to be offered with compassion and understanding, no matter how much time has been spent detailing the action plan for which the question is being asked.

### Focus on Continuing

A good start is just that. What does your client need to stay the course? How will she deal with setbacks? What will keep her going when the end seems so far away? And the end itself is more imaginary than real; it is rarely the final point. How does your client solidify and nurture what she has gained?

As noted in our discussion of the TTM, continuing action for at least six months brings a person to the stage of maintenance—and maintenance can go on for a lifetime. Consider exercise, or healthy eating, or not smoking, or stress management. Do we ever fully enter a zone where what needs to take place happens automatically, like breathing?

Within the coaching relationship, a focus on continuity is about ensuring that the desired changes and new patterns are sufficiently established and that the client has awareness and skills to address any relapses or setbacks. In essence, the achievement of a goal is just a marker along the way. When

Michael Phelps won his six gold and two bronze medals in Athens in 2004, his training days were far from over. He went on to win eight gold medals in Beijing in 2008 and four gold and two silver medals in London in 2012, ultimately becoming the most decorated athlete to compete in the Olympic Games.

We offer more guidance on how coaches support continuity in chapter 11 when we discuss the 11th ICF core competency of managing progress and accountability. For now, we will drop in on our two clients for one final look at their coaching experiences.

**Appreciating Bob's Likelihood of Continuing**    Six months have passed since you first met Bob. He reports great satisfaction with his progress and is likely to end the coaching relationship shortly. "When I first met you, I thought it would just take a couple sessions to get me back on track," he tells you. "But, the whole thing was much bigger than I realized." Bob notes how he struggled with the fitness classes at first and how he turned the corner by challenging some of his old habits. He has found one class that he particularly likes and is experiencing a growing confidence in his abilities there. And he has been back on the court for a month now, enjoying the game and the camaraderie almost equally.

"I don't think of myself as getting older," Bob says, "but I am. That doesn't mean I should just lie back and take it easy, but it does help me appreciate that what worked for me once doesn't necessarily fit my lifestyle now." He beams when discussing the lovely afternoons he has spent with his wife at a café following a good workout. He is also happy about having connected with the seniors' league for basketball. "I don't think I would do too well playing basketball until 11 p.m. and then going out for a few beers—not the way I live these days." He also comments that he goes about training in a kinder and gentler way that he is beginning to appreciate. "I even tried a few classes in qigong. The old Bob would never have done that," he notes.

You sense that Bob has a clear map of his current reality that will guide his choices for quite a while. It's a different map than the one he had at the beginning of the coaching relationship, and it's one that yields fulfilling experiences. "I feel good in my body . . . not much weight around my waist these days. And I love what I'm doing and what it brings me."

Setbacks may come, but so far there are no warning signs on the horizon. Bob is grateful for the insights he has gained through coaching and seems able to talk to himself "the way you and I talk in our sessions."

REFLECTION 4.12

Bob has learned so many things through coaching. He is now at a place where he has met his initial goals and seems on his way to pursuing his dreams. Take a moment and reflect on his process. What is the trajectory that he followed to achieve the changes he wanted? In what ways was coaching beneficial for Bob? What do you think about his readiness to end coaching? Is there anything else he needs to achieve before you complete your work together?

It is likely that should Bob struggle with other dilemmas in his life, he will be less hesitant to find a coach who can get him moving forward again. For less complex issues, he seems to have gained an internalized coach; he now dialogues with himself in the way that he did with his coach during his sessions. This will permit him to stay on course and to make adjustments when needed.

From the initial meeting onward, it didn't seem that continuing would be much of an issue for Bob. However, part of the reason for this derives from the quality of coaching he received. Had he forced himself to just do the same old things in the same old ways, he might have ended up discouraged. His emerging plan and the guidance he received throughout enabled him to chart a new course that encompassed his lifelong passions with his unfolding way of life as a semiretired man.

### Appreciating Amy's Likelihood of Continuing

It has been close to a year since Amy began her coaching relationship. Some things turned out differently than expected. She was downsized from her job in spite of her best efforts, but she immediately landed a new position involving far less travel. A few romances came and went—by her choice. She looks different and worries less. "My sons have to grow up, too," she notes in one of her sessions. "If they had to go to a local college they'd make it. We gave them the foundation, and the rest is up to them."

Amy did run the half marathon and she discovered that it wasn't her thing. "I'm glad I did it. I proved something to myself, but I'm not a hard-core runner by nature. Maybe a dancer," she adds with a glint. She seems to have made peace with her ex, at least inside herself. There has been almost no mention of him in months.

"What was really challenging," she remarks, "was the meditation program. I discovered how noisy my mind was and how negative I could be about so many things. That was hard to digest. I just wanted to quit." You ask, "How did you keep going?" She reflects back to the meditation instructor she found as a result of an action plan you collaboratively designed. "That instructor made a difference, but I wouldn't have thought of doing that unless we had really unpacked what was bothering me."

Amy's home gym is fully equipped. "I don't use it as much as I first did," she says. "I actually like going to fitness classes and being at the gym, but that may change." Her work schedule allows her to be in town more, so fitting in regular exercise has become a nonissue. You note the absence of self-consciousness when she talks about being at the gym.

"I've always been determined and I think you've seen this in me during the past year," she remarks. You support this perception and ask her whether this comment was leading somewhere. She says, "I think I'm reassuring myself that having taken hold of what wasn't working for me in my life will give me confidence that I can make changes when they come knocking at my door in the future."

Amy has learned so many things and grown so much through coaching. She has more than met her initial goals and seems keen on continuing the journey. What comes through in this segment is her ever-widening scope of change: One thing leads to another. Amy arrived with an agenda of exercising and doing something to relax. A year later, she has consistently exercised and meditated, changed jobs, developed a new outlook on her responsibilities, started dating, made peace with her divorce, and developed positive body esteem that allows her to exercise comfortably in gym settings. Changing one part of ourselves influences all other parts.

Her half-marathon experience was positive in terms of what she learned and the confidence she

REFLECTION 4.13

When you consider *continuing* in Amy's case, are you looking at just her exercise and relaxation practices? Take a moment and reflect on her process. What trajectory did she follow to realize the changes she wanted? How did her initial goals morph throughout the coaching relationship? How was coaching helpful for Amy? What's your sense of her readiness to end coaching? Do you have any hunches about what might be next for her?

gained. It would be inappropriate to see it as a false start just because she didn't stick with it. Coaching involves experimentation. With competent guidance, clients learn to extract relevant messages and principles from all their engagements.

Not surprisingly, meditation proved to be a challenge. Amy got to listen to all her internal chatter, and some of it was difficult to hear. But, she stuck with it, partly because she acknowledged her difficulties and effectively engaged in problem solving with her coach. What seemed to open up for her over the year was the awareness that learning to relax involved more than a few routine meditation exercises.

Although we didn't clearly indicate the shifts in Amy's intentions and the related recontracting that she would have engaged in with her coach, the likelihood is that in many coaching relationships such as Amy's, the agenda and the coaching contract evolve over time. What distinguishes coaching from a somewhat open-ended counseling or therapy process is that coaches endeavor to keep their focus on the agenda for which a client has hired them until the client redefines what she wants to work on. As we leave Amy in this final meeting, it is not entirely clear to us, though it is probably quite clear to Amy and her coach, which agendas are being managed and tracked for progress.

The focus on continuity may become more or less central in coaching, depending on the degree to which clients struggle with follow-through. Clients often enter coaching with a far-reaching agenda. Innumerable tasks and personal development requirements may be embedded in these agendas. Based on the skill sets and resources with which they begin their journeys, the process may be more or less prolonged. When clients struggle, coaches are proactive. They explore the sources of difficulty, they examine other paths to the same objectives, they uncover hidden resources and opportunities, and they search for deeper meaning and motivation.

Some clients have clearly articulated goals at the outset of the relationship. However, they know from personal experience that their habitual patterns are strong, and although they haven't been able to be reliable to themselves, they believe that being accountable to someone else will work for them. In other words, if they have to report to coaches about their progress, they stand a better chance of succeeding. If their coaching relationship is only about this, it is a faint shadow of what coaching can be. As we have seen with Bob and Amy, the initial agendas were expanded and topics that were thought to be straightforward touched upon multiple dimensions of these clients' lives.

There is an aspect of continuing in virtually every coaching session. Clients plan action, commit, and then engage in various processes in between meetings with their coach. At some point in each session, a review of progress takes place. When engagement is chronically inconsistent or even absent, the viability of coaching for this particular client comes into question. More fundamental matters may need to be addressed before the person can wholeheartedly pursue significant change efforts. Put differently, coaching does not intentionally work on core personality change processes. Though personal transformations often emerge through coaching, an explicit request for such a goal is perhaps more appropriate for counselors and psychotherapists. Referring clients to other helping professionals does not imply failure or that the clients don't want to change. There are building blocks to change processes, and sometimes the deep structures need to be more firmly established.

At some point, the coaching relationship will end, and if the work has taken root, the clients will continue on their path with skills to address predictable and unpredictable experiences that may derail them on their journey. Over time, whatever it is they have achieved or are pursuing may need adjustment—or perhaps a new intention signaling a new journey will arise. The waters will spill over in a new direction.

# COMMENTARY

Coaching relationships address significant matters in clients' lives; they are rarely focused on trivial concerns. Clients want something badly enough to go through the effort of finding a coach, telling their story, and challenging old habits and approaches to how they normally do things. It is essential to honor clients' courage in embarking on the journeys through coaching.

At the beginning of the relationship, clients often express energy and enthusiasm. They have taken the first step, or at least an important new step. The flow model of coaching provides both a useful metaphor and practical guidelines for working with clients as they apply action to the fruitful pursuit of their dreams.

Too often people live in a world of wishful thinking. Their hopes and aspirations come and go without evidence of realization. We know of the inestimable capacity of human beings to make dreams come true, and we also know that the dreams-into-reality process is rarely fed by idle thought alone. Actions are needed. But what actions are best?

At the beginning of a relationship, it takes time to understand who the client is, what her intentions are, how her life is configured, what resources she has, and how actions need to be sequenced to best facilitate the realization of her wishes in a fashion that endures over time. Gaining insight, understanding patterns, and identifying resources provide the basis for action planning. Without these, there are limits to how much energy clients can bring forth, how long they can endure, and how many setbacks they can sustain before they stop, turn back, or sit down in bewilderment.

Embodying the metaphor of flow in their work, coaches may want to privately reflect at various moments in their sessions with clients: "Am I flowing? Is my client flowing? Is there movement forward? And if not, how can I generate a sense of flow that is so essential to this work?"

As we address core competencies of coaching in the upcoming chapters, we invite you to keep the flow model of coaching in mind. The core competencies we will discuss are intimately connected to the creation of flow.

# 5

# SETTING THE FOUNDATION FOR EFFECTIVE COACHING

## *I*n this chapter, you will learn how…

- solid foundations are created to ensure progress in a coaching relationship;

- self-awareness and mindfulness are necessary for effective coaching;

- core moral principles pertain to virtually all helping relationships;

- ethical concepts permeate the work of lifestyle wellness coaches;

- coaching boundaries are strongly related to a coach's role, resources, and circumstances; and

- contractual agreements are indispensable in coaching relationships.

The time will come
When with elation
You will greet yourself
Arriving at your own door

—*Derek Walcott*

In this chapter, we commence a systematic discussion of the ICF's 11 **core coaching competencies** (ICF, 2011c) (see ICF Core Coaching Competencies). The metaperspectives offered in the first four chapters of this book provide a broad framework for coaching and the processes that clients experience in their work. Though the remaining chapters would seem to have a narrower focus on skill development, the order in which ICF has listed the competencies captures progression within a coaching relationship. Because of this, learning about core competencies will further solidify your appreciation of movement within and between sessions.

We can view the 11 core competencies from two levels: The first is as an identification of elements and processes of a single coaching session; the second is as a map of progression in the overall work of the coaching relationship.

From the perspective of a single session, you can easily grasp that coaches need to listen well and ask questions while being fully present and fostering trust in the process. You can also recognize that they need to communicate directly and work with clients so they attain greater awareness of their topics. Of course, it is pivotal that coaches and clients plan and codetermine action in each and every session. Managing progress and accountability can be found in coach-initiated reviews of previous action agreements with their clients, which might then lead to shifts in the coaching contract itself. In brief, all 11 competencies should be readily apparent in the unfolding dialogue between coach and client within a single session.

When considered over the course of the entire relationship, certain core competencies may emerge as more central in certain phases of coaching. For instance, building trust and intimacy is crucial early in the coaching process, whereas in later phases coaches may rely on the existence of trust and intimacy while engaging in more challenging discussions with clients about awareness and direct communication. It is also true that there comes a time when clients are reasonably in flow toward their dreams and the focus is more on managing actions and ensuring accountability. From this perspective, the competencies provide a sketch of the coaching relationship over its temporal duration.

In this chapter, we present in-depth coverage of the first two ICF core competencies categorized under the heading of setting the foundation for effective coaching: meeting ethical guidelines and professional standards and establishing the coaching agreement.

## ICF Core Coaching Competencies

A. Setting the foundation
   1. Meeting ethical guidelines and professional standards
   2. Establishing the coaching agreement
B. Cocreating the relationship
   3. Establishing trust and intimacy with the client
   4. Coaching presence
C. Communicating effectively
   5. Active listening
   6. Powerful questioning
   7. Direct communication
D. Facilitating learning and results
   8. Creating awareness
   9. Designing actions
   10. Planning and goal setting
   11. Managing progress and accountability

International Coach Federation 2011

# MEETING ETHICAL GUIDELINES AND ESTABLISHING THE COACHING AGREEMENT

The ICF (2011c) defines its first core coaching competency of meeting ethical guidelines and professional standards as the coach's understanding of coaching ethics and standards and ability to apply them appropriately in all coaching situations. The ICF further states that to meet the exigencies of this competency, an ethical coach is one who

- understands and exhibits in its own behaviors the ICF standards of conduct (see appendix C);
- understands and follows all ICF ethical guidelines (see appendix C),
- clearly communicates the distinctions between coaching, consulting, psychotherapy, and other support professions; and

- refers the client to another support professional as needed, knowing when this is needed and the available resources.

International Coach Federation 2011

By way of introduction, let's consider a wonderful parable about a monk traveling back to his monastery. As he crosses an open field, a fierce samurai warrior suddenly confronts him. The samurai blocks the monk's path with his hand menacingly poised above the hilt of his sword. In a threatening voice, he asks the monk three questions in staccato fashion: "Who are you? Where are you going? Why are you going there?" Somewhat stunned by this unexpected turn of events, the monk regains his composure and responds with a question of his own: "How much does your shogun pay you to stand on guard here and ask these questions of all travelers?" The samurai, slightly taken aback by the question, replies, "Two bags of rice each month." The monk smiles and says to the samurai, "I will pay you three bags of rice a month if you will ask me these same three questions every day."

Clients who embark on the journey of coaching explore these three questions—Who are you? Where are you going? Why are you going there?—over and over again with the help of their coaches. What this parable brilliantly illuminates is the interrelationship of goals, motivations, and personal identity. Though coaching is ultimately a goal-driven, action-oriented methodology, effective coaches continually strive to appreciate who their clients are in the context of their yearnings and dreams.

A more practice-based rendition of the monk and samurai parable appears in the work of Jeffrey Kottler (2008), who offers three questions for clients to consider: Where are you going? How will you get there? How will you know when you have arrived? These questions allude to the fact that clients need to enter the coaching relationship with a statement of intention. They also have to discover their unique path toward their goal and clearly identify criteria for knowing when they have arrived.

When contrasted with other forms of helping such as counseling and psychotherapy, coaching clients typically begin the relationship with goals that are widely framed. As noted in the previous chapter, the agendas that they initially present typically evolve over time. In this respect, they have at least a preliminary answer to the first question that Kottler (2008) proposes: Where are you going? The work of coaching then fills out this answer, while giving ample focus to the two remaining questions.

The ICF rightly positions ethical considerations as the first of its 11 core coaching competencies. Ethical discussions may seem abstract, but a central and practical ethical question is whether the client's request for help is something that the coach can competently and efficiently address. When we find ourselves amid the multiple challenges of living and growing, the list of potential helpers can be perplexingly long: psychoanalyst, therapist, counselor, mentor, member of the clergy, psychic healer, coach, and so on. By analogy, if your car breaks down, you know immediately that you need to find an auto mechanic. In coaching, the responsibility for determining whether the person seeking help is in the right place rests squarely on the coach's shoulders.

Virtually all professions have explicit codes of conduct and ethical guidelines. In some cases, they may appear as a list of dos and don'ts, but more likely these codes are framed as broad guidelines for responsible professional engagement. Based on Kottler's (2008) questions, coaches need to understand and embrace the nature of their role—what they can do, what they cannot do, and what their process of working with clients looks like. Moreover, they need to be able to express these ideas articulately and unequivocally so clients have no misunderstandings at the outset.

The second of the ICF's 11 core competencies, establishing the coaching agreement, focuses on agreements or contracts that coaches and clients determine together. It is easy to see how this competency is intricately interwoven with that of ethics. In a sense, a coach's ability to determine with her client the terms, conditions, and objectives of their working relationship needs to be founded on an ethical examination of what coach and client can reasonably do together that will be positive and forward moving.

# DISTINGUISHING AMONG VALUES, MORALS, AND ETHICS

Most of us have a personal understanding of the term *ethics.* Occasionally, we may get our definition mixed up with other concepts that seem similar to ethics. Three terms that are sometimes used interchangeably are *values*, *ethics*, and *morals*. Admittedly, there is a fine line differentiating these terms; however, they can have different and even contradictory implications. Corey, Corey, and Callanan (2011) provide a thorough review and consideration of ethical concerns within the helping professions, and they offer this clarification of the three terms in question: **Values** concern beliefs and attitudes that provide us with direction in everyday living, whereas **ethics** pertain to the beliefs we hold about what constitutes right or wrong conduct. More specifically, ethics represent moral principles adopted by an individual or group to provide rules for conduct. **Morality** is concerned with perspectives of right and proper comportment and involves evaluating actions on the basis of some broader cultural context or religious standard.

## Values

Values are personal principles that are not necessarily about right or wrong. They are individually held beliefs and attitudes that guide action. Sometimes people talk about friends who have good values. By implication this means that someone can have bad values—but bad according to whom? Experts (Ivey, Ivey, & Zalaquett, 2010) believe that parental interactions, religious upbringing, and traumas such as accidents, wars, and personal violations are primary factors in shaping our deeply held values. Viktor Frankl (1969), a prominent psychiatrist who wrote about his experiences as an inmate in a Nazi concentration camp, argued that human behavior constantly raises issues of values. Life is about choice. As we express our choices, our values become evident. Values are learned to such an extent that some theorists argue that one can make a child value virtually anything if that child is raised and reinforced in particular ways (Gladding, 2009; Hackney, 2000).

Part of a coach's work is to enable clients to clarify their values. Discovering clients' values enables coaches to better align courses of action with intentions. Interestingly, client values may present serious challenges for coaches. In the domain of health, wellness, and fitness, one might presume that the vast majority of client intentions represent positive values. After all, what could be wrong with eating well, getting fit, and pursuing a healthy lifestyle? But what if your client wishes to pursue such objectives at all costs and without restraint? What if she wants to make changes through methods you don't value? What if she wants your help in doing something that you personally think is wrong? For example, what if she wishes to lose weight by any means so she can look just like a cover girl, but you think these role models misrepresent healthy body proportions?

Values have implications for ethical behavior, but they are not exactly the same thing as ethics. You can have substantially different values than those of your clients and yet work with your client toward goal attainment in an entirely ethical manner. Therefore, as long as the goal of the would-be cover girl doesn't ask you to violate professionally recognized health standards, there should be no issue in helping her achieve that goal. Of course, clashes of values between coach and client may mean that the fit between the two is not conducive to a harmonious coaching relationship. In such cases, the coach might refer the client to another coach who may be a better fit. There is no guarantee that clients will be perceptive enough to fully appreciate what the coach's values are early in the relationship, so coaches bear responsibility for identifying any value differences that may influence the effectiveness of the coaching relationship.

Values are important in other ways. When clients' choices fail to reflect their values, they are likely to feel unhappy (Brown & Srebalus, 2003). If a client places a high value on wealth, he may direct great effort toward making money. This value may serve to justify any means for obtaining it. Here, we can see that a value does not imply good or bad, right or wrong. Of course, if you ask most people what they value, they will probably recite things such as wisdom, friendship, freedom, happiness, equality, or world peace (Parrott, 2003). Yet, as guides to action, good indicators of a person's values are the things that she chooses, the ways that she acts, and her behavior toward others.

As a lifestyle wellness coach, can you be value free? The simple answer is no. Taking good care of your body, exercising regularly, and eating well are expressions of your values, as are most other choices that you make in life. So, if you can't be value free, to what extent do you reveal your values to your clients? Answers to this question move us closer to ethics, especially if we consider attempts to influence clients toward your own value system.

Another perspective on values is that they form an integral part of our **personality** (Parrott, 2003) and therefore are inseparable from who we are and how we approach the tasks of coaching. As with other personality traits we possess (see Five-Factor Model of Personality), values influence our outlook on life and color the way we approach people.

Values are like a pair of glasses through which we see the world. A reflective professional (Schön, 2003) devotes time and effort to understanding his own values as well as any personal issues that may affect his work with others. To do so, he must work

## Five-Factor Model of Personality

Five major traits have been identified within the five-factor model of personality. The Big Five are (1) openness versus closedness to experiences, (2) high conscientiousness versus low conscientiousness, (3) extroversion versus introversion, (4) agreeableness versus antagonism, and (5) neuroticism versus emotional stability.

The Big Five model of personality, often referred to by the acronym *OCEAN*, conceives of each personality trait as spanning a continuum from one end of a spectrum to the opposite end. Just as attention to a client's learning style (discussed in chapter 2) helps the coach adjust to the uniqueness of each client, awareness of personality orientations can be invaluable in your ability to communicate with and assist your clients.

Here's a little more detail on OCEAN to enhance your understanding:

1. **O**penness versus closedness—This factor refers to interest in culture and openness to new ideas and novel experiences. At the open end, scores imply being highly creative and curious and seeking new experiences, whereas scores toward the closed end suggest that one is more traditional, practical, and reluctant to try new things.

2. High **c**onscientiousness versus low conscientiousness—This factor refers to how people engage in goal pursuit. High scores reflect a person who exhibits strict self-discipline, organization, and extreme goal orientation, whereas low scores point to patterns of being more laid back, disorganized, and indifferent to high achievement.

3. **E**xtroversion versus introversion—This factor refers to preferences for how one engages in social situations. One end of the range identifies people who are highly sociable and talkative, whereas the other end characterizes people who are exceptionally reserved and deliberate in expression.

4. **A**greeableness versus antagonism—This factor refers to how people interact with others. One end represents characteristics of being good-natured, forgiving, and trusting, whereas the other end suggests a pattern of unfriendliness, skepticism, and a highly competitive manner.

5. **N**euroticism versus emotional stability—This factor refers to thought patterns and ways of experiencing emotions. One end suggests a pattern of nervousness and insecurity with a propensity to experience negative thoughts and emotions, and the other end reflects a manner of being calm, relaxed, and secure.

(See Widiger & Trull, 1997, for a comprehensive review and assessment of the model.)

---

steadily to increase his self-awareness, a process that is viewed by many as a key to success. A reflective professional is one who seeks to cultivate a keen sense of who he is as a person, what makes him tick, and why he does what he does in the world.

Johnson (2009) defines **self-awareness** as "paying attention to and being aware of oneself" (p. 391), while Goleman (1995) suggests that "self-awareness refers to a self-reflective, introspective attention to one's own experience, sometimes called mindfulness" (p. 315). Self-awareness, often connected to the popular injunction to know thyself, has been identified as a cornerstone of **emotional intelligence** (Goleman, 1995). Noticing, witnessing, and being with one's experience as it occurs are all approaches to the development of self-awareness.

Coaching relationships may derail because the coach is insufficiently self-aware and mindful. Poor awareness of values, feelings, and behaviors can result in the coach's failure to appreciate how his values influence the questions he asks, the assumptions he fails to challenge, and the choices he promotes. Ultimately, coaching without self-awareness deprives clients of the insights they need in order to achieve their goals.

If values are part of the coach's personality, attempts to come across as value free in coaching are doomed from the outset. Having values does not mean that one should impose them on others. Ideally, the values that a coach advocates are ones that reflect positively on her character and approach to helping. Being mindful means changing values

---

**REFLECTION 5.1**

An important step here may be to reflect on your values and see how well they represent the way you want to be in the world. Reflecting on your values will provide clues about how you generally look at things and how your assessments influence your coaching practice. To guide your reflections, you might ask yourself, what makes me happy, satisfied, and fulfilled? What gives me energy? What am I proud of? What do I most aspire to achieve? You might also want to reflect on how experiences in your life have shaped your attitudes and beliefs. What are the values of your culture? What life events were most significant in forming your values? Can you relate early life experiences to the values that guide your actions today? To further your reflections, you may want to complete the VIA survey of character strengths found at www.authentichappiness.org.

---

that are contrary to effective human relationships and the promotion of well-being (Silsbee, 2010). For instance, a person who drinks excessively or who has a habit of smoking tobacco or other substances would not be the best role model for clients working on health behaviors.

## Morals

Moral development seems to flow from a variety of social and cultural standards, shaping our understanding of how behavior should be evaluated (Jaafar, Kolodinsky, McCarthy, & Schroder, 2004). Moral codes underlie the values we see expressed within various communities and cultures. Nagy (2011) identifies a number of principles for professional behavior that commonly appear in the ethical codes of most North American professional societies (e.g., psychology, law, medicine). These principles include beneficence and nonmaleficence, fidelity to professional responsibility, justice, and respect for people's rights and dignity or autonomy. Let's see how these principles speak to your work with coaching clients.

### Beneficence and Nonmaleficence

Beneficence, or doing good, refers to promoting the welfare of clients. Nonmaleficence, or doing no harm, means actively avoiding identifiable risks or damaging actions. Though coaches intend to help their clients through an egalitarian professional

relationship, it may become evident that they either cannot help a particular person or that the actions a client is contemplating will not enable her to reach her goal. Furthermore, clients may not be cognizant of the potential effects of certain programs or actions, and they may not know about the issues that might emerge in discussions of goals and objectives. Although coaches cannot foresee all possibilities, they need to be vigilant to the risks of harmful processes and actions. The principle of beneficence and nonmaleficence requires that coaches assess, to the best of their abilities, their competence to help clients. It holds coaches responsible for ensuring that their actions will be beneficial and will cause no harm.

### Fidelity to Professional Responsibility

This moral principle is about making honest promises and honoring commitments. It speaks to truthful and honest conduct. Guiding principles of professional responsibility involve striving for truth in advertising and ensuring that clients know what to expect as they enter a coaching relationship. In particular, clients must be informed about fees, cancellation policies, and limitations to the relationship at the onset. Coaches must be proactive in informing clients about dimensions of the coaching relationship of which clients may not have full knowledge. In this regard, they must discuss the limits of confidentiality and spell out what coaching is and what it is not. For instance, coaching is not therapy, and clients—not the coach—are responsible for the results they achieve.

Fidelity is also about ensuring that qualifications and areas of competence are marketed accurately. It asserts that coaches are trained to do what they advertise, that they are trustworthy, and that they strictly abide by the code of ethics in all professional activities. In other words, coaches need to be above board regarding all aspects of their work. The principle of fidelity to professional responsibility requires consistently having the best interests of clients at heart. The coach is expected to avoid taking advantage of her relationship with clients and to make full disclosure where potential conflicts of interest may arise (e.g., being a shareholder in the client's business). She also has an obligation to refer her client if she deems that another professional could be more helpful.

### Justice

Justice refers to providing equal treatment to all clients. This concept does not mean that coaches have to be equally skilled in working with all types of people or in all issues that people might bring them, but rather that within the range of their expertise, they treat all clients fairly, without discrimination, and with sensitivity to their unique backgrounds and issues. Where feasible, this principle also carries an expectation that approaches and processes will adapt to the unique needs and characteristics of their clients.

### Respect for People's Rights and Dignity or Autonomy

This principle requires that clients' privacy be respected through strict adherence to confidentiality. It also implies that coaches recognize the uniqueness of their clients and fully respect their cultural norms, values, and beliefs. To do so, they are expected to develop self-awareness of biases and prejudices that could affect their coaching and work diligently to minimize them. This principle necessitates the promotion of clients' independence and self-determination in the practice of coaching. Paradoxically, dependency may be an important component in the beginning phases of the coaching relationship, yet as the relationship develops, greater self-sufficiency should strongly emerge.

Moral principles remain constant across the various helping professions. At root, they speak to the need to do what is right, to anticipate and prevent potentially harmful actions wherever possible, to be honest, to be fair, to respect clients, and to actively prepare them for solo flight.

---

**REFLECTION 5.2**

Take a moment to reflect on your moral standards. The coaching profession offers guidelines for ethical conduct. However, your understanding of morality is subjective. Even the moral code you may have adopted as a guide to your daily actions, be it the Bible, the Koran, the Vedas, the Four Noble Truths and Eightfold Path, or others, is subject to your own interpretations. To help your reflections, you might ask yourself the following: What behaviors characterize a moral person or moral conduct in my culture and in the communities I associate with? What is my definition of *moral character*? How do I ultimately determine what is right or wrong, good or evil? How might my moral standards affect my coaching practice?

---

## Ethics and Ethical Codes

There are many helping professions and innumerable forms of one-to-one relationships. The bonds that unite the various types of helpers are likely to include their deep and compassionate concern for others and their profound desire to be supportive. In this light, it might seem that ethical behavior would come naturally: Helpers want to be helpful. So, why have we, along with the ICF, chosen to address ethics as one of the first coaching competencies? There are multiple answers. Probably the most central one has to do with a desire to establish the foundation of your coaching relationships. Long before you ever meet your first client, you will want to do some serious self-examination and then test yourself against a number of demanding standards for coaching excellence. Wanting to help isn't enough. Being a good and moral person isn't enough. Having fabulous communication skills isn't enough. Even putting all of these together, there is much to learn in order to ensure that your good intentions are fully respectful of the character and perspectives of each unique person you will encounter.

Coaches do not have a standard academic curriculum that they have all followed in preparation for their careers. As noted earlier, coaches come from all walks of life and have varying degrees of preparation and life experience. Some may think that helping means telling people what to do based on their personally gained wisdom; others may believe that there is a recipe book of solutions for various issues. Many practitioners have had other careers before finding their passion in coaching work. They may have been psychologists or business leaders, for example, and many will have dabbled in various occupations before discovering a home base in coaching. Although the desire to help may be widespread, what it means to be helpful will be individually interpreted.

The ICF requires as little as 60 hours of instruction for its first level of certification (associate certified coach—ACC). That's not a lot of time to ensure that coaches have fully embraced what it means to coach and what the limits of their role might be. For instance, one of the ethical principles in the ICF code of ethics (see appendix C) is to not knowingly mislead or make false claims about what clients will receive from the coaching process. Another informs coaches to not give clients information or advice they know or believe to be misleading or false. As you read these two statements, you're probably thinking, "Of course I wouldn't."

So, then, what would you say to your new client? "I'm going to help you!" Well, no, you can't say that. You could say, "I'm going to try to help you," but now you may need to tell the person how exactly you are going to do this. So you say, "I'm going to listen to you carefully and then we're going to figure out together what would be best for you to do." That sounds okay—until it comes time for you to offer your opinions. You wouldn't intentionally offer false or misleading information, yet you might not have all the facts about an issue and might inadvertently suggest something that is simply incorrect or unintentionally harmful. Are you beginning to feel a little anxious? Hopefully so! Helping another person is a big responsibility.

Coaching is not about advising clients what to do based on your accumulated wisdom. It is a partnership between equals where both the coach and client are responsible for agreements that they make. The core of ethical responsibility is that professional helpers do nothing that will harm the client, the community, or society in general (Nagy, 2011). Clients who seek help may be vulnerable and susceptible to undue influence. We assume that people who train to be coaches want to do the right thing. In a classic description of ethics, helpers might be described as people who seek to be virtuous (Gelso & Fretz, 2001). *Virtue* can be defined as a disposition to do what is morally right (Beauchamp & Childress, 2009). According to Parrott (2003), virtue is anchored deep within the self, yet good intentions alone do not necessarily translate into ethical behavior. Helpers need to get beneath the lofty language of ethical codes to concretely identify what it means to be competent to help another person with a specific concern or desire.

Professional societies formulate ethical matters into codes of conduct representing critical values that members need to demonstrate in their practice (Gibson & Mitchell, 2008). Though legal considerations are certainly relevant to ethical codes, laws typically define the minimum standards that society will tolerate (Corey et al., 2011). Ethical codes speak more to *ideal standards*, to the highest aspirations of a professional group for member conduct and relationships with clients.

Although it is implied, all codes of ethics require practitioners to act in accordance with relevant governmental statutes and regulations. Occasionally, ethics and the law may be in conflict. For instance, what occurs in helping relationships is often bound by a client's right to confidentiality, yet some circumstances—such as when working with minors or with people who reveal that they are about to harm

themselves or someone else—may require a professional to breach this ethical principle. Whenever such conflicts are identifiable, ethical guidelines require professionals to inform clients of conditions under which rights of confidentiality do not apply.

> ## REFLECTION 5.3
>
> Take a moment to read and reflect on the ICF code of ethics (appendix C). Do you have questions about any of the 25 points covered in the four sections of this code of ethics? If so, please note these questions. You may want to visit the ICF website for further explanations or discuss them with an ICF-certified coach.

# IMPLICATIONS FOR ETHICAL CONDUCT IN LIFESTYLE WELLNESS COACHING

The ICF code of ethics is a well-formed and comprehensive guide to ethical behavior within a professional coaching relationship. There are also other associations and professional groups whose ethical codes are conceptually and structurally aligned with the ICF's as it applies to lifestyle wellness coaching (see Associations With Ethical Codes Relevant to Coaching).

As discussed previously, the ethical codes for the helping profession are likely to manifest significant overlap and communality. Even so, the uniqueness of coaching requires that as the profession develops, special materials (e.g., books and articles) will need to be offered with case studies that help unpack the practical applications or interpretations of ethical concepts (Fisher, 2012). We will take a moment now to present relevant ethical areas for lifestyle wellness coaches.

## Proper Training and Ongoing Education

To be of benefit to clients and to ensure the absence of harmful interventions, proper training and continued education are mandatory. Chapter 12 explores this topic more extensively.

## Client Rights

If clients are to be self-determining, they must fully understand the parameters of the coach–client

## Associations With Ethical Codes Relevant to Coaching

Organizations such as the ICF have made significant efforts to formalize certification requirements for professional coaches. Becoming an ICF-certified coach carries the requirement of adherence to its code of ethics. However, a number of other organizations related to coaching and other helping professions have detailed ethical principles that are well worth reviewing. The following organizations or associations may provide guidance:

- American Association for Marriage and Family Therapy: www.aamft.org
- American Counseling Association: www. counseling.org
- American Psychological Association: www. apa.org

- Association for Counselor Education and Supervision: www.acesonline.net
- Executive and Business Coaching Network: www.execcoach.net
- International Association of Coaching: www. certifiedcoach.org
- Life Coaching—United Kingdom: www. uklifecoaching.org
- National Board for Certified Counselors: www. nbcc.org
- Worldwide Association of Business Coaches: www.wabccoaches.com

See also www.peer.ca/coachorgs.html#profs for a list of other coaching organizations.

relationship. It might not be optimal for a client to self-determine an exercise or nutrition program without expert guidance, yet coaches need to be vigilant for indications that clients are complying unwillingly with programs professionals offer them because they believe they have no choice or because they think that the consequences for noncompliance would be significant.

## Exceptions to Rules of Confidentiality

Certainly, coaches need to assure clients of their rights to privacy and the confidential nature of the coaching relationship, and therein lies a responsibility for coaches to inform clients fully of all matters pertaining to their agreements, actions, and aspirations. Common sense tells us that in a life-and-death emergency or in the event that a coach has information that might save a client's life, the coach would have reason to breach confidentiality agreements. This principle extends to such unlikely situations as a client's revelation that he is intending to end his life or that he plans to harm someone else. Similarly, if there is clear evidence that the client is abusing or neglecting minors or elderly or disabled people, the coach must assume her civic and legal responsibilities and breach the confidentiality agreement. Legal statutes also stipulate other conditions under which a coach must make records and conversations with clients available to the courts.

## Caring

At times, caring for someone within a coaching relationship slips into more intimate feelings from the perspective of either the client or the helper. Caring is always viewed in relation to the contract and the nature of the work occurring between coach and client. A coach may become concerned about a client's health or well-being, especially if she sees him intentionally putting himself at risk. Yet to intervene in such cases, the coach needs to frame her actions within the legitimate bounds of the profession and the contractual nature of the relationship.

## Referrals

Coaches may refer clients to other professionals or other services. Two forms of referral can be identified. In the first, the coach completely ends her relationship with a client and refers all matters to another professional that the client chooses. In the second, the coach retains an overseeing or facilitative role with the client and cocreates topic-specific referrals that will advance the client's objectives. To illustrate, a coach may deem it inappropriate or ineffective to continue working with someone and therefore may suggest that the person consider working with another professional. The coaching relationship then officially ends, even though the client may not have reached the intended objectives. In the second type of referral, the coach may discuss with the client certain ancillary activities, perhaps through work with other people. These may be allied health professionals, or they could be other service providers, such as lawyers, realtors, or financial planners. Of course, the way in which referrals are made would incorporate principles of free and informed choice. In practice, this might mean letting the client look for a service provider on his own, or it might mean offering a list and suggesting how he might obtain independent assessments of these professionals' competencies.

# Boundaries

Forming ethical agreements is intricately related to the concept of boundaries. What are boundaries? A football field has boundaries. You clearly know when the ball is out of bounds. The same applies for lifestyle wellness coaching. Boundaries serve as guides for making calls about what is within limits and what is out of bounds, and in this respect boundaries are closely tied to professional ethics. In sport as in life, the rules of the game are intended to be clear. Subjective elements related to boundaries can be problematic. The more effort you invest in clarifying role and relational boundaries, the more readily you can identify out-of-bounds behaviors.

Professional boundaries stem from definitions of your role, job skills, and responsibilities. Professional boundaries evolving in the coaching field will help guide your actions in a wide array of situations, but they can never cover all events that you are likely to encounter in your professional career (Williams & Davis, 2007). In discussions of boundaries, a useful distinction has been made between a **boundary crossing** and a **boundary violation** (Zur, 2009).

## Boundary Crossing

**Boundary crossing** refers to behaviors that have the potential to create conditions for eventual misconduct but are not inherently wrong. Examples of such behaviors include accepting a token gift from a client, giving a client a hug after a victorious experience, or regularly attending meetings of community organizations that your client also attends. It is important to remain attentive to matters of diversity and cultural differences here; what may seem to be a completely innocent expression on the part of one person may assume meaning of far greater proportion by the other. Nevertheless, some writers (Smith & Fitzpatrick, 1995) argue that such actions pave the way to boundary violations and to breaches in ethical conduct. Others (Lazarus & Zur, 2002; Zur, 2009) suggest that when the client's well-being remains a priority, certain types of boundary crossings can sometimes engender healthier relationships.

## Boundary Violations

The more serious matter, **boundary violations**, is universally understood to be unethical (Zur, 2004). Overstepping these parameters is problematic in most helping relationships because it blurs professional role definitions (Welfel, 2010). An obvious example of a boundary violation is having sexual relations with a current client. We suggest you consult the ethical guidelines for coaching in appendix C to determine what other behaviors might represent boundary violations. If you think of boundaries as limitations to thought, action, or even the expression of feeling, what might guide the establishment of limits?

**Your Role**   As a lifestyle wellness coach, you have a particular domain in which it is legitimate for you to practice. Your training, contracts with clients, personal characteristics, and limitations help to define your scope of work. Moreover, although you may be competent to administer a certain service, legal limitations imposed on professional groups may restrict the activities of members of your profession. For instance, you may be an insightful and skilled communicator with a graduate degree in psychology and extensive knowledge of psychological issues, yet it would be unethical for you to switch into a psychotherapeutic role with a coaching client even though you might be able to do it well.

**Your Resources**   Even with all these demarcations of professional action, at times you will have to make a judgment call. When your personal resources are at low ebb, you may better serve yourself and your client by not taking on a particular activity. An example might be a client request for an additional session when you are tightly booked and need time to address your own needs.

**The Situation**   At times, situational dynamics may supersede normal boundary limitations and require intervention. Most rules have exceptions that apply in unusual circumstances. Imagine that a client breaks down and cries uncontrollably in the midst of a session because she has just experienced the ending of a long-term intimate relationship. This issue may not be part of your contractual agreement, but because of the severity of the matter, it would be appropriate to listen with great empathy. In any case, if you find yourself making so many exceptions that customary role behaviors become the

**REFLECTION 5.4**

To explore your sense of boundaries as a coach, take time to reflect on the following questions:

- What do I consider the limits of my professional role as a lifestyle wellness coach—what's in and what's out?
- What are my responsibilities?
- What would I consider to be examples of boundary crossings?
- What would I consider to be examples of boundary violations?
- What are areas of my personal and professional life where I have difficulty asserting my boundaries?
- What steps could I take to enable me to maintain appropriate boundaries at all times?

exception, you may want to examine your criteria for exceptional circumstances.

## Malpractice

Even when you believe you are fully adhering to the ethical code for coaches, things can go seriously wrong. A client may believe that you have harmed him through your coaching and may accuse you of malpractice. *Malpractice* is a legal term that involves unethical conduct and negligence resulting in injury or loss to the client. In cases of malpractice, the coach has failed to render appropriate professional services or has failed to exercise the degree of skill or expertise that would ordinarily be expected of similar professionals in the same situation. As summarized by Corey et al. (2011), malpractice generally falls into six categories, which have been modified here for lifestyle wellness coaches:

1. The coach used a procedure not considered within the realm of accepted coaching practice.
2. The coach used a technique or method for which she was not properly or adequately trained.
3. The coach failed to use a technique or procedure that would have been more beneficial to the client.
4. The coach failed to warn others about a violent client and thereby did not act to protect these people.

5. The coach failed to obtain or properly document the client's informed consent about coaching activities.
6. The coach failed to explain to the client the possible consequences of coaching interventions.

In malpractice cases, the burden of proof generally rests with the client. Four elements must be demonstrated to prove that a coach is guilty of malpractice: (1) A bona fide professional relationship existed between the coach and the client, (2) the coach acted in a negligent or improper manner or deviated significantly from the usual standards of care in the coaching profession, (3) the client suffered harm or injury from acting on the coach's recommendations, and (4) a causal linkage exists between the coach's negligence or breach of conduct and the actual injury or damage presumably experienced (Corey et al., 2011).

Discussions of malpractice may seem more pertinent to medicine or psychiatry, yet all professionals must be vigilant about these matters. In isolated cases, practitioners deliberately set out to harm their clients. In most instances, harm or injury results from some oversight, a moment of inattention, or unconscious neglect.

# COACHING AGREEMENTS

The second core competency, establishing the coaching agreement, is defined by the ICF (2011c) as the ability to understand what is required in the specific coaching interaction and to come to agreement with the prospective and new client about the coaching process and relationship. In this case, an effective coach

- understands and effectively discusses with the client the guidelines and specific parameters of the coaching relationship (e.g., logistics, fees, scheduling, inclusion of others if appropriate);
- reaches agreement about what is appropriate in the relationship and what is not, what is and is not being offered, and about the client's and coach's responsibilities; and
- determines whether there is an effective match between his coaching method and the needs of the prospective client.

International Coach Federation 2011

Clients hire coaches because they want to achieve something. They have a goal in mind and they believe it would be more reliably realized with the help of a coach. As discussed when we outlined the flow model of coaching, it often takes investigation to get to the real topic that the client wants to address. Initial formulations of the goal may be expressed concretely as an objective of losing a certain amount of weight, running a marathon, or sleeping peacefully through the night. As topics are explored, something else may emerge as the overarching purpose that clients want to realize. It may not be weight loss as much as it is feeling good about one's body. Perhaps an initial goal of running a marathon evolves into an objective of sustaining a high level of wellness over time. Likewise, sleeping peacefully through the night may translate into simplifying life so that anxiety and stress are not one's daily diet.

Whether initial intentions or derivatives of these intentions become the focus of the coaching relationship, clients have something they want to get out of their investment of time, money, and effort. Coaches need to clarify what the client truly wants and then determine whether they can help. Assuming a clear topic is identified and the coach believes she is competent to help this client reach her goal, the discussion necessarily must turn to the specifics of the agreement: How will the coach and client work together? What will the coach do, and what won't she do? What is expected of the client? What happens if the coach or client doesn't live up to the terms of their agreement? Who else might be involved? How confidential is the relationship? How long will the relationship continue? How much will it cost? And on it goes until all questions are answered, all terms are agreed upon, and all boundaries and limitations are identified as best as possible!

The evaluation that takes place when articulating an agreement is ideally two-sided. Both coach and client are engaged in determining its elements; they are both involved in reviewing expectations and assessing whether the coach's methods are appropriately suited to the stated goals. A client may have an objective pertaining to an area where the coach is richly experienced and knowledgeable. Based on personal experience, the coach believes that she can help. But the client has expectations that the help will take a particular shape. For instance, the coach will write out a prescription that he will unfailingly follow. Even when coaching evolves into a more commonly understood professional field, some clients will continue to arrive with expectations that simply do not fit the model to which the coach adheres.

Ultimately, there is a question of match or fit. Will this client work well with that coach toward the achievement of this particular goal? Will using that method of coaching be effective? Will this coach be able to work with that client who has this particular style of behavior and set of expectations toward a specific outcome within a defined time frame? An essential question about fit can be simply put as follows: Is there chemistry between coach and client?

## Signed Agreements

We define an *agreement* (see appendix B) as a mutually determined understanding of commitments. The terms *contract* and *agreement* are often used interchangeably, though contracts are more official in a legal sense. We can agree to do something, but does that carry the same weight as signing a contract? That is not clear. The existence of a written and signed agreement doesn't make it unalterable; rather, it provides a formality that calls for both coach and client to pay full attention to what they are committing to do. Elements of agreements can always be modified with mutual consent. Written agreements help clarify the coaching relationship and give it direction; moreover, they protect the rights, roles, and obligations of both parties and thereby increase the probability of a successful relationship (Gladding, 2009). Let us also remember that the ICF code of ethics prescribes that client records must comply with the law and that they must be maintained, stored, and disposed of in a manner that preserves privacy.

We believe clients benefit from the structure of a written and signed agreement rather than a verbal agreement. This gives them an opportunity to revisit their commitments and review the terms of the work they are doing with the coach. Signed agreements remove the element of doubt or question about what was said at the outset. In the first coaching session, when agreements are typically determined, clients may be preoccupied with the issues they are presenting and less so with the processes and terms that the coach is describing as part of their contractual working relationship. It may come as an unwelcome surprise when they are informed, for instance, that they have to pay for a missed session. The prevailing wisdom is that the terms and conditions of helping relationships should be agreed upon as early as possible (Brammer & MacDonald, 2003), and we would encourage that a written agreement be reviewed in the first session or that a draft document be sent to the client before the second session.

A signed agreement serves as a road map that provides general directions for getting from one point to another and confirms that both coach and client have explicit intentions to move in the same direction (Shebib, 2010). Contracts add to the clients' sense of ownership of and responsibility for agreed-upon objectives and methods. An often-overlooked value of signing an agreement pertains to the specification of terms and conditions for ending the relationship. Coaching relationships are more likely to be time limited than open-ended. Having agreements concerning how and when the relationship might end focuses both coach and client on benchmarks of progress and the identification of probable points of termination or renegotiation.

## Psychological Contracts

The concept of **psychological contracts** was originally offered by Levinson (1976). These are the assumed agreements that people often bring to professional relationships. Clients have rich histories of experiences with professionals and perhaps formal and informal helpers. Based on these histories, they enter professional relationships with certain expectations. Think of your expectations of teachers when you were in high school. As you moved on to other educational experiences (e.g., university coursework, professional training and seminars), how were your expectations confirmed or disconfirmed? And how did that affect you?

Psychological contracts constitute a two-way street. Both coaches and clients initially meet with separate sets of assumptions. Clients may believe that coaches have the answer or that coaches should make them feel better each time they come for a session. Novice coaches in particular often expect that clients are fully motivated to take on the challenging engagements of a change process. Coaches may assume that they will enable their clients to succeed no matter what. Clients may also believe that now that they are in professional hands, results are practically guaranteed.

The fewer unexpressed assumptions that there are in a coaching relationship, the better off both parties will be. Even when coach and client are clear at the outset about the terms of their relationship, behavioral patterns may be interpreted to suggest that the contract has been implicitly renegotiated. That is, the psychological contract may evolve differently from the written agreement. Let's look at a few situations where this may happen:

- Imagine an instance where the coach serves coffee at the first three meetings. What might the client come to assume is part of the working arrangement?
- The client repeatedly shows up 5 to 10 minutes late for appointments and the coach always gives him the contracted 45-minute session. Could the client not reasonably assume that he is entitled to the full session no matter when he shows up?
- A client answers his cell phone during sessions without comment from the coach. Even if sessions end at the agreed-on time, what is the implied agreement about calls during the session? Might they not be seen as taking precedence over the coaching agenda?

These situations all have one thing in common: People observe behavior and infer the rules or agreements. Regardless of what you say, actions often speak louder than words. Each time a deviation from the agreement occurs without comment or discussion, it holds the possibility for altering what was formally agreed upon. Over time, both coach and client may come to assume that their agreement is different from what was originally stated. This is not to say that agreements should remain fixed; rather, the parties need to acknowledge variations or changes explicitly and either define them as exceptions or incorporate them into a revised agreement that is then signed by both parties.

Most coaches have a standardized agreement. At a minimum, this covers the basic terms of the working relationship, and it may also make explicit not only the ways of working but also the boundaries of the relationship and its implications. Even in more detailed contracts, some issues may be missed. A critical skill for effective coaching is the ability to surface unexpressed assumptions and expectations that clients might have about the professional relationship and its objectives. Embedded elements

---

### REFLECTION 5.5

If you have been working with clients in a helping role, reflect on some of the assumptions they have formed, perhaps as a result of your actions or because you have failed to act. If you have not yet started working with clients, think of family and friends and how they have come to expect certain things from you because your actions or inaction gave them permission to do so. How have you contributed to the assumptions people have made about your agreements with them? How have these assumptions affected the relationships? What has happened when you tried to correct some of these assumptions? In a professional context, how might you keep your written agreements aligned with your psychological contracts?

of the client's unexpressed psychological contract may take weeks to identify. It is important to remain alert to the possibility of a misalignment between client expectations and the realities of the coaching experience. When the evidence is clear, an effective coach will respectfully present her impressions so they can be mutually explored.

## CRITICAL ELEMENTS OF AGREEMENTS IN LIFESTYLE WELLNESS COACHING

As we have repeatedly noted, the client's agenda as stated in the first session may evolve over time. It may become more focused or even more complex. For this and other reasons, agreements are not commitments to goal attainment within specified time limits. Agreements have more to do with the process and terms of the working relationship. There may well be an initial statement of the client's objectives for coaching, and beyond that there would be descriptions of how coach and client will work together, responsibilities for actions, fees and pay schedules, length and frequency of sessions, and expected duration of the agreement, among other things. Some critical elements of a coaching agreement are as follows:

- Meets the legitimate needs of coach and client; both parties perceive the agreement as fair.
- Contains concrete, descriptive statements of expectations for both coach and client.
- Describes arrangements for reviews of how the agreement is working and how terms and conditions can be renegotiated when necessary.
- Clearly stipulates exchanges of resources, materials, and fees. These should be based on objectively justifiable principles. For example, fees, meeting schedules, terms of working together, and limits of the working relationship should be based on principles of professional expertise, industry norms, mutual respect, and scientific evidence.

Reaching an agreement requires great attention to small and large matters. As detailed as it may be, it can nonetheless energize the relationship by providing clients with solid ground for their work. It can be seen as a relationship-building engagement that strengthens the abilities of coach and client to work cooperatively and come to fruitful resolutions of differences.

## EXPLORING THE COMPONENTS OF AGREEMENTS

The coaching agreement should detail the rights and responsibilities of both coach and client in implementing the agreement. An important framework for understanding the elements of coaching agreements can be found in the questions *who, what, when, where, how,* and *why.*

### Who?

Who is involved in the coaching relationship? It may be just coach and client, although lifestyle wellness coaching might include a team approach in collaboration with a medical doctor, nutritionist, personal trainer, or other allied health professionals. This variation would be represented in a multiparty agreement. In other instances, coaches may provide group coaching or may be hired by an organization that pays their fees to provide coaching to employees. In this case, the name and responsibilities of the sponsor are outlined in the agreement and the client is cleared of the financial element of coaching to the extent agreed upon with the sponsor.

### What?

What is involved and what is not involved in coaching? What is contracted for? Exactly what services are provided? What are the boundaries of the relationship? What are the coach's responsibilities? What are the client's responsibilities? What are both parties expected to do to live up to these responsibilities? What are they expected to do between sessions?

### When?

When will coaching take place and for how long? If a client hires a coach for one hour a week, the agreement stipulates not only the length of a session but also the minimal duration of the contract, such as six weeks. Another critical aspect of this question concerns when the terms of the coaching relationship might not apply. Clients may want to discuss their issues during unscheduled meetings or phone calls. Is this acceptable? How often and at what times are you willing and available to accept such unscheduled conversations? What is the time frame for responding to e-mails? Finally, agreements need to outline the cancellation policy. What is the client's obligation in terms of cancelling an appointment? When can sessions be made up? What if the coach needs to cancel a meeting?

## Where?

Where does coaching take place? In an office? At the client's home? In a fitness facility? Over the phone? What are unacceptable venues for coaching (e.g., coffee shops, casual street encounters)?

## How?

What does the working relationship look like? Some health, wellness, and fitness professionals may enact their responsibilities in a hands-on manner rather than while sitting and talking. What methods or assessment tools will be used? What training and certifications need to be signified in order to legitimately use these approaches and tools? How will clients inform the coach that something is not working for them? How will coaches let clients know of issues affecting the relationship?

## Why?

Though this question comes last in this chapter, it is really the first one that needs to be addressed. Through the rapport-building process of detailing a client's interest in achieving certain goals, coaches can begin to understand the reasons behind intended actions. Why is this goal so important that the client is willing to devote time, money, and effort toward its accomplishment? Too often, the *why* is assumed rather than made explicit. You may assume that an overweight client asking for guidance and support in maintaining an exercise program may hardly need to be asked why, yet the value in doing so can be substantial. Is the motivation coming from the client or from others? Does a larger issue need to be addressed while the client is undertaking a specific lifestyle change?

---

### ACTIVITY 5.1

Given the benefits of a written and signed contract, think about a client with whom you have worked and imagine what a coaching topic might be for this person. If you are not yet working in one-to-one relationships, create a fictitious client who comes to you for coaching. Review the coaching agreement provided in appendix B. Once you have done this, try to complete the *who*, *what*, *when*, *where*, *how*, and *why* questions for your coaching client.

---

# COMMENTARY

Within societal parameters, people are free to choose their goals and to pursue them by legitimate means. When they elect to work with lifestyle wellness coaches, professional considerations and ethical codes define the range of goals, the types of processes, and the nature of the relationship.

For some people, goal statements resemble ungrounded fantasies. In working with coaches, amorphous intentions are shaped into specific objectives and ultimately described in contractual ways. Only in moving from abstract to concrete or from general statements to specific objectives can coaches fully understand what is expected of them and whether such expectations are reasonable and within their scope of practice. A core requirement is that coaches be completely aware of what they have been contracted to do and whether they are fully capable of the work that has been negotiated. This can best be achieved through ongoing learning, practice, reflection, and supervision. The material reviewed in this chapter will serve as an indispensable tool for your success as a coach. We have offered it as a guide for achieving high-quality coaching relationships rather than as a litany of arcane rules and regulations. Excellence in practice stems from a vision of your being of the greatest possible service to clients rather than from a defensive stance of guarding against malpractice.

# 6

# COCREATING THE COACHING RELATIONSHIP

## In this chapter, you will learn how...

- coaching is founded in relationship building, as evidenced in the ICF's theme of cocreating the relationship;

- emotional intelligence and awareness of feelings help establish trust and intimacy in coaching;

- genuine concern for the client, empathy, personal integrity, intimacy, and deep respect foster solid coaching relationships;

- issues of competence, power, transference, and countertransference need to be considered in the working alliance with clients; and

- coaching presence is achieved through practices that create an open mind, open heart, and open will.

It is as though he listened
and such listening as his enfolds us in a silence
in which at last we begin to hear
what we are meant to be.

—*Laozi, 2300 BC*

Life is about relationships (Cashdan, 1988). Whether as a professional, friend, family member, or citizen, we are shaped by our social lives. To some degree, we know who we are through others' impressions of us. Coaching is first and foremost about relationships. The bottom line is that without relationships, there is no coaching. With good reason, then, this chapter delves into aspects of coaching reflected in the third and fourth core coaching competencies under the ICF theme of cocreating the relationship. More specifically, these competencies are establishing trust and intimacy with the client and coaching presence. In many ways these competencies are inseparable dimensions of a coach's way of serving clients' intentions.

The third core coaching competency, establishing trust and intimacy, is defined by the ICF (2011c) as the ability to create a safe, supportive environment that produces ongoing mutual respect and trust. In this regard, an effective coach

- shows genuine concern for the client's welfare and future;
- continuously demonstrates personal integrity, honesty, and sincerity;
- establishes clear agreements and keeps promises;
- demonstrates respect for the client's perceptions, learning style, and personal being;
- provides ongoing support for and champions new behaviors and actions, including those involving risk taking and fear of failure; and
- asks permission to coach the client in sensitive new areas.

International Coach Federation 2011

Coaching is a distinctive form of helping in terms of the relationship qualities it nourishes. For instance, consider the relationship that might exist between a surgeon and a patient. Though bedside manners may be relevant, most patients are more concerned with the doctor's surgical skills and track record. Viewed from another angle, the surgeon isn't primarily engaged in dialogue as the form of treatment, whereas in coaching, communication skills, interpersonal qualities, emotional connections, and other processes of mutual engagement heavily affect the outcome of the work. The coach's skill base is founded in relationship dynamics. In this respect, the surgical skill of the coach, so to speak, relies greatly on her capacity to connect in a way that builds trust and creates realistic hope for meaningful change.

Most of us are involved in helping relationships every day (Miars & Halverson, 2009). Some of these relationships occur informally, whereas others are typically more formal. Accordingly, our expectations of helpers vary based on whether the person is a family member, friend, or professional. We expect certain types of support and advice when we share concerns with friends, whereas professional helping carries other expectations. In general, professionals bear greater responsibility throughout the helping process, and we expect them to be objective, purposeful, and knowledgeable.

# ESTABLISHING TRUST AND INTIMACY

Relationships constitute a fluid, complex, and powerful realm in our lives. Daniel Goleman's (1995) notion of emotional intelligence provides a unique angle on how we function in relationships. According to Goleman, emotional intelligence refers to the ability to manage ourselves and our emotions effectively, along with relating well to others. Critical elements of emotional intelligence include the

---

**REFLECTION 6.1**

Identifying your feelings (i.e., becoming emotionally literate), taking responsibility for how you feel, and expressing your emotions appropriately are ways to develop emotional intelligence. For the next few days, momentarily stop what you are doing and take your emotional pulse on at least three occasions during the day, preferably when you become aware that something is up with your emotional state. Feelings just are. There is no need to attach judgment to them and you do not have to justify how you feel. So, simply notice without judgment. To help you understand your feelings, you might want to complete this sentence: "At this moment, I feel_____."Once you have identified your feelings (e.g., happy, sad, angry, content, proud, grateful, anxious), reflect on how you want to express them. Do you need to talk to someone? Do you need to journal? Do you need to go for a run? Exactly what do you need to do to manage your feelings appropriately so that you don't become emotionally overwrought?

degree to which a person has self-awareness, is able to regulate personal behaviors, is self-motivated, is capable of experiencing and expressing empathy, and can readily access personal resources to care about self and others. Emotional intelligence also reflects how much the person is able to establish rapport with others, how competent he is in creating an atmosphere of trust, and how well he can influence others appropriately.

## Trust

Trust is a quality that is more or less present at any moment in a relationship. It is not static; rather, it ebbs and flows. Small actions may have major repercussions. People in a relationship can trust one another, that is, they can both be trusting. However, placing trust in another person presumably would be based on the fact that the other person seems trustworthy. Otherwise, trust would be misplaced. As a core competency, building trust and intimacy is viewed from the perspective of what coaches need to do in order to be perceived as being trustworthy. In the following sections, we highlight key elements that foster trust in a coaching relationship: intimacy, genuine concern, empathy, personal integrity, and respect. It might be assumed that coaches are trusting by nature, though in reality we know that sometimes our ability to trust others may be challenged.

---

**REFLECTION 6.2**

What creates trust for you? Before you continue reading, take time to reflect on the experiences you have had in a variety of helping relationships, such as with doctors, lawyers, accountants, teachers, counselors, and other helpers in situations where you were the person in need of help or guidance. What led you to believe that these professionals could help? What qualities or behaviors fostered trust? What qualities or behaviors detracted from your confidence in their abilities to help? What helper behaviors empowered or disempowered you in these encounters?

---

## Intimacy

As an emotional bond between coach and client, intimacy is one of the necessary conditions for gaining traction concerning client dreams and visions. The term *intimacy* in the context of professional relationships may seem misplaced, yet to work effectively with clients as a coach, you need to ask questions and discuss information that goes deeper than merely surface knowledge. A normal human response to revealing personal information is to feel vulnerable. To encourage and develop trust, appropriate self-disclosure is often advised as a way of leveling the field. Suitable self-disclosure (see chapter 9) reduces clients' uneasiness and allows positive connections to evolve in the relationship (Bloomgarden & Mennuti, 2009).

How intimate are coaching relationships? That may be hard to define, but it certainly stops far short of physical contact, and it does not encompass discussions unrelated to the coaching topic. However, that still leaves a fair amount of leeway. The danger is to push for too much intimacy or, conversely, to come across as too clinical. A coach may have strong needs for intimacy and, as a result, may probe deeper than necessary for the contracted agenda. On the flip side, if the coach is tentative about emotions, he may behave in a manner that precludes clients from talking about necessary topics. For example, to avoid strong emotional content in sessions, a coach may prevent clients from expressing such emotions as anger and sadness.

Deep fears of intimacy or strong emotionality can be a liability in coaching relationships. A coach who remains consistently objective and aloof may dampen clients' emotional expressions or their willingness to experience vulnerability through self-disclosure. This may allow the coach to feel safe, but if the client's topic includes significant emotional themes that aren't explored, the effectiveness of the coaching process will be impaired.

## Genuine Concern for the Client's Welfare and Future

Carl Rogers (1961), one of the founders of humanistic psychology, wrote extensively on relationships and the qualities of helpers that nourish clients' growth. One of his central themes was the belief that people are always in a process of becoming. In other words, no matter what age, people can change—they are not bound by their past. Rogers' position represented a dramatic shift in beliefs about human nature derived from an earlier Freudian perspective (Freud, 1964). Rather than treating people as products of their past and incapable of altering their behavior, Rogers and his followers, Carkhuff (1969) and Truax (Carkhuff & Truax, 1967), urged helpers to appreciate clients as having strength, potential, inner power, and the capacity for self-realization. In a Rogerian perspective, coaches' attitudes and genuine concern toward their clients are as important in determining outcomes as their technical skills or theoretical knowledge.

A classic tale of helping that Rogers (1961) described was of a man who successfully completed counseling after having had an unsuccessful previous experience with another counselor. When the second counselor inquired why the client was able to work through his issues so successfully this time, the client responded that the second counselor had done about the same things as the first, but that in working together the client felt that this counselor really cared about him. Although some of Rogers' (1957) reflections about effective helping relationships have become almost prescriptive, his profound concern for the client and the quality of the relationship formed by a helper's thoughts, feelings, and actions can be framed in simple questions that coaches might ask themselves:

- How can I act so my clients perceive me as trustworthy?
- How can I cultivate attitudes of caring and interest toward my clients?
- How do I demonstrate deep empathy for my clients' feelings and their perspectives?

The Latin phrase *sine qua non* ("without which nothing") captures the importance of relationship dynamics in helping. For many, the relationship is the principal medium by which clients bring forth significant ideas and feelings that form the working agenda (Lambert & Barley, 2001). It is the quality of the coaching relationship that determines whether successful results are achieved. High levels of healthy, appropriate interactions between coach and client positively influence client outcomes (Crits-Christoph, Connolly Gibbons, & Hearon, 2006). Coaches who exhibit trust, flexibility, and empathy engender positive relationships with their clients (Ackerman & Hilsenroth, 2003).

A coaching relationship empowers clients to maximize their potential. As coaches, we hold positive beliefs about clients and about humanity in general. No matter what clients have experienced or what limiting self-beliefs they might present, genuine helpers remain confident that there is much unrealized potential and capability in each person with whom they work.

## Empathy

In our effort to build trusting coaching relationships, we can never overestimate the power of empathy and the generative effects of fully appreciating clients' concerns, interests, and needs. Once again, we call upon the wisdom of Carl Rogers, whose definition of **empathy** has gone virtually unchanged for more than 60 years. He described an empathic helper as someone who takes on "insofar as he is able, the internal frame of reference of the client" (Rogers, 1951, p. 29). This is often described as seeing the world through the eyes of another. In being empathic, one must demonstrate an ability to express awareness of the other person's reality. To further clarify the concept of empathy, we have created some hypothetical client statements and corresponding coach responses. We offer a critique of each response to highlight the difference between those who demonstrate empathy and those who somewhat miss the mark.

---

**CLIENT STATEMENT 1:** I'm not very good at exercising. I've never been able to do as much as I'd like to on a regular basis.

---

### Response from coach A

"Well, I think you're a success story about to happen!"

### Response from coach B

"I can sense how this upsets you—wanting to feel good about exercising regularly and being concerned that, once again, you simply won't be able to do it."

### Critique of responses

The coach provides the client with reassurance (that may be unfounded) and in so doing may prevent the client from further exploration of feelings.

The coach empathizes with the client and thereby allows opportunity for further exploration of the matter, should the client decide to do so.

> **CLIENT STATEMENT 2:** Ugh, these past weeks have been so difficult. I tried to follow the plan but I couldn't do it. It was a good plan—I simply failed.

### Response from coach A

"Don't say you failed! You tried! You'll do it! Cut yourself some slack! It happens—sometimes you just need to back off, regroup, and then try again."

### Response from coach B

"I hear you. It's been difficult, you believe that you failed, and you don't see a clear reason for this. How can we explore this so you can understand it better?"

### Critique of responses

The coach's comments are encouraging, almost cheerleading. They override the client's personal feelings and reactions, substituting what the coach wants the client to think and feel. Exploration and insight are largely blocked by this response.

The coach captures the core client messages and connects with her inner world, as unsettled as it may be. The coach notes the client's belief that there was no solid reason for what happened and opens the door to exploration.

---

Three levels of empathy have been identified within helping relationships (Carkhuff, 1969; Rogers, 1961; Truax & Carkhuff, 1967):

1. Basic empathy—A helper's responses carry roughly the same meaning and are essentially interchangeable with those of the client.

2. Additive empathy—A helper's responses acknowledge aspects of the client's communications that were perhaps implied, communicated nonverbally, or inferable from other things that the client said and add these elements to a basic empathic response.

3. Subtractive empathy—A helper's responses delete significant elements of the client's communications or even distort their meaning.

Helping professionals are sometimes reluctant to get too close to the emotional world of their clients for fear they may become trapped in their clients' feelings. Rogers (1961) was keenly aware of the risks involved in stepping into the world of others sufficiently to feel and appreciate their experiences. Such willingness takes more than courage; it also requires a strong sense of self. Entering a client's reality could provoke feelings of confusion or identification if the coach is currently in personal turmoil or if her self-awareness is less than clear. Identifying with another person is different from empathizing.

In empathy, one retains one's separateness, whereas **identification** means that one person takes on the feelings and reality experienced by the other as if they were her own. When a coach identifies with her client, there is no separateness. Perhaps more critically, there is no coach! The coach has become the client and there is a kind of symbiotic quality to the relationship. When empathizing, however, the coach is able to verbalize her understanding of clients' inner worlds so that they experience a caring reflection of the reality that they live.

Consider a simple example: A coach says to her client, "I know exactly what you're feeling," and thinks to herself, "This is the same stuff I've been

---

**REFLECTION 6.3**

Carl Rogers (Rogers & Sanford, 1984) refers to the importance of unconditional positive regard, or consistent acceptance and warmth toward another (Mearns & Thorne, 2007). Take a moment for reflection. How would this translate in a personal relationship? How would it be represented in a coaching relationship? How would you consistently show warmth, empathy, acceptance, and respect to your clients? What attitudes and behaviors would demonstrate your keen interest in them? How different would it be from the way you approach the world now? What do you need to do to nurture the development of these qualities?

going through for years!" The coach is so caught up in remembering her own experiences that she is no longer listening. What she is hearing is her own story, and she may be unconsciously forcing the client's reality to fit her own. At a certain level, she becomes her client and begins projecting her own experiences, feelings, and solutions onto the client. This is the essence of identification.

## Personal Integrity, Honesty, and Sincerity

Coaching is a partnership—an agreement to collaborate in working on an agenda defined by the client. As a helpful coach, it is crucial to demonstrate personal integrity and act in highly consistent ways. When we experience another person as communicating through filters or from behind masks, our willingness to be open and trusting with that person diminishes. Some coaches engage in their professional relationships as if they were performing on stage, while others navigate the boundaries between private citizens and professionals in a smooth and virtually seamless manner. Of course, a coach's actions with clients would not be expected to be the same as with intimate friends and family, even though the qualities of his presence may be virtually indistinguishable. A professional who shows caring, empathy, and sensitivity with clients but then switches these qualities off as soon as sessions end will invariably reveal leakage between these separate identities. Our core nature reveals itself in time.

Being genuine may not happen easily or automatically. Someone who is deeply genuine is likely to speak with integrity and to be perceived as congruent. The renowned spiritual teacher Don Miguel Ruiz (2001) suggests, as one of his four agreements, that we must be impeccable with our word; we must speak with integrity and say only what we mean. Saying what you mean and speaking the truth will go a long way toward building trust. The first of his four agreements, being impeccable with your word, is built on efforts by coaches to raise their emotional intelligence and to persistently cultivate self-awareness.

The quality of **congruence** also refers to the person's authenticity and not simply behaving according to the rules of her role or doing what she is supposed to do according to society's definitions of a professional (Carkhuff & Berenson, 1977). A congruent coach understands her own values and

motivations; she knows when she is aligned at all levels of her being. Her nonverbal communication is consistent with her verbal messages. What she says is an accurate reflection of inner values and beliefs. People easily sense insincerity. When someone smiles because it is a programmed role response, we know it isn't genuine. When someone pretends to be fine because she believes it's required by her role, she will eventually lose credibility and be seen as untrustworthy. Consistently demonstrating integrity, congruence, and sincerity means that clients know they can expect honesty even in difficult matters.

> ### REFLECTION 6.4
>
> There is little possibility that one can fake integrity, congruence, honesty, or sincerity over the long term. These qualities exist as the bedrock of a person's character, which implies that they are revealed in coaching relationships and pervasively in the coach's life. As you interact with others or engage in helping relationships, are there times when speaking your truth is particularly challenging? What are those situations? Can you identify what makes this challenging for you? Is it the topic, the person, the situation, or some combination of these? How might you strengthen your practice of being impeccable with your word? Who might support you in asking hard or perhaps unimagined questions?

## Respect for the Client's Perceptions, Learning Styles, and Personal Being

Respect pertains to valuing others and holding them in positive regard simply because they are human. Embedded in the concept of respect is a capacity to minimize judgmental attitudes. However, not only is it impossible to remain without judgment, certain types of judgments are essential. We need to assess situations, and we must use judgment to evaluate people, circumstances, and conditions to determine whether they will support us or threaten our well-being. These kinds of judgments differ from being judgmental, which suggests being disparaging, negative, or disapproving.

Respect requires that rather than acting on assumptions and biases, we strive to approach people and situations with an open mind and an open heart. Along with being empathic, to be respectful means communicating in thoughts, words, and actions a deep sense of appreciation and regard for the client irrespective of differences in background, attitudes, or behaviors. We live in an increasingly diverse world. We sometimes think of the term *diversity* in relation to cultural sensitivity, yet it is much more than that. It also encompasses gender, age, physical attributes, religion, sexual orientation, language, education, economic status, intellectual capacity, beliefs, values, preferences, and, as we have seen previously, learning styles and personality traits.

Appreciating and respecting diverse others require more than awareness and experience; it calls for willingness to value differences and to commit to learning about people with traditions that are different from our own. What it does not mean, however, is constantly walking on eggshells because we aren't sure how to address some aspects of the person's diversity. When in doubt about something, it is better to be upfront rather than jump through hoops not to offend someone. Simply ask the person respectfully for guidelines regarding how he would prefer that you address the particular situation that puzzles you. Respect for diversity also requires learning new skills based on a growing knowledge of differences and an exploration of how various people are likely to perceive the coach with her own diverse attributes.

Expressions of judgment extend to phrases such as "She's a good person." If we speak of *good*, we implicitly frame our remarks with awareness of its polar opposite—*bad*. When speaking with clients, rewarding phrases such as "That's great" or "You were wonderful" are double-edged. While praising the person, you also position yourself in the relation-

ship as a judge. Clients may wonder, "This week she thought I was good, but what will she think if I don't perform the same way next week?"

# THE WORKING ALLIANCE

In the coaching literature as well as in the broader literature of helping and counseling, the term **working alliance** can provide perspective for understanding what needs to happen between coach and client in order to maximize trust and thereby the effectiveness of a supportive relationship (Bordin, 1979; Horvath & Greenberg, 1994). It is important that coaches have a certain level of expertise related to their clients' topics, yet it will ultimately be the quality of the working alliance that most strongly influences outcomes (Rogers, 1961; Sexton, Whiston, Bleuer, & Walz, 1997). Unlike the surgeon we referred to earlier, coaches must connect in appropriate ways and at an emotional level suited to the client's style and agenda. Three necessary elements of the working alliance are represented in (1) agreements on goals, (2) agreements on tasks, and (3) the emotional bond between coach and client. We have already addressed the essential elements of agreements in the previous chapter; here we discuss the emotional bond that fosters trust in the relationship.

As noted earlier, many people carry implicit definitions of professional behavior characterized by a cold and distant demeanor. Carl Rogers (1961) urged helpers to trust that it is safe to express warmth in professional relationships and to let clients know that you care. As Mehr and Kanwischer (2011) point out, warmth requires accepting clients as being of equal worth. Clients express more willingness to try new behaviors and to accept the risks of failing because of the openness and acceptance that they experience from their coaches. In simple words, warmth sends the message "I am trustworthy. You don't have to be afraid of me. It is safe to be vulnerable with me, just as I will allow myself to be vulnerable with you." Demonstrating warmth in no way precludes dealing with difficult issues or confronting clients when needed. In fact, confrontation (see chapter 9) becomes more productive when clients are aware of the genuine warmth their coaches express toward them.

Moving a bit deeper, we also know that whenever two people get together for some purpose, each party's history in relationships has bearing on the success of the working alliance. Focusing on the coach's behavior, we would like to consider four

---

**REFLECTION 6.5**

Make a list of all the aspects of your own diversity—jot down as many attributes as you can. How might each of these unique characteristics act as a lens through which you see others? What would enable you to become more fully aware of your judgments of others and to minimize any potential judgmental elements in your perceptions? What would strengthen your appreciation for the diverse others with whom you may be walking alongside as a coach?

patterns that can derail this professional relationship (Brems, 2001):

1. Coaches may have needs for intimacy that are either excessive or insufficient to form effective alliances with clients.

2. They may have needs for approval that sometimes constitute a reversal of roles.

3. They may be too transparent in disclosing personal information or they may be too private, thereby causing clients to feel treated like an object rather than as a person. Although an emotional bond must be present between coach and client, the coach's level of emotional expressiveness may not be appropriate to the client and her agenda.

4. Finally, there may be issues of dependency. As the relationship develops, the coach may become dependent on clients for a sense of accomplishment, or he may foster dependency by presenting himself as indispensable to their welfare and growth.

There are no simple guides to self-understanding or to knowing what clients are going to evoke in you as they present intimate details of their lives. There is, however, one clear requirement, which is to be awake to all that is happening in powerful helping relationships. No training program or teacher can tell you what you will experience personally when you begin coaching. You will learn from your own practice by examining it regularly, thoroughly, and candidly. The literature on helping offers useful guidance concerning three dynamics that are frequently present in the working alliance:

---

### REFLECTION 6.6

Considering the deeper levels at which the working alliance operates, can you identify motivations, needs, or your ways of being in relationships that might interfere with your effectiveness as a lifestyle wellness coach? Specifically, how do you experience your own need for intimacy? When you do something well, what are your expectations about approval from others? How transparent are you in relationships? What are your experiences with dependency? Have you noticed any of these dynamics in personal or professional relationships over the years? How might you work to change patterns that could be problematic in coaching?

---

competence, power, and transference (Brown, 2007; deVaris, 1994; Norcross, 2002; Weiner & Bornstein, 2009;). In truth, these might factor into all your relationships. For now, let's see how they play out in coaching.

## Competence and Trusting Your Inner Knowing

No matter how many degrees you have or how many certifications you pursue, an expanding knowledge base in coaching and the health, wellness, and fitness professions places you on a never-ending journey of learning. Ironically, what you know now may serve as impediments to the acquisition of new learning, especially when what is new represents a **paradigm shift** in knowledge or understanding.

Developing technical competencies can be comforting at times. Being able to enlist the aid of formulas or technology in determining answers helps reduce ambiguity about potential solutions. Blood lab analyses, $\dot{V}O_2$max assessments, and formulas for body composition offer some degree of concreteness and may allow you to feel expert in your judgments. Yet, as you move away from technical analysis into coaching, certainty diminishes and the quest for knowledge to reduce ambiguity multiplies. The more deeply you work with clients, the more likely you are to encounter dilemmas and imponderable questions. Because coaching is an action-oriented process, you might feel the urge to move efficiently from assessments and analysis to decision making and engagement. In moments such as these, you may want to stop and exercise self-awareness and mindfulness. You can choose to remain open to not knowing and express curiosity about what the client is saying or not saying. Having internalized the structures of a coaching session, as described in the flow model of coaching, you know it is important to continually demonstrate presence as you listen to your inner self and access your personal wisdom. Your ability to be fully conscious, alert, and available will allow your clients to explore previously unfamiliar territory, generate new insights, and discover novel avenues for action.

As you launch into the soft sciences surrounding lifestyle wellness coaching, you may experience nagging doubt and second-guessing. Should you have done something differently? Was your choice of intervention the wisest? Understanding how you assess your own competency allows you to estimate your vulnerability to doubt, negative self-beliefs, and self-criticism. Some patterns of response to these reactions, such as owning your feelings, working with a mentor coach, or researching the literature, can be helpful, while others may be counterproductive. Denial, blame, minimization, and catastrophizing are rarely helpful when striving for excellence.

Rather than hope that things never go wrong, you might make contingency plans for occasions when things do not go as you had hoped. This doesn't mean waiting for something to go awry. It means appreciating how you have responded in the past when things didn't turn out well. Acknowledging your patterns of dealing with less-than-stellar results allows you to put in place supportive practices and options. How you manage these moments in your career will affect how well you thrive in this challenging line of work and how compassionately you are able to assist others. After all, if you are not a good coach to yourself, how beneficial can you be to others?

---

**REFLECTION 6.7**

We all make mistakes; they are unavoidable. However, when they occur in your personal life or your work, how do you respond? How do you treat yourself? When you are working with others and you believe you have not served them well, how do you feel? What are your thoughts? How do you behave? What do you do to regenerate confidence and forward movement in moments like these?

---

## Power and Influence

One thing is certain—there is a clear difference in the power bases of coaches and their clients. Clients may be highly successful in many domains of life, yet in the particular topic for which they are seeking your help, they are likely to feel inept. They look to you for knowledge and guidance, and in these regards you will be seen as having power. Power isn't a bad thing or something to be denied. Indeed, power differences exist in virtually all relationships. When acknowledged and appropriately understood, they facilitate the achievement of objectives and the cohesion of the people involved.

Ideally, a coaching relationship is created so that a sense of equality is experienced, yet there exists this paradoxical difference in power. Take, for example, the matter of asking questions (see chapter 8). To move forward, the coach needs to ask questions, some of which can be very personal. Within a short time, she knows a lot of information about her client, but the client knows far less about her. If knowledge is power, as the dictum goes, does the coach offer to tell the client as much about herself to balance power in the relationship? For the most part, the answer is no. However, creating opportunities for the client to ask what he needs to know often makes sense. The trick is determining what constitutes a need to know.

Our lives are embedded in a context of power relationships. We have all had experiences where we might have felt we had too much, too little, or maybe just the right amount of influence over another person and vice versa. Discomfort with power may lead to minimizing attempts at influencing clients and perhaps failing to intervene even when such action could help. At the opposite extreme, power can be misused through the conviction that because the coach has the knowledge, he necessarily has the power, or that because he is the coach, his advice should be heeded. Without self-monitoring, those who assume that they know what is right for their clients are likely to misuse the power that comes with their role.

Social scientists (Knapp & Daly, 2002) readily acknowledge that most communication is about influence. However, the term *manipulation*, which is synonymous with *influence*, tends to have more negative connotations in Western society. In actuality, we frequently manipulate one another with words, actions, and nonverbal communications. Simple requests such as "May I have that newspaper next to you?" represent low-level manipulations. We also know that some people tend to be exquisite manipulators, while others are easily manipulated. What elements of character, presence, or relationship allow one person to be more influential than another? If a particular person easily influences you, does that mean that she will be equally influential with others? You might want to explore your understanding of how manipulation occurs and how you feel about it as either the one being manipulated or the manipulator.

The agenda for coaching derives from the client. On this point, most practitioners and writers seem to agree (Coach U, 2005). They also concur that the client needs to willingly embrace actions that he has designed with his coach. So where does influence—or manipulation—come in? Clients are motivated to change or to pursue a goal, yet they need help unearthing the reasons, values, needs, and personal dynamics that pertain to their wishes.

They may require assistance in formulating plans that are robust and realistic. Once engaged in action, clients typically benefit from support, and although coaches should not be the sole source of support, they can provide invaluable aid by assisting in the creation of support systems. If clients could do everything on their own, they probably would not need to engage in a coaching relationship. This doesn't imply fault or inadequacy. Most coaching professionals regard their clients as individuals who are well functioning, successful, and strongly motivated to pursue their goals (Auerbach, 2003; Biswas-Diener, 2009). From this perspective, influence is rather straightforward and appropriate in coach-client relationships. Simply put, the coach is there to influence. She is not a passive witness to a client's musings.

In their exhaustive textbook, *Intentional Interviewing and Counseling*, Ivey, Ivey, and Zalaquett (2010) devote major sections to two classes of skills. They define one roughly as attending and the other as influencing (see Attending Skills and Influencing Skills). The interweaving of these skills in helping relationships is based on the notion that the helper first obtains the client's story (through attending) and then works toward influencing change. In coaching, the interconnection between the coach's attending behaviors and her use of influencing skills is generally shaped by input and feedback from the client. A common recommendation is to continue building rapport through the use of attending skills until two conditions have been met. The first is that

coaches have sufficient information to begin the process of influencing the client, and the second is that they have an adequate basis of rapport. That is, the **core relationship conditions** of trust and intimacy have been sufficiently established.

Perhaps we can reframe this apparent conflict between power differences in the coaching relationship and the goal of creating an equal partnership. Both coach and client choose to work together and to adhere to certain definitions and responsibilities of their roles. The client is doing his job answering questions and exploring his inner world and dreams, while the coach is doing her job asking questions and trying to cocreate meaning and

## REFLECTION 6.8

You might gain insight about power dynamics in coaching by reflecting on how power issues play out in your personal life. Consider your patterns and responses to power dynamics throughout your school and work history. Are you aware when power is becoming an issue? What is your experience with influence? How do you appreciate others' influence on your life? What do you not like about others' attempts to influence you? How do you use power in relationships? How does it feel when you know you have influenced another person to act in a certain way? Are you conscious of how you may influence people unintentionally?

## Attending Skills and Influencing Skills

Two broad categories of communication skills used in the helping professions are attending and influencing. Some attending skills, such as asking questions, can also represent efforts to influence the client. Depending on the client's state of mind, skills such as reflection of meaning can be experienced as a profound level of attending by the helper— or it might come across as an effort to change the client's thinking. Details about these skills are presented in the upcoming chapters.

| Attending skills | Influencing skills |
| --- | --- |
| Nonverbal support | Questioning |
| Minimal encouragement | Feedback |
| Questioning | Confrontation |
| Reflection of content | Instructions, information, and advice |
| Reflection of feeling | Reflection of meaning |
| Summarizing | Interpretations |

the basis for forward momentum. Each person is contributing, and throughout the relationship each retains the right to request that certain rules and roles be renegotiated. As long as such requests safeguard the boundaries of the coaching contract and relationship, all is well. At certain moments, the coach will intentionally try to influence the client and the client will hopefully open himself to this influence. So far, all of this seems on track—things appear equitable, even with the display of different expressions of power. Clients show power by cooperating, resisting, or inquiring for information; coaches demonstrate power in what they say, the questions they ask, the feedback they give, and so forth. Power expressions disturb the relationship's equilibrium when one or both of the partners' problematic histories with power, personalities, needs, values, or even their unconscious selves come into play. For instance, even though the client has hired the coach to help, she may express strong resistance toward any kind of feedback. If both parties were totally conscious and completely evolved beings, we probably wouldn't have to worry about any of this. But, after all, we are human.

# TRANSFERENCE AND COUNTERTRANSFERENCE

The phenomena of transference and countertransference are sometimes considered mystifying elements of relationships that apply strictly to psychological counselors, social workers, psychotherapists, or psychoanalysts. This perception is fundamentally flawed and probably arises from a mistaken assumption that these dynamics are necessarily negative or even pathological. Virtually all social behavior is influenced by past experiences. When we meet someone, we enter into the relationship with the fullness of our personal histories. For many, this history is exactly what allows us to be trusting and open, and this dynamic represents a form of transference.

When people are in intense, intimate relationships over a period of time, some predictable processes begin to occur. Patterns of communication and a unique language evolve, and each person's identity may become more linked to that of the other. Traditionally, this dynamic has been labeled **transference**. Although this technical term has its origins in psychoanalytic literature (Freud, 1949; Jung, 1969), its relevance to coaching relationships is unmistakable.

## Transference

Most of us have met someone new who reminds us of another person in our past. From the outset of this new relationship, we may need to be conscious about how our previous relationship is affecting the development of the current one. Appearances, mannerisms, or some other aspect of the new person can trigger associations to older relationships. Recognizing physical similarities is easier than identifying a resemblance that occurs at a psychological level.

People have different preferences for levels of intimacy. For instance, someone who seems content in a friendship may begin acting strangely once the relationship turns a corner toward a more intimate connection. Common wisdom suggests that perhaps this person is reacting to previous experiences. For instance, someone who has known pain and loss in intimate relations may begin to distance himself when signs of closeness increase. This scenario represents another face of transference.

Transference in coaching is a process whereby a client projects onto the coach thoughts, feelings, or attributes that she experienced in relation to other significant people in her life. Kahn (2005) suggests that it is extremely common in helping relationships. He sees it as a natural reaction to the stress that people experience as they explore issues. A more practical way of looking at transference is that the client focuses more on the helper than on herself (Young, 2009). In so doing, she avoids the necessary work of coaching. Watkins (1986) discussed five patterns of transference that seem common to helping relationships. These patterns have been reframed for your work as a lifestyle wellness coach:

1. **The perfect coach.** Because you are perceived as being perfect, the client begins to imitate your behavior, including modes of dress and manners of speech. He is complimentary of anything you do or say. Although flattery and imitation may be gratifying to the ego, a signal of transference is that you eventually begin to feel irritated with the adulation or you begin to worry about the excessive influence you have on the person's attitudes and behaviors.

2. **The great wizard coach.** The client sees you as having all the answers, as being all knowing and flawless in judgment. Conversely, she acts in a self-denigrating manner, criticizing her own judgment and knowledge. In the event that you continually receive such high praise, you may begin to worry about the potential of failing and begin to focus on making mistakes. Usually, the transference process

can be felt in the quality of overblown positive feedback.

3. **The divinely caring coach.** The client sees you as a loving and nurturing person with whom he feels totally safe and secure. The coaching relationship becomes a private haven where the client can open himself to all feelings; however, he confides that this all-embracing nurturance happens only with you. This kind of response may encourage you to give excessively out of a desire to be even more helpful. Over time, however, you might begin to feel depleted, experiencing an energy drain occasioned by the client's neediness.

4. **The obstructive coach.** The client acts as if you are standing in the way of her progress, either through questioning, planning, or requesting action. She sets up various tests and expresses a thinly veiled mistrustfulness. You can easily become caught in a kind of **self-fulfilling prophecy** in which the more the client mistrusts you, the more uneasy and cautious you become. Invariably, this exacting awareness may cause you to trip, thereby proving the client's misgivings about you.

5. **The irrelevant coach.** The client uses the coaching session in an aimless, goalless, and unmotivated manner. Although physically present, he blocks progress by undermining your efforts to focus conversations or direct action. Because you are being paid, you may begin to feel useless and come to doubt your own competency. You may experience growing resentment and annoyance as these clients continue to thwart your efforts to help them.

Although it may never be entirely clear whether a client's strong emotional reactions to a coach represent transference or honest and appropriate responses to perceptions of her behavior, the following strategy (Young, 2009) can increase the likelihood of positive outcomes.

## Step 1: Express Acceptance Without Retaliation

When transference is operating, clients may eventually erupt with strong feelings toward the coach. Especially when these expressions are unwarranted, the coach needs to communicate empathy and a genuine appreciation for the reality of the feelings experienced.

**CLIENT:** This is a waste of my time and money. Where are we going with all this? I think your ideas are simply unworkable.

**COACH:** I can hear how upset you are with me, and at the same time I'm glad you're willing to let me know how you feel. Now that you've brought it up, I can't think of anything more important for us to do than to take time to understand what's happening. Would this be okay with you?

## Step 2: Explore the Client's Thoughts and Feelings

In the face of the coach's accepting attitude and behavior, the client will be less likely to retreat into feelings of shame, hurt, or fear of retaliation. The coach's role at this point is to encourage further expression and clarification of the sources of the emotions.

**CLIENT:** I simply don't think this is working out. I keep coming here and I get the feeling that my lack of progress is completely my fault.

**COACH:** Thanks for telling me this. Are you aware of any messages coming from me that sound blaming or make it look like it's completely your fault?

## Step 3: Work to Find New Patterns for Expressing Feelings and Getting Needs Met

By maintaining a reassuring, accepting attitude throughout the dialogue, the client is likely to feel an increased sense of safety in expressing emotions and working through complaints without having to wait until an emotional buildup has reached uncontrollable proportions. Even when the client has legitimate issues, her manner of expression can be the focus of new learning. If the coach at any point turns to self-justification or efforts to prove his effectiveness, this learning opportunity will likely be lost.

**CLIENT:** No, I think it's me feeling like I'm not doing enough, and I guess I took it out on you.

**COACH:** That sounds like an important awareness. No matter how it came out, I'm glad we've reached this point of understanding. So, there are two things we might discuss now. The first is what brings you to feel you're not doing enough, and the second is how to more comfortably express your feelings about our work in the future. Do these sound like useful avenues for discussion?

If you believe that you carry no conscious bias toward a client, if you have behaved compassionately and supportively, and if you have lived up to your end of agreements, then persistent client concerns about your behavior may represent unresolved issues emanating from their past relationships (Kahn, 2005). With some of the skills that we will review in upcoming chapters, you can caringly discuss these matters, always with the client's agenda and welfare in mind. Of course, you need not confront all transference projections; some of them may simply be information that you make note of for potential future conversations. Moreover, not every concern voiced by clients will be evidence of transference; not every feeling will be a projection. We do form new relationships. We do like some people a lot and have difficulty with others simply because of our experiences with them.

## Countertransference

Of course, relationships are two-way streets; coaches may also project attitudes, feelings, or thoughts onto their clients. This phenomenon is known as **countertransference**. Gelso and Hayes (2007) articulate how, when mismanaged, these projections negatively influence the helping relationship. Alternatively, as Luborsky and Barrett (2006) have noted, when helpers take time to consider the feelings and attitudes behind these projections, they can learn much about themselves and their clients that they would otherwise miss (see Transference and Countertransference Case Histories).

---

## Transference and Countertransference Case Histories

To gain familiarity with the concepts of transference and countertransference, read the following case histories. Be sure to consider the questions that follow each case.

### Henry

Henry has been your client for over a year. Though you have made great progress with him in terms of his goals for personal change, you are aware that he is nowhere near ready to work independently. In fact, the more progress he makes, the more questions he brings to you and the higher he sets the bar for his own achievements. Although he is respectful in scheduling appointments and phone check-ins, he seems to save all his decision making for times when he can talk with you. He says, "You have such good advice. You're a genius. Without your input, I simply wouldn't know what to do."

- What do you think is going on with Henry? How do you understand his behavior?
- How might you discuss Henry's behavior with him?
- What might it imply about your coaching style if you have had a number of clients with similar patterns?

### Carla

Your client, Carla, has become increasingly critical of your work. She implies that you are sloppy and disorganized and that you act in a robotic manner. You have considered her feedback and asked some of your colleagues for their opinions about your work. You also know that your other clients do not share similar views. So far, Carla's remarks seem baseless. You are beginning to dread your meetings with her.

- What do you imagine might be going on with Carla?
- Do you think it would be appropriate to talk to her about her remarks and your feelings? If so, what exactly would you do and say?

### Ben

Your client, Ben, is successful in his work and seems to have a wonderful family. He is so good at what he does that you often wonder why he needs you as a coach. You find yourself judging Ben's success, attributing his accomplishments to his wealthy family or sheer luck. When you are coaching him, you are aware of looking for flaws in his plans, emphasizing what isn't working for him, or simply not congratulating him when he does something well. In your own family, you always defined yourself as the underachiever, especially compared with an older sibling.

- What do you think might be happening in your relationship with Ben?
- What do you believe an appropriate plan of action might be?
- Do you think it would be appropriate to talk to Ben? Do you think it would be helpful for you to talk to someone else?

All intimate helping relationships include both overt and covert personal dynamics that play out at varying levels of conscious awareness (Horton, 1996). For instance, you may work with a client who is extremely conscientious about her program, who is never tardy, who always takes your advice without resistance, yet who irks you for some inexplicable reason. A common way of reacting to this might be to discount it or attribute it to some quirk of your own. You certainly don't want to tell this outstanding client how irritating you find her! If you have behaved professionally and compassionately, an irritation that keeps surfacing is a signal that something deeper may be occurring. Let's assume you have no ax to grind with this client, yet you often feel triggered by what you describe as her perfectionist ways. Exploring your own history might reveal stories of being in school with classmates who always were prepared and got things right, while you struggled to stay afloat. Realizing this piece about yourself could help you name your countertransference and get on top of it. As a result, you would increase your capacity to be present and appreciative of your client's efforts and progress rather than hold back or feel mildly annoyed.

The bottom line is that when you have done your personal work to be a clear receiver and thoroughly professional, your awareness of clients and reactions to them may be fed by an ability to tune into a different frequency of interpersonal communications. So, before you toss out the data, spend a little more time exploring their potential meanings.

# CREATING A SAFE SPACE

Has someone ever approached you with a perplexing human drama or an all-consuming problem? Most of us have been present for friends, family, or even relative strangers who simply needed to talk about their experiences and wanted nothing more than for us to listen. In reflecting on such experiences, you might remember how you wanted to say something, to come up with just the right words to make the person feel better, yet you realized that nothing you could say would achieve this result and, in fact, that there was little that anyone could say to resolve the drama or emotions expressed. So you simply listened—with all your heart and soul. At the end of this encounter, the person probably thanked you profusely for being there, and you might have felt bewildered, thinking to yourself, "But I really didn't do anything."

To understand the structure of helping and, thereby, the function of a coach, one needs to grasp the significance of **containment,** or the creation of a **holding environment** (Winnicott, 1958). Experts such as Kohut (1984) and Hendrix (2008) offer insight into the healing capacity of safe spaces we create for others to express their realities. In a world of action and doing, it is important to recognize the power of simply being—without compulsion to do something. Just as day makes sense in relation to night, doing gains significance in its connection to being. When someone comes to us for help, our immediate thought is often about doing: "What can I *do* that will make this person feel better?"

Though coaching is intended to facilitate forward movement, it must begin with understanding the client's story. To promote storytelling, you want to be as inviting and supportive as possible. To reveal all the critical elements of their story, clients need a safe environment where their thoughts, feelings, and behaviors can be contained respectfully and without judgment. Manifesting such an environment is not always easy. When people feel unsafe, the story that gets told may be replete with distortions, deletions, and misinformation (Dilts & DeLozier, 2000).

To contain another person's story requires that you be fully present, that you open yourself to that person's felt meanings, and that you allow yourself to experience what it might be like to have lived his story. This task implies not only a readiness to listen but also an ability to convey back to the person evidence that he has been heard within the safe boundaries of the relationship.

This discussion of holding environments highlights two important issues. The first is the matter of how one creates the conditions whereby clients believe that they can safely disclose information. The material previously discussed on trust and intimacy was intended to help you with this. Moreover, the next section on coaching presence will hopefully add to your understanding of how to create safety for your clients. The second issue pertains to the dynamic of identification, which we discussed earlier in this chapter. Although lifestyle wellness coaches are not likely to engage in relationships as deep as those of psychotherapists, the intensity will nonetheless be sufficient to stir their emotions and activate their own musings about life.

Consider these examples: A young mother who once was quite active but now is managing a household and young children complains to you about a lack of support from her partner as she discusses plans to resume exercising. A busy executive talks to you about feeling so stretched by work that he neglects his friends, his family, and even his own needs. In both instances, you may identify with the client's story and feel uneasy about your own patterns. The closer the client's story is to your reality, the greater the probability that you may experience personal emotions. When this happens, it is best to try to regain perspective. Talking to other coaches or to someone who is supervising your work could be beneficial. Particularly in the early years of your coaching career, it would be wise to form learning and support teams with other coaches doing similar work.

# COACHING PRESENCE

The fourth ICF core competency is that of **coaching presence**. It is defined as the ability to be fully conscious and create spontaneous relationship with the client, employing a style that is open, flexible, and confident (ICF, 2011c). According to the ICF, a coach who demonstrates presence

- is present and flexible during the coaching process, dancing in the moment;
- accesses her own intuition and trusts her inner knowing, going with her gut;
- is open to not knowing and takes risks;
- sees many ways to work with the client and chooses in the moment what is most effective;
- uses humor effectively to create lightness and energy;
- confidently shifts perspectives and experiments with new possibilities for her own action; and
- demonstrates confidence in working with strong emotions and can self-manage and not be overpowered or enmeshed by clients' emotions.

International Coach Federation 2011

Imagine you are sitting across from an intimate friend and listening intently to his story. You are fully present—mind, body, and spirit. You have no agenda other than to be there. You have no need to change him; you simply want your friend to experience how available you are to him. How wonderful and rich this moment is!

The concept of *presence* is not easily captured in a brief definition. Coaching presence reflects the way a coach engages in relationships, including his physical presence, openness, spontaneity, flexibility, and creativity. As the fourth of the ICF's core competencies, coaching presence is tied to the theme of trust as one of the ways in which coaches evidence trustworthiness. It is also linked to our previous discussion about emotional intelligence, which includes the capacities to work confidently with strong emotions, to engage deeply without becoming enmeshed with clients' feelings, and to manage oneself with grace and compassion amid the sometimes tumultuous moments of change experiences.

The notion of presence can be traced through a number of Eastern and Western philosophical traditions and is often associated with awareness, **mindfulness**, and being in the now (Kabat-Zinn, 2005; Senge, Scharmer, Jaworski, & Flowers, 2004; Tolle, 2004). If you think about meditation practices, they often involve bringing your attention fully into the present moment. Sometimes your breath is used as an anchor to help you focus, while other methods involve repeating mantras or observing your mind without attachment to any of the ideas that emerge. The difference, of course, is that meditation is a solitary process, whereas coaching involves another human being. How can you bring forth a focused presence with your clients?

The ICF's definition of *presence* highlights key indicators of this competency in coaching. As in meditation, presence involves a highly awakened state of being. The coach tunes in on all channels—sights, sounds, emotions, intuitions, and beyond. As in a state of flow described by Csikszentmihalyi (2008), the coach is open to all that is present to her, including her own special ways of knowing. There is nothing formulaic about a coach's way of being in the relationship. Even though there is an intention to assist the client in moving forward, the process is never scripted in advance.

## Presencing

*Presencing* is a concept related to coaching presence that has gained widespread attention over the past decade. It derives from the works of Otto Scharmer (2007) and Peter Senge and colleagues (2004). In *Theory U: Leading From the Future as It Emerges*, Scharmer (2007) explains how presencing represents the blending of two words: *presence* and *sensing*. It means to "connect with the Source of the highest future possibility and to bring it into the now" (p. 163). Presencing is central to Scharmer's Theory U, so labeled because of the U-shaped flow of experiences whereby people become increasingly more capable of creating their highest future possibility. The state of presencing lies between heightened awareness of all that is available in the moment (e.g., facts, impressions, feelings, intuitions) and movement toward actions that will bring the highest future possibility into being. From this perspective, the concept of presencing captures what effective coaches do in conversations with their clients.

To build on Scharmer's (2007) ideas, coaching presence is reflected in the way a coach sits with clients and listens to their stories. Think of a professional sitting with a new client as she tells the story of what she wants, why she wants it, what she has tried, how she has experienced herself, and a myriad of other things connected to her deep desire to change. A typical process of helping would be to listen to all the facts, feelings, and other data; compare them against protocols and best practices; and offer a solution, usually in the form of a prescription. In such a model, help is formulaic; in coaching, however, it is not.

Coaching presence requires a very different way of being than usual. To begin, no matter what the downloaded data from the client, the first requirement is to remain open: open mind, open heart, open will. Scharmer (2007) explains the process as follows:

- Keeping an *open mind* requires that you address your own internal *voice of judgment*. It means that you consciously release your evaluations and judgments about the client's story based on your past experiences. Suspending judgment implies that you open yourself to a new place of wonder and curiosity.

- As you sit with full attention on your client's words and expressions, you then cultivate an *open heart* by releasing your *voice of cynicism*. This is the voice that represents all acts of emotional distancing. As we described earlier, empathy allows you to know the richly textured qualities of a client's landscape. As you open your heart, all the bountiful resources of your client's emotional reality become available. Similarly, the profound wisdom of your own emotions becomes accessible.

- The last part entails an *open will* that comes with the release of your *voice of fear*. The voice of fear limits options by avoiding what is new, unknown, or untested. It is a voice that focuses on potential embarrassment, the need for security, and playing it safe.

With all this effort to remain fully open, you will experience the true meaning of coaching presence. You are not playing a role. You are not a mindless human mechanic fixing a diagnosed problem. You are not even a wizard with an infinite bag of tricks. You are in a magical flow of moment-by-moment experiences, accessing wisdom far more profound than you knew to be available. Images and ideas float through your mind, and the dialogue with your client becomes a cocreative process. You build on each other's offerings and something new emerges. Even if it sounds simple and mundane, the rightness of it, the truth of it for your client, energizes the space between the two of you.

The process of working collaboratively with clients is energizing. Journeying so far into another's world brings profound gifts and untold riches of understanding that often apply to the coach's own existence. The powerful cocreations made possible through coaching presence would evaporate if coaches were operating from a stepwise process or checklist.

Coaching presence is a challenging aspiration for your work with clients. The wonder of this competency is that through its nourishment, everything is new, time after time.

## The Somatic Side of Presence

Consider once again the experience of meditation. An image of meditation that may come to mind is of a person in an upright posture who is simultaneously relaxed and alert. The head is held erect but not stiff, the spine is long, the shoulders are at ease, and the breathing is full. Now, let's come back to a coaching scenario. What does presence look like somatically? Wouldn't it resemble in some ways the posture of someone in a meditative stance?

When we discuss active listening in chapter 7, we will delve more deeply into nonverbal ways of expression. However, to address coaching presence without representing its embodied attributes would be incomplete. In order to access all your senses in a coaching relationship, you need to be fully awake. Having an open mind does not imply that you are intensely examining and analyzing every spoken word; rather, it suggests you are trusting that as your attention is riveted in the moment and not ruminating about things uttered a while ago, you capture the client's core messages in the now.

Somatically, an open mind is seen in a peaceful yet attentive facial expression.

An open heart also has a somatic representation. Try folding your arms across your chest and crossing your legs. Not only does this convey a sense of closure to someone sitting across from you, it is also likely to restrict the flow of your own energy. Arms held across your chest close down your breathing, depriving you of a fundamental source of energy—your breath. An open heart calls for a long spine and relaxed belly. Muscles in the face, arms, chest, and belly are peacefully awakened. The feet are comfortably placed on the floor, with legs uncrossed whenever possible so as to keep your energy moving throughout your body.

Finally, there is a clear somatic translation of a body without fear and anxiety. Hands are open and easy in their movements. Body gestures are soft and inviting. There is a relative absence of physical tension in all areas of the body. This isn't the same as being sleepily relaxed. Being awake, alert, and attentive is not represented in a tight or intense body. As you coach, tension may unknowingly creep into your somatic being. With awareness you can learn to release it and, in so doing, open yourself further to all your special ways of receiving and knowing yourself and your client in the moment.

As you begin to consciously adjust your patterns and bring more somatic presence to your personal and professional relationships, subtle changes may become evident. Your friends or clients may experience you differently and they, too, may begin to alter how they present themselves to you somatically.

Becoming more mindful of your somatic presence is an important part of the learning agenda for coaching. Here are some other ways of understanding your somatic self. As a health, wellness, or fitness professional, you are likely to be physically active on a regular basis. Most physical activities require that you use your body well in how you participate in sports or activities. Yet, you have no doubt seen countless people playing sports, running, swimming, and even doing yoga or Pilates with poor form. Good alignment and posture in physical practices support your ability to show up with a strong and supportive somatic presence when you are coaching.

Rather than suggest that all coaches do yoga or meditate, we believe that most physical activities can support somatic awareness in coaching if you engage in them mindfully. Somatic presence relies upon relaxed diaphragmatic breathing. Whether you are running or doing yoga, you will need to foster good breathing techniques in order to do your activity well. Learning how to breathe properly in your regular physical activities will reinforce your ability to do so when you are sitting with your clients and holding the space for their stories.

## COMMENTARY

Action is a hallmark of the coaching field. It's not coaching unless there is action that is planned and reliably engaged. We are in full accord with this perspective, and we would add that these actions are forged within a special and supportive relationship that empowers clients to ride the waves of change.

We are relational beings. We live and thrive in relationship to others. Yet, coaching differs from friendships and family connections. In order for us to work effectively with our clients, something more is demanded of us: We need to step out of our skin, at least temporarily. We need to see the world through the clients' eyes, understand it through their mental filters, and feel it through their senses. This is not easy, and it doesn't come naturally to most of us. We have to work at it.

If you believe that we transmit energies to one another or even if you prefer to say that we have strong nonverbal ways of messaging, then you are cognizant of how important it is for us to show up fully—mind, body, and spirit—in our coaching relationships. We like the term *presence*. It creates a picture of how we want to be as coaches. It offers a mind-set that is welcoming and awake as clients speak to us. It allows us to relax into that deepest place of knowing from which we can draw all the necessary resources for compassionate and effective work with our clients.

---

**REFLECTION 6.9**

We invite you to create video recordings of some of your coaching sessions and review these recordings with the sound turned off. Watch your body. What is it saying? How present do you seem? How available do you appear to your client? What do you notice about your breathing? Where are you holding tension? Do you tend to slouch? Are there somatic patterns that characterize your presence? Do you gesture or fidget a lot? Jot down your observations and list areas where you might be able to enhance your embodied presence in coaching.

There is nothing mechanical or rote about an effective coaching relationship. In this respect, it can be exceptionally demanding. We have to be awake and self-aware! We need to know our triggers and learn to deactivate them whenever possible. We need to avoid the trap of a quick fix and continue to dialogue with our clients until ideas emerge that resonate with affirmation from both sides.

# 7

# THE MAGIC OF LISTENING

## *In this chapter, you will learn how...*

- nonverbal communication needs to be appreciated in all its forms: kinesics, paralinguistics, proxemics, environmental features, and the use of time;

- active listening is represented in the use of minimal encouragement, reflections, and summaries;

- simple verbal and nonverbal encouragers can support clients' unfolding of their stories;

- reflections of content allow clients to sort through their stories and determine elements they most want to pursue;

- reflections of feeling expand clients' emotional intelligence and surface energy for goal-directed behavior; and

- summarizing provides ways of concluding discussions, shifting perspectives, or opening up new topics depending on the coach's intention and the client's need.

> To be in a life of our own definition, we must be able to discover which stories we are following and determine which ones will help us grow the most interesting possibilities.
>
> —*Dawna Markova*

oaching communications have a delicate and distinctive rhythm that develops through the unique dynamics of who the client is, who the coach is, and what agendas they are addressing together. Clients begin from varying places of trust and openness and then unfold into the relationship at varying rates and intensities. As described in previous chapters, there are phases of development of the coaching relationship, and each of these calls upon certain competencies more so than others. Active listening, the fifth ICF core competency under the broad heading of effective communication, is arguably the most difficult of the competencies to master even though it appears simple. It requires crucial skills that remain significant throughout the coaching process.

The ICF (2011c) defines *active listening* as the ability to focus completely on what the client is saying and is not saying, to understand the meaning of what is said in the context of the client's desires, and to support client self-expression. A coach who listens actively is one who

- attends to the client and the client's agenda, and not to his agenda for the client;

- hears the client's concerns, goals, values, and beliefs about what is and is not possible;

- distinguishes among the words, the tone of voice, and the body language;

- summarizes, paraphrases, reiterates, and mirrors back what the client has said to ensure clarity and understanding;

- encourages, accepts, explores, and reinforces the client's expression of feelings, perceptions, concerns, beliefs, suggestions, and so on;

- integrates and builds on the client's ideas and suggestions;

- understands the essence of the client's communication and helps the client get there rather than engaging in long descriptive stories; and

- allows the client to vent or clear the situation without judgment or attachment in order to move on to the next steps.

International Coach Federation 2011

An extensive literature documents the centrality of active listening in helping relationships (Brew & Kottler, 2008; Egan, 2010; Smith, 2007). Maintaining focus on the client's agenda requires that you show up in all the ways that coaching presence entails (see chapter 6). It necessitates listening and responding in a manner that doesn't draw the client's attention to the coach's world or toward things he thinks are important. As Carl Rogers demonstrated throughout his career, there is profound power in listening well (Rogers, 1980; Rogers & Farson, 1995).

# UNDERSTANDING THE UNSPOKEN

The ICF core competency of active listening encompasses both what is said and what is not said. According to Mezirow (2000), effective communication "requires that we assess the meanings behind the words; the coherence, truth, and appropriateness of what is being communicated; the truthfulness and qualifications of the speaker; and the authenticity of expressions of feeling" (p. 9). Of course, what is not said might simply be at the client's unconscious level, or there may be particular aspects of his story that he deliberately conceals. Unveiling what is not openly spoken relies on messages that are transmitted nonverbally.

Nonverbal communication holds a prominent place in coaching. It has been formally defined as "communication effected by means other than words" (Knapp & Hall, 2010, p. 5). Early research in this area estimated that nonverbal behavior conveys from 65% to 93% of the meaning of a message (Birdwhistell, 1970; Mehrabian, 1981). Before client and coach exchange their first words, nonverbal communication feeds impressions. In some cultures, nonverbal messages outweigh the significance of verbal content (Sue & Sue, 2008). An important feature of nonverbal messaging is that it operates at a more unconscious level than verbal remarks.

As a lifestyle wellness coach, you will benefit from increased awareness of and sensitivity to nonverbal communications. You may notice various nonverbal expressions and interpret their meanings. These working hypotheses about meanings can be verified either through direct questioning or further observation. In the early stages of the coaching relationship, you may choose simply to remain alert to nonverbal cues. As the relationship develops, you may be able to discuss hunches developed from clients' nonverbal behaviors and thereby add depth to the coaching experience. In most cases, it is best to tread lightly when interpreting nonverbal messages, avoiding strong attachment to the meanings you have derived.

Five dimensions pertaining to the nonverbal domain have been identified: kinesics, paralinguistics, proxemics, environmental factors, and time. Let's see how these can guide our appreciation of clients' messages.

## Kinesics

**Kinesics** refers to body motions and includes facial expressions, eye movements, gestures, posture, touch, and body movements (Knapp & Hall, 2010). According to some experts (Birdwhistell, 1970), kinesics may also include unchanging aspects of the body such as height, weight, and physical appearance. In isolation, a single observation of kinesics may have limited value. Over time, however, patterns that seem correlated with certain subject matter or emotional content seem to emerge. Knowing what is being communicated in these moments will greatly enhance your ability to be of service. Kinesics provides additional clues to the meaning of a person's verbal messages. Just as the same word can have more than one meaning, so too do nonverbal gestures vary in significance according to context. Though research on kinesics provides general ideas for extracting meaning, there is always a risk of overinterpreting or misinterpreting body movements. Let's consider some selected areas of focus concerning body messaging.

### Eye Movements

Much of what we sense about another person comes from the eyes. The way people's eyes appear when we engage in conversation offers hints about their inner states. Do they look at you when speaking? Is there deeper meaning in someone's raised eyebrows or furrowed brow? Does the person blink often, or is her gaze more of a stare? Being aware of subtle eye movements provides clues about how best to respond to client needs.

If the person easily reciprocates your attentive eye contact throughout the coaching conversation, it would make sense to interpret this as an expression of interest and interpersonal comfort. However, when a client shifts her eyes from side to side or looks down rather than directly at you, she is not necessarily conveying avoidance or disinterest. In some instances, this could reflect cultural norms; for example, lowering the eyes while speaking may be a way that members of certain cultural groups show respect and deference in conversations. Although many white North Americans might equate eye contact with listening, people from other cultures may interpret eye contact as bold and confronting (Knapp & Hall, 2010; Sue & Sue, 2008).

Communication experts in the area of **neurolinguistic programming (NLP)** (Andreas & Faulkner, 1996; Grinder & Bandler, 1976) argue that eye movements correspond to neural thought processing (see figure 7.1). They suggest that whether a speaker's eyes move up, down, or side to side can explain how information is being processed and what types of thoughts the person may be having.

For instance, when a person's eyes move on a horizontal level from side to side, NLP theory suggests that she is accessing verbal information. A movement that is horizontal and to her left indicates she is trying to remember the words of past conversations, while one that is horizontal and to her right means that she is constructing new sentences in her head. Eye movements up and to one side or the other mean she is either accessing visual images that are from the past (to her left) or she is creating in the moment (to her right).

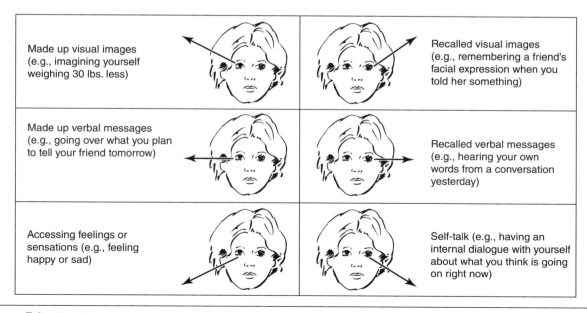

Made up visual images (e.g., imagining yourself weighing 30 lbs. less)

Recalled visual images (e.g., remembering a friend's facial expression when you told her something)

Made up verbal messages (e.g., going over what you plan to tell your friend tomorrow)

Recalled verbal messages (e.g., hearing your own words from a conversation yesterday)

Accessing feelings or sensations (e.g., feeling happy or sad)

Self-talk (e.g., having an internal dialogue with yourself about what you think is going on right now)

**Figure 7.1**    Neurolinguistic programming.

Eye movements down and to one side or the other reflect either an internal dialogue in which she is talking to herself (to her left) or the experience of a significant emotion such as joy or sadness (to her right).

A straightforward implication of this theory is simply that clients may move their eyes to access internal information that a coach may be requesting. For instance, if you ask someone to imagine himself doing a sport, he may create a visual image (eyes up and to his right) or remember a time when he participated in this activity (eyes up and to his left). In either case, NLP would argue that this person's eye movements parallel the information that he is trying to obtain.

## Facial Expressions

Scientific studies of facial expressions and emotion (Cohn & Ekman, 2008; Ekman, 1993) have confirmed much of what you may intuitively sense when looking at another person. Although the face is something that people usually learn to control, in unguarded moments all of us may reveal more than we want. It would appear that specific facial areas tend to convey specific emotions. You can usually see anger in the brows and lower face, for instance, and fear appears in the eyes. The mouth and jaw tend to display surprise, happiness, and disgust. For the most part, cultural differences are not thought to influence basic emotional responses shown in the face.

When a client is not speaking, the expressions of the lips and mouth may communicate a great deal. A person who is tight-lipped may be conveying experiences of control, anger, frustration, or repression. Biting the lips may express tension, and when the edges of someone's mouth turn down, you might be witnessing sadness or disappointment.

## Head

What does it mean when someone tilts her head or plays with her hair? Although playing with one's hair has been linked to nervousness, some (Fast, 2002) believe that angling one's head to the side suggests a questioning or doubting attitude about the matter in discussion—or it could simply indicate that the client has a hearing impairment. A rigidly held head can reflect anger or tension, whereas hanging one's head down may imply disappointment or sadness. It is a convention in Western culture that nodding one's head up and down displays agreement or compliance, and shaking the head from side to side means disagreement. Interestingly,

people often perform these movements without awareness.

## Upper Body

Your client opens the door and walks toward you. As you greet one another, you have already learned a lot about her from the way she stands. Her posture will reflect attitudes of assurance, rigidity, dependency, or self-esteem (Dychtwald, 1977; Kurz & Prestera, 1976). A slouched posture with a protruding abdomen may indicate dependency or lack of assertiveness, whereas a rigidly erect posture could convey defensiveness and a controlling attitude. A rounded spine may imply lack of confidence and low self-esteem.

From a seated position, leaning into the conversation may express interest and attention, while leaning too far forward could convey aggression. How does the client occupy her chair? Is she sitting on its edge? Is she crumpled into it with a look of resignation? Or is she bolt upright, as if she is ready to spring into action?

Shoulders are another part of the body that might be telling you something about the client. Shoulders that are sloped downward may indicate disappointment or depression, whereas shoulders turned inward toward the chest may represent nonreceptivity. Shoulders elevated toward the ears may indicate fear or anxiety (Dychtwald, 1977), and a shrug of the shoulders could convey doubt, uncertainty, or indecision.

People also communicate a great deal with their hands. Though some cultures use hand gestures as a normal way of emphasizing speech, tension or anger may be evident in hands that are tightly held or clenched into fists. Fidgeting motions of the hands may also indicate that a person is feeling anxious or worried. Arms tightly folded across the chest generally represent a self-protective or closed attitude. Easy arm movements could signify openness and involvement, whereas rigidly held arms and hands may be a sign of anxiety or self-restraint (Dychtwald, 1977; Kurz & Prestera, 1976).

In our discussion of coaching presence from the previous chapter, we mentioned the importance of posture. Just as it is important for the coach to sit with an awakened spine and open body, so too is it important for the client to present herself in a way that enables her to work effectively with the coach. In the first few sessions, posture will be something you observe in order to increase your understanding of the client and her issues. Later on, you may actually suggest that she alter her body position so she can access more of her personal resources for the discussion.

### Total-Body Movement

Often outside our awareness is the synchrony of body movements as we converse with another person. As you sit with clients during a coaching session, your body's movements may display varying degrees of harmony with your clients'. When your body moves easily in a rhythmic pattern in relation to their movements, you are likely to sense synchronicity in the relationship. Equally, when you display very different forms and degrees of total-body activity, this might suggest disharmony or conflict and potentially a power dynamic in which the more mobile body conveys greater discomfort (and less power) than the body that exhibits limited and steady movement.

Ekman (1993) discusses how a person's overall body movement is descriptive of his current internal experience. Body touching, scratching, rubbing, or other repetitive body movements may reflect the person's psychological state. You may observe someone stroking his arm when describing a difficult situation, suggesting that he is soothing himself as he talks.

### Touch

A final dimension of kinesics is the extent and manner of touching that occurs between helper and client. In depth-oriented helping relationships such as counseling and psychotherapy, most forms of touching are likely to be problematic, but health, wellness, and fitness professionals may engage in various kinds of touching, sometimes for corrective purposes (e.g., postural alignment) and other times in more spontaneous expressions (e.g., celebrations of achievements).

Coaches usually work with fundamentally healthy and well-functioning people; as such, they are not likely to avoid appropriate physical contact. Even so, touch can have so many connotations, especially when we factor gender and culture differences into the mix. It is wise to observe how clients initiate physical contact. A person who likes to give you a full embrace at the beginning and end of each session may simply be expressing himself the way he normally does with most people he knows. However, as his coach you need to be attuned to how this affects you and whether it crosses any of your boundaries. You also need to consider how this may influence your ability to work with him in a manner that competently addresses his agenda.

## Paralinguistics

When we listen to people, we are not only attuned to their gestures and words, we also hear the music of their speech. How loudly do they speak? Where are their intonations? That is, what words or expressions do they emphasize? Is their speech fluid or staccato? Does their voice quaver? Although these aspects of **paralinguistics** may characterize a person's general speech pattern, they may also vary depending on the topic or emotional shifts in the relationship. The flow of conversation in any relationship mirrors the styles and internal experiences of the speakers. Some people have a rapid-fire conversational style, while others are slower and more measured. Perhaps this comes from cultural background or personality. You will need to identify your clients' patterns so that you can recognize fluctuations in how they speak. Changes in paralinguistics signal a shift in their internal world, and accurately identifying these shifts increases your professional resources for promoting change.

Silence or pauses in speech can convey much meaning. A refusal to answer, hesitation before responding, or respectful silence following another person's self-revelation may communicate much more than words. A person hesitating before answering a sensitive question may reveal the truth before she speaks. Silence can be a means of control or a way of creating space for the other person to reflect.

Each culture has norms about silence (Sue & Sue, 2008). In general, North Americans interpret a pause in the conversation as disruptive or indicative of discomfort. It is common to avoid the void and fill the gap; we disallow a pregnant pause. To effectively use silence in service of clients' agendas, it is important for you to be comfortable in the absence of verbal communication and to learn how to use conversational pauses to deepen the communication and help clients shift perspectives. Many people experience discomfort with silence. In the early phases of the relationship, an overuse of silence by coaches can unduly spike client anxiety. Later on, when rapport and trust have been established, clients may welcome silence as an opportunity to reflect.

## Proxemics

How close is too close? What is your comfort zone? You know intuitively at what physical distance from another you feel most comfortable. When someone moves beyond the boundaries of your personal space, you may experience anxiety, fear, a desire for greater intimacy, or a need to keep conversation informal (Hall, 1966, 1976; Sommer, 2007). In a North American helping relationship, physical distance of 3 to 4 feet (90-120 cm) between helper and client tends to be experienced as comfortable (Trenholm, Jensen, & Hambly, 2010).

**Proxemics** involves both the consideration of personal space and the arrangement of environmental space. If you meet clients in person rather than over the phone, you need to be intentional in how you arrange the space in which you coach. You may place chairs face to face with no obstructions in between, or you may work at tables or desks, either side by side or across from one another. There is no such thing as a neutral environment. Everything in your office offers itself to interpretation, and your clients will extract messages from your coaching environment. It is important to take extra care in preparing your space before each session. Create an environment that is most likely to facilitate transition from the world outside to this unique world of unfolding opportunity.

## Environment

In considering proxemics, we addressed the arrangement of the coaching space. Here, we want to discuss where that space is located. Some of the spaces available to you may be shared or have multiple uses. Where you meet your clients has meaning and conveys intended or unintended messages. Health, wellness, and fitness professionals traditionally operate at health facilities, wellness centers, spas, physiotherapy offices, or sport complexes. As a lifestyle wellness coach, you may choose to base your practice in one of these locations. Given the potentially sensitive nature of coaching conversations, you will need to create a safe and private environment.

Coaching sometimes takes place in clients' environments, such as in their homes or places of business. What conditions do you need to negotiate for the venues to be viable? For instance, a client's office may be an appropriate place for coaching. However, if she allows interruptions by coworkers or answers phone calls during the session, it is your responsibility as a coach to create clear boundaries about how you will work together in this space so as to maximize the effectiveness of the coaching relationship.

The growth of coaching can be partly attributed to the versatile environments it employs. Coaching by phone significantly increases accessibility. Internet options further propel communication through the transmission of materials and the availability of quick updates and check-ins. Though there are pros and cons to each coaching context, the ability to readily adapt communication environments to circumstances is a hallmark of the industry. If coaching sessions take place by phone, a clear agreement stipulates boundaries for times of contact and the inviolability of the session. If a client is multitasking (e.g., working on a computer, driving a car, sorting through papers) while talking with you, the effectiveness of the session will be diminished. If you conduct web-based coaching through systems permitting voice and video contact (e.g., Skype or FaceTime), the physical environment where the session takes place remains important. You may want to ask yourself ahead of time what your client will see on and around you during the video call. Is this the message you want to convey as a coach?

Novice coaches may be concerned about the downsides of phone contacts when contrasted with the richness of face-to-face communications. Experience indicates that excellent coaching occurs over the phone. To some degree, it may be a matter of preference and practicality.

## Time

The nonverbal dimension of time exhibits significant cultural differences (Gielen, Draguns, & Fish, 2008). In this section, we address time in a number of ways. First, time can pertain to when and for how long the coach and client meet. Second, it may be seen as a boundary that is respected or violated. Finally, it may be understood in terms of where coaching conversations are located—in the present, past, or future. Each of these meanings of time offers a unique lens to understanding clients beyond the spoken word.

Questions of time can be found in scheduling preferences. How often does the person want to meet? Over what duration—measured in weeks, months, or even years? Is he able to schedule well in advance, or is his life so unpredictable that sessions can only be set for the imminent future? Most often, the duration of each session is set in the coaching agreement; this is not to say that clients are without preferences. What meaning can be found in a client's desire to contain discussions to no more than 30 minutes? In contrast, what sense can be made of a client's message that an hour is never enough to cover what he wants to cover? The first may be overwhelmed with other demands on her time or she may afford little importance to her stated agenda, while the latter may have more latitude in terms of scheduling or may be lonely and relish the time spent with his coach.

The second sense of time is about respecting agreed-upon meeting schedules. Is the client habitually punctual, or is she consistently late? Does she push to end early, or does she want to extend the session by bringing up loaded topics in the last few minutes? How about cancellations? What messages can be found when a client lives up to the contract by cancelling at least 48 hours in advance and yet cancels sessions almost as often as they are scheduled? For business reasons and to ensure the viability of the coaching relationship, clear guidelines regarding meeting times and session length are necessary.

Respect for the client requires that you be exactly on time except for truly uncontrollable situations. We even suggest that you be ready at least 5 minutes before the predetermined start time. This will give you an opportunity to sit quietly, take a few deep breaths, hold your client in your thoughts, and ground yourself in the present moment. You may also want to review any notes you've made about the previous session with the client so as to be fully prepared. A word of caution is essential here. A coach who is truly engaged in active listening will attend to the client's agenda rather than to her own objectives during the coaching relationship. Reflecting on the notes from previous sessions or reviewing a preparation form sent to you by the client, you might develop ideas concerning the direction of the forthcoming session. The fifth ICF core competency calls for you to put aside your own considerations and remain fully open to whichever agenda or topic the client wishes to address as she embarks upon each new session.

Another perspective of time concerns your responsibility for respecting the coaching contract regarding the length of the session. You may ask, what if your client gets highly engaged or emotional toward the end of a session? Should you allow the session to go over? Although rigidly enforced time boundaries may adversely affect client perceptions of the coach's care and support, lax boundaries are problematic in other ways. One interpretation of a relaxed attitude toward session length is that the relationship is more like a friendship than a professional engagement. As a rule, when all the stages of the flow model pertinent to this session have taken place, the client is satisfied with the robustness of her action plan, and she appears ready to jump into action, coach and client may consensually agree to end the session early. What about the opposite

scenario where a session runs over the agreed-upon time limit? In such situations, we recommend that you acknowledge the time issue and ask the client's permission to pursue the session for another few minutes. Be mindful that clients might feel short-changed when their sessions consistently end prematurely, and, conversely, they might experience annoyance with the coach's inability to effectively manage sessions when they always end late.

A final consideration of time centers on where coaches and clients locate their discussions—in the present, past, or future. A hallmark of coaching is its emphasis on the present and future rather than on the past. Knowing what a person has experienced, what has happened to him before the coaching relationship, or what has previously worked well can be critical for successful goal pursuit. However, as alluded to during our discussion about the differences between coaching and therapy, it is important to move efficiently from historical analysis toward future-focused planning.

Lingering discussions, historical reviews, or rambling commentaries are a poor fit with the philosophy and methodology of coaching. Yet, clients sometimes need to tell lengthy stories. For some cultural groups, historical considerations carry such significance that narratives of the past play a significant role in moving forward (Gielen et al., 2008). At the end of each session, however, robust

---

**REFLECTION 7.1**

In exploring nonverbal communication, we invite you to examine what you communicate nonverbally. In order to do this, arrange to be recorded on video during a simulated coaching session for at least 15 minutes. It would be best to do this in the place where you most often coach. Then, view the segment twice. First, look at the video with the audio turned off. Simply notice your nonverbal behavior. What do you observe? What patterns can you identify? Are you sitting straight? Do you smile and laugh often (nervously?) or do you frown and remain stern throughout? Do you lean forward? Do you touch your client? What do you see in the environment, and how might your clients interpret this? Reflect upon what you might be communicating nonverbally. The second part of this exercise is to view the video with the audio turned on. What do you observe now? Is your nonverbal communication congruent with the words you are saying? What attitudes are you communicating through your paralinguistic communications?

plans of action need to be articulated so that the client's agenda is clearly addressed and movement toward her goal is encouraged.

# THE ACTIVE NATURE OF LISTENING

Most of us believe we are good listeners, and no doubt we are at certain moments. However, the ICF core competency of active listening is worlds apart from the common conception of listening. In this context, it represents an appreciation of the multilayered nature of human experience and ensures that all relevant dimensions of a person's story have been brought forth. It means attending so deeply that the other gains profound self-awareness and insights. Active listening is a process that relies on trust and support to facilitate the client's movement from more peripheral subjects to the heart of the matter. It requires clearing our internal space and quieting the incessant chatter of our minds to be fully present.

Active listening is often distinguished from other skills by its unwavering respect for following and feeding the flow of the client's story without deliberate efforts to provoke shifts in direction. A coach listens with a kind of map, not of the content of what the person is saying but of the range and robustness of the story as it is told. Human experience is composed of thoughts, feelings, desires, values, actions, morals, and a myriad of other elements. Knowing what might be missing in the person's story requires that the coach appreciate what needs to be there, not out of personal curiosity but from awareness of elements that will elevate the tale from a simple recitation of facts to an expression that can nourish movement and growth.

It's not easy to sensitively listen and guide a client's unfolding into her desired future without taking control of the story. In discussing active listening, we borrow four skill designations from the field of communication (Evans, Hearn, Uhlemann, & Ivey, 2010; Hall & Hall, 1988). These skills are commonly known as minimal encouragement, reflection of content, reflection of feeling, and summarization. There is also another type of reflection, reflection of meaning, which we discuss in an upcoming chapter on creating awareness.

## Minimal Encouragement

As listeners, coaches need to provide feedback to their clients to guide their process of stating their agendas. An effective way to accomplish this without taking over the direction of the material disclosed is to use minimal encouragement. Ladany, Walker, Pate-Carolan, and Evans (2008) define a **minimal encourager** as a verbalization that echoes "the exact words" of the client or provides "some notable indication that [they] should continue" (p. 226). Often you will find yourself using minimal encouragers without realizing it when you are listening intently to someone's story. Almost under your breath, you utter, "Uh-huh." With more awareness, you might respond with expressions such as "Yes, I hear you," "Right," or "Okay." A body posture that reflects attention, a nodding head, or a repetition of key words normally accompanies such expressions. Minimal encouragement has the magical impact of supporting clients without interrupting their flow, thereby allowing them to explore their topic in greater detail (Sharpley, Fairnie, Tabary-Collins, Bates, & Lee, 2000).

Coaches know when they are listening, but clients may not know that they are being heard. Perhaps more importantly, they may not know *how* they are being heard, that is, whether the coach is listening critically, judgmentally, or empathically. In your efforts to be nonjudgmental, your face may appear masklike and, paradoxically, this may convey an impression opposite of that intended. Although you might believe that your quiet nonverbal presence adequately demonstrates your interest, clients who feel anxious in disclosing intimate details often need overt signs of support and encouragement.

In a North American context, most people use minimal encouragement liberally and without much forethought or awareness. In coaching, however, you need to be exceptionally aware of your perhaps unconscious way of encouraging others to speak. For example, the timing of your minimal encouragers may have a pattern. They may tend to coincide with certain content areas of client stories or certain facets of their self-disclosures, such as when they are talking about feelings. Perhaps when people talk about their success or positive happenings, you typically respond with an enthusiastic "Mm-hmm" while otherwise remaining relatively silent. This sends a clear message to clients about where your interests lie.

If we take behavioral conditioning principles to heart, your response pattern may unintentionally reinforce presentations of particular themes or types of content. If, for example, you respond to key words connected to success with minimal encouragement, your clients may begin to dredge up any remotely connected story of achievement in their histories to get the reward of the minimal encourager. Another point to bear in mind is that because minimal encouragers act as behavioral reinforcements, they can influence not only the direction of a conversation but its depth as well. You can drive a client's conversation into deep terrain by focusing on self-disclosures that are more intimate. Incidentally, a nonverbal behavior such as nodding or smiling will have a similar effect of encouraging people to say more about whatever is being discussed in the moment.

Some caveats about the use of minimal encouragement are fitting here. Three areas in particular need attention when using this communication skill:

1. Minimal encouragement needs to be paced according to the client's speech patterns. Paralinguistic features of speed or volume may lead to misinterpretation. Saying, "I hear you" loudly and quickly will have an entirely different effect than saying the same words softly and evenly.

2. The overuse or untimely application of minimal encouragers can easily communicate impatience or even boredom. Coaches who repeatedly say, "Mm-hmm . . . mm-hmm . . . mm-hmm," may seem to imply, "Okay, I've heard enough about this. Let's move on to something else."

3. The use of minimal encouragers as a prelude to speaking must be done thoughtfully. A coach may say, "Right," or "I hear you," just before interrupting the client's flow in order to provide feedback, instruction, or another kind of commentary. Clients may unconsciously adapt to the timing of these interventions by becoming silent as soon as they hear the cue that the coach intends to say something.

In coaching relationships, virtually everything you do influences your clients. The central issue is whether the direction of influence is advantageous for their growth and goal attainment. It is overly simplistic to say that the use of minimal encouragement demonstrates that you are listening; it is perhaps more accurate to state that minimal encouragers provide evidence of *what* you are listening to. As a coach, you are in the business of interpersonal influence. That's why clients have hired you. As an aware and self-reflective agent of change, you will want to continually examine your patterns of communication, especially those that are likely to be ingrained, habitual, and unconscious, such as minimal encouragement.

> ### REFLECTION 7.2
>
> Ready to view your recorded session again? This time we invite you to listen to all the minimal encouragers you used throughout your coaching conversation. What do you hear? Can you identify patterns? How do your minimal encouragers influence your client? What potential avenues of client disclosures do they reinforce? Do you respond to certain topics more than others? Do you tend to use certain forms of minimal encouragement to the point of potential irritation? Or do you use few minimal encouragers and perhaps seem aloof and distant in your sessions?

## Reflection of Content or Paraphrasing

Imagine yourself standing in front of a mirror. What do you see? The mirror reflects the side of you that you present to it. It doesn't afford a 360° view of the outside, and it certainly doesn't reveal what is on the inside. Client messages are complex constructions. At one level, content is expressed verbally along with some emotional elements that might be conveyed nonverbally. At another level, there may be other things that the person is trying to say but hasn't yet figured out exactly how to express.

Paraphrasing (Weger, Castle, & Emmett, 2010) and mirroring (Geldard & Geldard, 2008) are essential elements of active listening. Paraphrasing is feedback "that restates, in your own words, the message you thought the speaker sent" (Adler, Rosenfeld, & Proctor, 2004, p. 154). Though the term *paraphrase* is widely used, **reflection of content** is perhaps more precise because it describes the aspect of feedback specifically related to the content of a message. Another communication skill we discuss later, reflection of feeling, addresses the emotional dimension of the message. Together, these two types of reflection create a more complete mirroring of the client's message. The third form of reflection, reflection of meaning, offers an inside mirror of what the person has said.

Reflection of content is not a word-for-word reiteration: rather, it is a way of capturing the essential elements of what the person is communicating (Segal, June, & Marty, 2010). The coach takes the main words of the message and presents them back in a natural manner (see Effective and Ineffective Reflections). Good reflections are the antithesis of a formulaic repetition of words. They are offered

## Effective and Ineffective Reflections

| Client's statement | Reflection of content or paraphrase |
|---|---|
| I'll never be able to stop smoking! I've tried so many times but never lasted more than a week. I'm addicted! I come to the end of a meal and I have to have a cigarette. There are other times, too, when I automatically reach out and light up. It's just something I do. I also smoke when I'm stressed . . . I can't deal with stress without a cigarette. | **Effective reflection:** What I'm hearing is that it's hard for you to believe you can ever stop smoking. Though you've had small successes in the past, smoking has become so automatic that it's like an addiction. There are so many triggers to just light up. Quitting seems unimaginable. Is this right?<br>**Ineffective reflection:** You don't believe you will ever be able to stop smoking. You've tried so many times but never lasted more than a week. You think you're addicted. You smoke automatically at the end of meals and there are other times, too, when you automatically reach out and light up. It's just something you do. You also smoke when you're stressed. In fact, you can't deal with stress without smoking. Do I have it right? |
| My job is boring, my exercise program is off and on, my eating is out of control, I watch too much TV, and I keep arguing with my teenage son. I just don't have what it takes to pull myself out of this rut. | **Effective reflection:** I'm getting that you are dissatisfied with a number of areas in your life and that you feel powerless to change. Is this what you are saying?<br>**Ineffective reflection:** Your job is boring, you exercise off and on, your eating is out of control, you watch too much TV, and you keep arguing with your son. You don't think you have what it takes to pull yourself out of this rut. Am I right? |
| I am thrilled! I've done what I said I'd do last time we were together. I was able to run a full 10 minutes without stopping even though I wasn't sure I could do it. | **Effective reflection:** Sounds like you're both pleased and surprised to have accomplished what you planned to do!<br>**Ineffective reflection:** You are happy and you have done what you planned to do the last time we were together. You were able to run 10 minutes without stopping even though you were not sure you could do it. |

with ease, and as a result the client experiences an attitude of caring attention.

### Steps in Reflection of Content

As with all other elements of communication, reflections of content are adapted to our individual styles. Ivey and colleagues (2010) offer a four-step process for structuring this kind of communication.

1. **Consider timing.** The client's behavior determines the timing of the intervention. An effective reflection of content occurs close to the time when the person presents his thoughts, when he pauses, or when he appears to be seeking feedback. If the client's story is highly charged, a reflection could interrupt the flow. In this instance, minimal encouragers would likely work better.

2. **Use sentence stems.** A reflection of content is often initiated with a phrase such as "What you seem to be saying is . . . ," "Sounds like . . . ," "What I'm hearing from you is . . . ," or "You're telling me that . . ."

3. **Use the client's key words.** Listen for key words or expressions that the person has mentioned over the past few minutes and then capture them in brief phrases and sentences. When the client's words are ambiguous or have unique meaning, repeat

them exactly rather than use synonyms or seemingly similar expressions.

4. **Get confirmation.** Reflecting content can be risky. The client may not realize what she has said, and upon hearing her own words, she may reject the presentation as an inaccurate portrayal of the issues. Moreover, you may have used synonyms that failed to capture the intended meaning or even distorted the message. For reasons such as these, the fourth step is an accuracy check. The reflection might end with questions such as "Is this what you were saying?" "Am I hearing you accurately?" or "Is this what you mean?" Sometimes a client's nonverbal communications make such accuracy checks unnecessary, and at other times nonverbal behavior indicates that you are off track even before you have finished.

Just as we cautioned about attachment to your interpretations of nonverbal behavior, we encourage you to avoid holding onto your reflections. Even when you have perfectly mirrored a client's words, she may reject the paraphrase because hearing it aloud is too threatening or it is simply not what she intended to communicate. People have the right to change their minds and to say things differently. Creating that possibility is one of the many benefits of reflection.

## Upside of Reflection of Content

In Rogers' (1961) model of the helping relationship, reflections of content are a central skill of successful helpers. Elegant reflections foster the conditions for clients to discover their own meanings and solutions. When done well, the client may be mostly unaware that the coach is paraphrasing, yet she will feel buoyed by the conversation and encouraged to go deeper in self-discovery and clarity of vision. Reflections of content have greater impact than minimal encouragers in demonstrating active listening, and they do not direct the client to respond in a specific way as might occur when questions are used to explore a topic.

Reflections of content add to the coaching conversation since clients might reconsider their thoughts and modify, evaluate, or acknowledge them for what they are when they hear their own words reflected back. Until clients verbalize their internal world, they may not fully know it. Often the importance of our words takes on value only when they are expressed to another. In a process of self-discovery, many clients will find themselves

contradicting things they said earlier in a session as they come to fuller realizations of their deeply felt meanings. A further benefit of reflections of content is that they allow clients to focus on the issue of greatest importance to them. Sometimes they get so caught up in swirling thoughts that only through timely reflections can they stop spinning and move into a focused dialogue.

From the coach's perspective, reflections of content are crucial in a number of situations. At some point in a session, you may have so much information that you do not know which path to emphasize. A competent reflection allows you to identify all the leads that clients have put out and thereby place responsibility for direction appropriately on their shoulders. In a related sense, a coach who is highly oriented to action may feel compelled to do something or to make something happen, even while realizing that the timing is wrong. To slow the process, he can use reflections of content and help clients complete their stories or fill in missing pieces.

Reflection of content has one additional value worth noting. When coaches experience conflicts with clients, verbal exchange often accelerates at the expense of listening. Almost in an effort to prove who is right, each party details her evidence and impatiently awaits the termination of the other's litany to provide the conclusive argument. Even when the coach is factually correct, he must steer clear of proving his case and instead focus on listening. Fully hearing the client and reflecting content can take some of the steam out of the argument while also creating space for the person to hear her own words. By listening nondefensively, the coach is able to empathically take in what the client is saying and accurately paraphrase her thoughts and perceptions.

## Downside of Reflection of Content

When done poorly, clients can experience reflection of content as irritating, demeaning, or even mocking. Though the intended purposes of this skill are positive, reflections have problematic sides, such as the following:

1. **Slow rate of progress.** If clients have to discover all their issues, needs, goals, and action plans through an introspective process encouraged by reflective techniques, it may take more time than many are willing to commit. Overusing reflections of content may slow progress and consequently clients may become demoralized.

2. **Intervening too deeply.** Reflection supports clients in looking inward and understanding their

issues thoroughly. If you continually combine reflection of content with reflection of feeling, clients may become too introspective and coaching may begin to resemble psychotherapy. You only need to know enough about clients' histories and internal worlds to support the structuring and implementation of robust and viable action planning. An overuse of the reflective process can encourage clients to talk about issues far beyond what is required for coaching.

3. **Reflection as a defense.** You have surely been in a conversation in which you asked someone a question and the person responded with a question back to you. You probably experienced this as a defensive reaction. At times, rather than answer questions or respond to feedback, you may reflect the client's input, perhaps in the belief that it would be better for him to answer his own questions in order to understand more about his concerns. Though this misapplication of reflection does occur, it probably happens far less often than the opposite scenario in which coaches respond to questions when they should be reflecting them back to the client.

4. **Formulaic reflections.** When reflections are programmed, ill timed, or too frequent, they can be grating and ineffective. Clients may react to them defensively or simply come to see you as unhelpful.

## Reflection of Feeling

Whereas reflection of content pertains to the verbal part of the client's message, **reflection of feeling** is a restatement of the emotional, often nonverbal part of the story. In coaching, a distinction is made

---

### REFLECTION 7.3

We invite you to try reflecting content in some of your everyday interactions. Using the sentence stems we presented previously ("What you seem to be saying is . . .","Sounds like . . .","What I'm hearing from you is . . .","You're telling me that . . ."), practice reflection of content in three conversations with friends, coworkers, or family members. Notice how you feel doing it. (It may feel somewhat awkward if you are not used to it!) What is the speaker's reaction? Does the conversation shift? Where does it go? From what you noticed, what would be the impact of using reflection of content in a coaching conversation?

---

between emotions that are conveyed as part of the client's past experience (historical accounts of emotional states) and those that she is experiencing in the moment (account of present emotional states). To complicate this slightly more, another variation of feeling expression in a session occurs when a client says that she is experiencing a particular emotion while her nonverbal communications strongly suggest another emotion (conflicting emotional messages).

A historical account of emotional states may be accompanied by descriptive details that minimize their importance (e.g., "Oh, it was silly to feel that way") or distance the person from the emotion (e.g., "Well, that was a long time ago—it doesn't bother me at all now"). In these cases, the reflection of feeling may be more akin to reflecting content than to capturing the client's present emotional state. Here is an example:

**CLIENT:** I used to feel embarrassed about my weight, but I'm not sensitive about it anymore. Even so, I would like to lose about 30 pounds just for health reasons.

**COACH:** What I understand is that your motivation to lose weight is for health concerns, though at one point you felt embarrassed about your weight. Is that right?

Present emotional states are verbally expressed when the client describes a current feeling. This might happen as follows:

**CLIENT:** My desire to lose weight is primarily driven by health concerns, but ever since I can remember *(blushes, shows obvious discomfort)* I have been really uncomfortable about my body size.

**COACH:** I hear your concern and sense your emotions even as you talk about it now.

In this reflection of feeling, the emphasis is on the emotion rather than on the content of the communication. The rationale for this might be that by addressing feelings more fully, the client will be better able to make clear commitments and motivate himself to adhere to a program.

Conflicting emotional messages often demand more than a simple application of reflection of feeling. When clients verbalize one emotion while manifesting another nonverbally, we must choose how to deal with this information. Although both the words and the nonverbal behaviors can be reflected, the fact that these contain conflicting information is an indication that other skills might be more effective in addressing this matter. We will postpone this discussion until chapter 9, when we explore the core competency of direct communication.

Clients may experience emotions in coaching sessions without stating exactly what their feelings are. Even when they provide verbal descriptions, they may mask their genuine feelings by putting up a kind of verbal smokescreen (see figure 7.2). Feelings are just that, yet when people continually repress, deny, rationalize, or otherwise contain them, they may take on proportions far larger than the realities they represent. Growth and development rely on the capacity to give voice to emotional experiences that inform and motivate appropriate action.

Reflection of feeling makes clients' emotions explicit. The first step is for the coach to clearly identify the client's emotions. She must then decide whether it is appropriate to reflect the feelings—there needs to be a clear rationale for focusing on emotions. You will notice in the previous example of the client dealing with weight issues that the coach deliberately focused on the emotions without labeling them. Although she might have thought that the nonverbal cues represented emotions of sadness or a recurrence of shame, by not directly labeling the feelings, she provided the client with wide latitude to address his feelings at whatever level or depth he felt comfortable.

## Steps in Reflection of Feeling

Guidelines for reflection of feeling are similar to those for reflection of content (Brammer & MacDonald, 2003; Cormier, Nurius, & Osborne, 2009; Ivey et al., 2010). The structure consists of the following four steps.

1. **Consider timing.** The timing of reflections of feelings is critical. They need to occur close to the actual expression of the emotion. Unlike reflections of content, reflections of feeling may be effective when the coach inserts them in momentary pauses rather than when the client has more obviously finished a thought or a story. These reflections can be quick and supportive, such as "Ouch, sounds like that hurt!" or "Wow, I sense how happy you are." If a client is still in the midst of an emotion or the telling of an emotional story, nonverbal indicators (an understanding facial expression) or minimal encouragers ("I can sense that.") may better facilitate client expression. Sometimes, you may want to combine your reflection of feeling with a reflection of content to provide a more complete expression of what you have witnessed. Remember that reflections of feeling always need to be appropriate to the agenda that the client is addressing and his readiness to face emotions.

2. **Use sentence stems.** Introduce the reflection in a nonrepetitive manner that is congruent with your own style of speaking. Examples might include "Sounds like you are feeling . . . ," "What I'm hearing is that you are feeling . . . ," "I sense you are feeling . . . ," or "You're saying that you are feeling . . ." Note that these sentence stems are phrased in the present tense. Depending on whether the client is discussing past or present feelings, the tense of the verb needs to reflect the timing of the experience.

3. **Identify the client's key emotions.** Reflections of feelings require great care when clients report strong emotions or describe them in the present context. Using synonyms may inadvertently minimize

| Pseudoexpressions of feelings | may indicate the following | real expressions of feelings. |
|---|---|---|
| I'm feeling that you aren't really listening. | | I'm feeling lonely.<br>I'm annoyed. |
| I'm really feeling that you don't care about me. | | I'm feeling sad.<br>I feel rejected. |
| I feel like you're not going to help me. | | I'm disappointed.<br>I'm frightened. |
| I'm feeling that I'm never going to reach my goals. | | I'm worried.<br>I'm feeling hopeless. |
| I feel that everyone here is in a great mood. | | I'm happy.<br>I'm enjoying being here. |

**Figure 7.2**   Pseudo and real expressions of feelings.

or exaggerate emotional experiences and thereby diminish rapport. Sometimes using the client's exact words is safest. In instances when the person only hints at emotions or conveys feelings through nonverbal behaviors, it might be wise to be even more tentative than normal in reflecting feelings. In these cases, sentence stems such as the following may be preferable: "I can't be certain about this, but I'm getting the impression that you are feeling . . ." or "I have a hunch that you might be feeling . . ." Usually, when clients do not explicitly state their feelings and you decide to reflect nonverbal cues, slight underestimation likely works better than overestimation of the emotional level. Some clients might be resistant to owning emotions that they have not publicly stated, especially when the emotions are discomforting. Reflections that suggest stronger emotional experiences than they are willing to own could cause them to retreat into defensive intellectualizations or even outright denial.

4. **Get confirmation.** Reflecting emotion can be riskier than reflecting content. As noted earlier, clients may not be aware of their emotions, or they may not be ready to own them. Even if you accurately capture your client's emotional experiences, completing the reflection with an accuracy check may still be beneficial. The reflection might end with such questions as "Is this what you're feeling?" "Do I sense your feelings correctly?" or "Am I right about this?" The client's response may be to give nonverbal agreement or continue the discussion at a deeper level. When the reflection is inaccurate or the person is not ready to acknowledge his emotions, the feedback will provide clear guidance about how to proceed. In this instance, the client may want to clarify, justify, minimize, intellectualize, deny, or avoid. Rather than pursuing the subject or attempting to prove that your perceptions are accurate, follow the person's lead. This does not mean agreeing with denials or minimizations; rather, you might slow down the process so that the client can regain composure.

## Upside of Reflection of Feeling

Shining a light on clients' emotional experiences can be powerful. There are at least five reasons why a coach would choose to focus on emotions (Cormier et al., 2009). First, a reflection of feeling helps the client identify what her emotional experience (positive or negative) might be in a certain situation, with a particular person, or about a specific topic. Emotions are key sources of energy for movement. When people become more aware of their emotional

responses, they are likely to be able to make clearer choices concerning the future.

A second purpose of reflection of feeling is to increase the client's capacity to cope with and manage emotions. If someone believes that he cannot handle certain emotional states, he may fail to take action for fear of the feelings that might be aroused. If he is overly concerned by others' reactions to his emotions, he may be doubly guarded against creating situations where emotions might occur. As a result, this client may develop unrealistic beliefs about the consequences of emotional expression without having the opportunity to experiment safely with feelings. Although coaching is not counseling or therapy, it shares the objective of empowering clients through validating their experiences. As people express emotions in a coaching process, they learn how to release their feelings safely so that ultimately they feel less controlled by them.

A third purpose of reflection of feeling relates to the coaching relationship itself. At various times, clients may have reactions to the experience or to the coach. A common occurrence might arise when the client is not making progress and looks for someone to blame. Perhaps the coach has misjudged some critical elements, or the client has failed to comply with agreed-upon plans. As a defense against anxieties clients may feel in the relationship, resistance may arise (Patterson, 2000). Behaviors such as lateness for sessions, nonpayment of fees, unreturned phone calls or e-mails, or passive-aggressive reactions to the coach's suggestions are forms of resistance. By respectfully and supportively identifying evidence of emotional blocks or resistance, you can enhance your clients' capacities to manage their emotional world. When feelings about the coach or the coaching process remain unexpressed, clients are less likely to address the real issues standing in the way of their goal attainment. Eventually, they may terminate the relationship in dissatisfaction.

A fourth purpose of reflection of feeling is educational. If you ask a client how she feels, she may respond with a thought.

**COACH:** How do you feel about not getting the promotion?

**CLIENT:** I feel that my boss was totally blinded by [the successful candidate's] charm and didn't see what I had to offer.

Here, the person responds with a rationale for what happened and neglects to speak about her emotional response. Because this type of answer is so common, the risk is to continue by addressing why the client believes this about her boss rather than focusing on how she feels about the situation. Enabling the client to identify her emotions is both instructive and useful: The client develops her emotional intelligence while discovering energy with which to better address her concerns.

We can characterize feelings in a variety of ways (Ekman, 2003; Goleman, 1995; Hutchins & Vaught, 1997; Lazarus & Lazarus, 1994). Here, we have extracted four major categories: glad, sad, mad, and distressed. Within each category are levels with words representing degrees of emotional experiences (see figure 7.3). For instance, a person might express a low level of sadness as feeling *disappointed*. She might show a moderate level of sadness in words like *dejected* or *down*. Words such as *hopeless* or *crushed* might communicate a strong level of sadness.

As a coach, you can help clients differentiate among emotions they are experiencing, and you can work with them through reflections to identify the levels of feelings they are having. Some clients may not even have a vocabulary for emotion, and they simply spin in undifferentiated states of feeling without knowing what the implications might be or how to shift out of those feelings.

Although the coaching agenda is not directly about developing emotional intelligence (Goleman, 1995), such growth may be either a means to goal attainment or one of the ends itself. For instance, a client may need to be able to identify concrete feeling states about his experiences in various fitness activities (means), whereas another client may wish to become more assertive through physical training and as part of that work become able to differentiate among such emotions as anxiety, fear, and excitement (ends).

The fifth purpose of reflection of feeling is similar to one for reflection of content, namely, to convey empathy and understanding. Think of the norms for everyday greetings. We typically respond to the question "How are you today?" with the response "Fine. How are you?" Expressing real emotion allows others to see our inside reality; it is an intimate act. Even when we take risks and expose our feelings ("Actually, I'm kind of blue today"), the response we get may be minimizing or rationalizing ("Yeah, must be the weather" or "Don't worry, it will pass"). To be heard with empathy when we reveal emotions can be tremendously validating and often beneficial in enabling us to move beyond present feeling states.

## Downside of Reflection of Feeling

Emotions provide rich sources of energy and reinforcement for goal-directed behavior. Yet when clients bring up difficult or unpleasant experiences, reflection of feeling may encourage them to talk more about troubling emotions. Here are some downsides to keep in mind.

1. **Deepening the emotional agenda.** Clients of lifestyle wellness coaching are typically focused on positive life changes. Although any significant behavioral change is likely to have an emotional component, feelings are unlikely to be the central

| Level \ Type | Glad | Sad | Mad | Distressed |
|---|---|---|---|---|
| **Strong** | Ecstatic<br>Overjoyed<br>Delirious<br>Blissful | Depressed<br>Crushed<br>Disconsolate<br>Stricken<br>Tearful<br>Hopeless | Furious<br>Outraged<br>Enraged<br>Livid<br>Infuriated<br>Boiling | Frightened<br>Terrified<br>Scared<br>Dreading<br>Panicky |
| **Moderate** | Cheerful<br>Happy<br>Delighted<br>Joyful | Dejected<br>Cheerless<br>Sad<br>Down<br>Blue | Mad<br>Stormy<br>Angry<br>Antagonized<br>Incensed | Agitated<br>Frustrated<br>Upset<br>Flustered<br>Rattled |
| **Low** | Pleased<br>Glad<br>Content<br>Cheery | Low<br>Bored<br>Disappointed<br>Dour | Upset<br>Ticked<br>Displeased<br>Ruffled<br>Vexed<br>Disgruntled | Anxious<br>Apprehensive<br>Confused<br>Dismayed<br>Uneasy<br>Bothered |

**Figure 7.3** Types and levels of feelings.

theme of the client's agenda. By emphasizing emotional content, coaches implicitly sanction this focus in sessions. As a result, the person may believe that she *should* be talking about emotions or that she may experience some personal benefit from discussing her emotions. However, coaching is not a therapy. Clients will ultimately evaluate coaching experiences based on their success in achieving goals. Although they may feel better after talking about emotions, they will not necessarily reach their primary objectives through this means.

2. **Fostering emotional dependency.** When a coach proves to be trustworthy and caring, clients may feel encouraged to self-disclose at levels far deeper than necessary for achieving their stated goals. If a client has a number of emotional concerns and few outlets for discussing them, reflection of feeling can generate an environment of safety and support. Those who lack this kind of support may seek to continue the coaching relationship for covert emotional reasons. These remarks are meant to caution against overemphasizing this skill rather than to discourage you from offering reflections of feelings. You can sense that clients are implicitly shifting the agenda to a hidden emotional one when conversations linger around emotional themes or when they continually attempt to redirect the discussions to life matters that are clearly peripheral to the agreed-upon focus of the working alliance.

3. **Provoking resistance.** Clients might be willing to tell you what they want to achieve, how they want to achieve it, and what they are willing to do, yet they might discourage any attempt to move close to their emotional world. When coaches reflect emotional themes, they need to be prepared for the possibility that their input might be sidestepped. In a therapy relationship, such behavior would be identified as resistance. Resistance to exploring emotional topics may be entirely appropriate in lifestyle wellness coaching, however, and a client may send strong signals that she does not want to discuss her feelings. You have at least two choices at this point. The first and most probable one is to follow the client's lead, because your role is to work with her agendas so she achieves her objective. If the emotional content that the client is denying or avoiding has a strong link to the stated agenda, then you may need to address this matter using competencies described in chapter 9. Briefly, you may need to discuss perceptions and review alternative strategies for continuing the work.

4. **Poor timing.** Coaches can be right about the emotions that they detect but wrong about reflect-

ing them in the moment. Emphasizing emotions too early in the relationship may lead clients to believe that the coach is implicitly communicating that something is wrong with their emotions. Another sense of poor timing pertains to when the reflection is offered. The reflection may seem out of context—and irrelevant to where the person is at the current moment—if it is offered too long after the client has expressed the emotion. If you are fully present in each moment of the session, you will be in tune with your clients' emotions and know whether it is appropriate and timely to reflect.

---

**REFLECTION 7.4**

To reflect the feelings of others, you need to practice identifying your own feelings. Think back to reflection 6.1, where we invited you to identify your feelings as a means to increasing your emotional intelligence. How difficult was it for you to label your feelings? Did naming your feelings make a difference? Did it help you reframe the experience that gave rise to these emotions? How might adopting this practice benefit you as a coach?

---

## Summarizing

Sometimes you listen to a client for quite a while with the occasional interjection of a minimal encourager or a reflection. At a certain point, you begin to sense that the person needs to shift focus or that both of you need to step back and review all that has been said up to now. Summarizing the conversation that has taken place will help you do just that.

**Summarizing** can be described as a kind of reflection that occurs over a longer conversation (Evans et al., 2010). A summary may represent a periodic synopsis of the session to this point in time. For instance, the session may have been in progress for about 15 minutes and you want to pull together everything that has been presented thus far, so you offer a summary. Such summaries may be used to test the waters regarding whether it is time to shift to something else. They may also provide clients with opportunities to determine if any critical pieces are missing. In addition, a closing summary may be helpful at the end of a session, where the coach brings together essential points. Closing summaries may be used to detail agreements and action plans, or they may enumerate the aspects of conversation and work covered in the session. A summary may also be used to bring together a theme or topic that the client has mentioned across a number of sessions. For instance, a client may have repeatedly noted a theme of self-sabotaging change, and having tracked this theme, you might bring it into sharp focus by summarizing the various times it has been mentioned.

## Steps in Summarizing

Because summarizing can be somewhat longer than reflections of content or reflections of feeling, it needs to fit into the structure of a session. Depending on its purpose, a summary may occur at the beginning, middle, or end of a session. For instance, in bringing focus to a particular theme in the client's messages, you will need to position the summary in the session so that you have adequate time to develop the conversation. On the other hand, a closing summary needs to come shortly before, but not exactly at, the end of a session. If you offer a closing summary at the last minute, no opportunity will be available for client reactions or modifications. The following four steps provide a structure for summary statements (Cormier et al., 2009).

1. **Frame the summary.** Find a way to introduce the summary that is appropriate to the material that you are summarizing. If it is a closing summary, you could say, "I'd like to end our session with a brief synopsis of our work together. These are the main points that I can remember . . ." If you use the summary to focus the client on a recurring theme during the session, you might begin by saying, "I think I'm hearing a theme in what you've been telling me. It sounds like . . ." As with other skills, summaries must be offered tentatively so that the client can easily disagree with or modify your remarks.

2. **Identify key elements of the client's message.** When you focus on a theme that has emerged across a number of sessions, mental recall of details may be less precise than written notes taken during or shortly after sessions. When coaching has progressed to stages in which the client is actively implementing plans, records of progress can be helpful. These might include charts that are reviewed together at each session. The degree to which the summary is seen as accurate will affect your credibility. If you say that you are going to review the entire session, then you must account for the entire process, although you may represent large parts of the discussion as items on a list (e.g., "We discussed in detail your progress, and in your

estimation you're 80% on track"). If you focus on a theme, you would generally have at least two concrete instances of when this theme was presented. Note that detailing every instance in which the theme was mentioned may overwhelm the person and provoke a defensive reaction.

3. **Summarize content and feelings.** The messages that you choose to summarize must appropriately represent both the content and emotion expressed. The agreed-upon agenda, the client's receptivity to emotional data, the amount of time needed for processing the summary, and the purpose that it is intended to serve determine what is appropriate. It is unwise to consider summaries as topical checklists devoid of emotional content. You want to relate emotional dimensions of your clients' experience to the content so that the result is a well-rounded representation of their expressions rather than a unidimensional, strictly logical view. Part of a summary that demonstrates the weaving of emotion and content might sound as follows.

**COACH:** You focused some of your discussion today on further limiting your caffeine intake, though you sounded pessimistic about being able to do this.

An exception to this principle might occur when you are summarizing action steps that your client has agreed to. In this case, the listing of steps would be adequate because its function is primarily to reinforce the agenda in your client's mind.

4. **Get confirmation.** Summarizing can cover a lot of ground. Depending on how much material the summary represents, you will need to provide clients with opportunities to reflect on, react to, or modify it. They must also be encouraged to take an active role in the process. The responsibility for summaries and tracking progress is best shared. To achieve this, you may invite your client to think through what you have summarized so that she is not a passive recipient of lists of details. Here are some examples of such verification messages: "Well, that's how I would summarize the session, but I'm interested in knowing how you would capture it," or "Is this an accurate reflection of what you've said? Is there anything that doesn't fit or that you'd like to put another way?"

## Upside of Summarizing

Summarizing parts of sessions or recurrent themes across sessions can create new energy and understanding in coaching relationships. The effective application of summaries not only builds trust, it can also influence clients to change. People need to experience increasing levels of autonomy over the life span of the coaching relationship so that they are able to carry on independently and successfully afterward. Communication experts in the helping professions have identified several functions of summarizing (Evans et al., 2010; Kratcoski, 2004). The first is to confirm general understandings or validate assumptions during a session. Given that clients may present a range of information, presenting them with a review of issues or themes demonstrates that you have grasped their core messages. At the same time, the process affords them an opportunity to reflect on the whole of their communications and perhaps realize that an important element is missing. When you review major themes, clients can more easily perceive progress. Additionally, clients who express diverse ideas may have little clarity about their relative importance. Through a summary statement such as the following, they may have the opportunity to reflect and then continue the discussion with greater clarity.

COACH: Let me take a minute here to see if I've gotten all you've said about your reasons for wanting to work with me. As I recall, you mentioned that you have three goals. First, you said you want to feel better about yourself because right now you think you're in a "bit of a rut." Then you mentioned that committing yourself to a scientifically sound nutrition program would give you a sense of doing something positive for yourself instead of ignoring reality. The third thing I heard was that eventually you wanted to train for a 10K race, although you noted that was likely "way down the road." Were these the main points you made? Did I miss anything?

Note that in this example the coach is tentative in her summary and tries to repeat key words or phrases that the client used.

As previously mentioned, a second function of summarizing is to shine a light on a particular theme that the client has repeatedly mentioned in a number of sessions. When a statement or issue continues to emerge, you are likely to attribute additional weight to that topic. At an appropriate point, you may summarize the various references to this single theme and thereby enable the client to consider its significance and how it relates to moving forward. For instance, someone who has repeatedly

mentioned the influence of family members on her ability to adhere to an exercise program may need to explore this issue. Here is how you might summarize this theme.

COACH: I've heard you mention a particular issue a few times this session and in our last meeting as well. It sounded to me like you were saying that you have trouble thinking of yourself as a regular exerciser because of the expectations your partner and your parents have of you. You said just a minute ago that your aging parents were very needy and dependent on you. For you to be unavailable to them when they wanted you was unthinkable. Last session, I remember you saying that your partner might feel bad if you took up part of your free time to devote to a regular exercise program. Have I put this together accurately? Is this something you've been trying to tell me?

The function of summarizing a theme is for the coach to focus the client's attention on a particular point in greater detail; however, the client may not be open to addressing the matter at this time. In using thematic summaries, there needs to be adequate rapport and a solid rationale for raising the issue at this time.

A third function of summarizing may serve the coach's needs as much as it serves the needs of the client. When meeting someone for the first time, an overwhelming number of details may be presented. A coach may want to slow down the process both to allow time to think more clearly about what has been said and to give the client an opportunity to reflect and concentrate. Clients may be anxious and therefore speak rapidly and possibly without a great deal of coherence. Some may want to download as much information as possible so that the coach can quickly put things together in an action plan. The coach will find cues about exactly how to pace his summary in the paralinguistic dimensions of the client's speech. If the client speaks in a rapid, nonstop manner, the summary will have to be similarly fast paced and probably point by point. An example of the pacing and content of a summary for someone who has swiftly given a life review and five reasons for engaging in a coaching relationship might sound as follows.

COACH: Let me pause for a few seconds to make sure I've got it all. I heard you say you're generally healthy, happy, and highly motivated. You want to work with me for a maximum of six months, and you want to achieve these goals—one, lose 10 pounds; two, find an exercise plan you can stick to on your own; three, learn proper technique so that you don't injure yourself; four, improve your nutrition plan; and five, learn how to relax. Is this an accurate summary?

Here, the coach enumerates issues and gives a concise summary. The client wants to move quickly into action. And although this pattern may change as the relationship progresses, the coach is aiming to reflect the no-nonsense, let's-get-down-to-business attitude suggested by the client's initial presentation of her reasons for working with him.

Regulating the pacing of a session by summarizing might also occur in instances where clients seem scattered or are experiencing a high level of stress from life situations. Summarizing in this case might signal safety and ease pressure rather than just capture all the themes. Here is an example of such an exchange:

**CLIENT:** (*Speaking in a rapid, pressured way while showing nonverbal signs of tension and stress*) I'm sorry . . . I'm so sorry . . . I just couldn't do what I promised to do this week. My life has been totally out of control. My car broke down, so I had to take the bus every day. Things at work have been unusually busy, and my youngest child has been home sick. I'm simply overwhelmed. Please excuse me . . . what a waste . . . I really intended to train. I don't mean to dump this on you, but I couldn't do what I said I would do. I'm just feeling all over the place. I don't know if I'll ever be able to pull myself together to be regular about exercising.

**COACH:** I hear you. Can we just stop here for a minute and take a breath? It sure sounds as if you have had one heck of a week and you're really feeling overwhelmed. So many things going on and many of them unexpected . . . all of this leaves you wondering about what's possible in the future.

In this instance, the coach uses summarizing to slow down the process and give the client room to reflect without the pressure of moving forward. Rather than reiterate the elements of the client's difficult week, the coach provides an empathic and encompassing summary. In so doing, she conveys permission for the client to simply be with her experience for a few minutes before addressing the coaching agenda.

A fourth function of summarizing is to bring all the themes and issues of a session together toward the end. This review serves as a confirmation of what has been discussed, as a kind of progress note, and as an opportunity to launch the next step from this platform. Clients need to experience forward movement in coaching. A summary at the end of the session confirms themes so that they may continue to engage in action during the interval between sessions. You need to structure summaries in a manner that ties together diverse themes so that clients leave with an experience of coherence rather than with fragmented thoughts. Even though you may take notes during the session and thereby have reasonably complete lists of issues and concerns, until you summarize this information verbally clients may not be clear about what they said or whether they were heard. By summarizing sessions, they leave with a comprehensive review and a supportive sense of having been fully heard. It is also important to acknowledge that in this particular application of summarizing, it is best to cocreate the summary rather than act as the secretary for the session's minutes. We look at this point further in the next section.

## Downside of Summarizing

Effective summarizing requires a high degree of creativity, insightfulness, and accurate recording (mental or written); it is far from a rote process of detailing the elements of a conversation. Learning to summarize a session concisely or capture a theme across sessions consistent with the client's energy, pacing, and style takes a great deal of practice. Some of the more common pitfalls of summarizing are the following.

1. **Coach-led summaries.** If you always assume responsibility for detailing sessions or capturing themes, clients can become dependent on you. As a result, they may grow more passive and the coaching process may take on a lifeless quality. Summarizing must serve a specific purpose in a session. It should never sound like a checklist or recital of elements of the conversation. Sometimes clients will summarize of their own volition, a practice that is highly encouraged. It is beneficial to structure summaries as a mutual process where coach and client conclude their work by collaboratively reviewing the session. In this form, summaries are back-and-forth exchanges in which coach and client take turns identifying key elements of the session.

2. **Inconsistent applications of summaries.** Patterns emerge rapidly in relationships, and they

enable us to experience comfort and safety. If you use summaries at the beginning of a session (e.g., "I'd like to begin by reviewing briefly where we were at the end of last session") or at the end, clients may come to expect this behavior. Inconsistent use of summaries might then lead them to attribute meaning to this behavior. For instance, a client might think that not much happened in the day's session because you neglected to summarize her progress. If you establish a pattern of closing sessions with cocreated summaries, then this component needs to remain consistent unless there is good reason to omit it.

3. **Incomplete summaries.** Without intentionally deleting elements of what is being summarized, if you represent only part of the person's messages as a complete portrayal, your credibility and trustworthiness may diminish, and your client's faith in you as an accurate source of information or as a competent listener will decrease. When you are not sure that you have all the elements of a summary, you need only say so. The strategy of cocreating a summary can be valuable for closures; you might use this approach to ensure that your summary is complete. The following is a sample invitation to the client.

COACH: I wonder if we could end our work today by putting together a summary of what has occurred in this session. I have my own notes, but I think it works best if we can do this together. So, if I can start, the first area we covered was a review of your sleep pattern this past week, which you described as great. What do you remember as coming after this discussion?

A collaborative approach will probably be less appropriate when you are trying to bring focus to a particular theme. When you wish to do this, you need adequate details or information before you begin; otherwise the summary may be more confusing than helpful. For instance, the following illustrates a coach ineffectively summarizing a client's thoughts about body issues without sufficient detail to create awareness.

COACH: I think there is an important theme of body image in what you have been saying today. You mentioned earlier something about how you feel when you exercise, and then there was something else you said about a kind of unhappiness with how you look. Do you remember?

Here, the theme of body image may have been tracked at a subconscious level. At what seems to be an opportune moment, the coach tries to bring it to a conscious level through dialogue. Without the necessary details, however, it is likely to confuse and disorient rather than propel progress.

4. **Biased summaries.** Unlike the previous example, a biased summary has a sharper degree of intentionality and focus. Imagine that a coach identifies a theme and listens for evidence supporting her hypothesis or concern. Whenever the client mentions this theme or something related to it, she eagerly notes it. Intervening topics receive less detailed attention. When she offers her summary, key elements that contradict her statements may be missing. If the client is aware of these deletions or omissions, he may become rightfully concerned about the coach's objectivity. The capacity to develop and test hypotheses about client behaviors is a critical coaching skill, and it must be done intentionally. You need keen self-awareness of what you are paying attention to, and you need to be equally vigilant to search for evidence to the contrary. Sometimes it may make sense to explain your hypothesis to your clients so the search becomes collaborative rather than a game of catching them in the act.

5. **Argumentative summaries.** One final misuse of summaries can be likened to courtroom arguments in which evidence is marshaled to prove a point. Like everything else we discussed in this chapter, summaries are rarely offered in a conclusive manner. Their primary purpose is to promote rapport, understanding, insight, and action. Because coaching is by definition a collaborative venture, the use of argumentative summaries implies an adversarial relationship. The following is an inappropriate use of summarizing by a coach to prove a point.

## REFLECTION 7.5

To help you with the skill of summarizing, review your recorded coaching session one more time. Stop the video at significant points during the conversation and write a summary of what you have heard so far. Go back and check the accuracy of what you wrote. Should you wish to gain further practice, you can get creative by picking out a few films or TV shows where there are dialogues between two people. Pause your viewing at various points and try to capture in a verbal expression, as if speaking to one of the actors, a summary of what has transpired.

**COACH:** So far in this session, I've noted six times that you said equipment problems at your gym interfered with your program implementation. Three times the equipment was in use, two times it was during hours when use was restricted to 20 minutes, and the sixth time, the machine was in repair. It seems that you are blaming the machines rather than taking personal responsibility for not living up to your agreement.

# COMMENTARY

Active listening is a highly engaged process of attending to the client's words and behaviors with exquisite awareness and then expressing back in a timely manner the messages received. Its functions for the coach are to increase understanding of the client and to establish trust and rapport for the work that lies ahead. From the clients' perspective, active listening facilitates open and appropriate communication about issues that they wish to address; it enables them to perceive the viability of the coaching relationship as a means to their ends. Although the use of minimal encouragers, reflection of content, reflection of feeling, and summarizing may be highest in the early stages of the coaching relationship, they will remain essential ingredients of any coaching session. As clients encounter difficulties in implementing plans, they may show signs of resistance or become more emotional about their perceived failures. These reactions and feelings need to be acknowledged, and the competency of active listening will be immensely helpful in these matters.

Some of us have been told that we are good listeners by family, friends, and acquaintances. Although this kind of feedback can be gratifying, people in our personal networks may have different meanings for the term *listening*. They may mean that you agree with them; give them good advice; don't talk much, thereby allowing them to talk; or ask a lot of penetrating questions. Active listening as a coaching skill is not necessarily something that comes naturally. It often takes years of concentrated practice to deepen our capacity to see, hear, and feel the expressions of those who choose to share their realities with us.

Though active listening is rarely used in isolation from other coaching competencies, it is the bedrock of coaching. We encourage you to bring your attention to how well you are listening. You might do this by reviewing audio or video recordings of your coaching sessions or by holding practice sessions where peers or mentors can give you feedback on your mastery of this critical competency.

# CHAPTER

# 8

# THE POWER OF QUESTIONING

## In this chapter, you will learn how…

- curiosity as expressed through powerful questions is a magical gift that coaches have to offer their clients;

- specific types of questions—open, closed, indirect—serve specific functions in the coaching relationship;

- attention to critical details can prevent structural errors in the design of questions;

- reflections can be used in lieu of questions to elicit information when the client's comfort is at risk;

- questioning and other coaching skills need to be blended to facilitate movement forward; and

- powerful questions equip coaches with unique avenues to foster client insight and advancement.

> To talk with someone,
> ask a question first, then—listen.
> —*Antonio Machado*

f you want to know something, ask a question. A common way people express interest in one another is by asking questions. Where do you live? What do you do? What's your favorite food? The way you express your curiosity through questioning can fuel unparalleled growth or shut down communication completely (Strachan, 2001). Just as there are great questions and unique ways of framing them, there are also ways of inquiring that are problematic. As Antoine de Saint-Exupery (1958) tells us through his characters in *The Little Prince,* people may ask the wrong questions. Or, they may ask the right question but at the wrong time! In this chapter, we introduce the art of questioning. Continuing within the theme of effective communication, powerful questioning is the sixth ICF core competency, defined as the ability to ask questions that reveal the information needed for maximum benefit to the coaching relationship and the client (ICF, 2011c). A coach who effectively uses the skill of powerful questioning

- asks questions that reflect active listening and an understanding of the client's perspective;
- asks questions that evoke discovery, insight, commitment, or action (e.g., that challenge the client's assumptions);
- asks open-ended questions that create greater clarity, possibility, or learning; and
- asks questions that move the client toward what he desires, not questions that ask for the client to justify or look backward.

International Coach Federation 2011

Powerful questioning is a skill that remains essential in all aspects of the coaching process. Before presenting some of the unique styles that make questioning powerful, we will discuss the structures of questions, their effects, and the pitfalls that could derail a coaching relationship.

Questioning has many purposes and forms. It is a means of fostering rapport, understanding the client's perspective, and deepening the relationship. Asking powerful questions is a potent way to develop insight and guide change. Although questions are essential to coaching, as Kottler (2008) remarks, "Asking questions is a mixed blessing. It does get you the information you want in the most direct fashion, but often at a price" (p. 77). He suggests that if you cannot get the information that you need by another means, then ask a question, almost as your last resort.

If you have been to a job interview recently, you might recall how frequently interviewers ask questions and how it feels to be questioned. You may also have memories of being cross-examined, grilled, interrogated, or otherwise required to answer a seemingly endless list of pointed questions. As a result you might have developed extreme sensitivity to being questioned. Interviewers may gather a great deal of information with their questions, but at what cost? They might use trick questions, leading questions, biased questions, closed questions, or questions to which they already know the answer. When a person asks you a leading question (e.g., "You like this job, don't you?" or "You are going to do something about this situation, aren't you?"), you are likely to assume that the questioner already has made up her mind, that she expects a certain answer, or perhaps that the situation is a bit unfriendly. In this light, how does questioning serve as a supportive, trust-building, awareness-generating, action-promoting empathic skill?

Clients expect you to ask questions; they more or less open themselves to this process. Yet the experience of being questioned can move the client in so many directions—some of them beneficial, others not. No doubt, your desire is to be helpful, and surely you intend to probe delicately and caringly. Nonetheless, when you ask certain questions, your client may say, "Ouch," and you may retreat a step or two. Sometimes, however, your client will say, "Ouch," and you will decide to continue to ask. Questioning is an art! The job interviewer referred to earlier has it easy by comparison. She typically has a preset list of questions and areas to cover, and she isn't necessarily interested in building a relationship. In coaching, you are an explorer in an uncharted world. Asking the wrong question can bring you to the edge of a precipice; asking the right one can reveal new worlds.

# GENERIC TYPES OF QUESTIONS

The two most prevalent types of questions are closed and open questions. A third type, the indirect question, occurs when people make statements that imply a need for response.

## Closed Questions

**Closed questions** lead the client to respond in a word or short phrase rather than an expansive

**REFLECTION 8.1**

Before continuing, arrange to have a 10-minute recorded conversation with a friend or a colleague who agrees to work with you on this short experiment. First, ask your friend to talk to you about something big he would like to do in the next 6 to 12 months that he is not doing right now. Then inform him that you will only be asking questions for the whole 10 minutes. When the 10 minutes are over, ask your friend how he experienced the process. Did he feel heard? Did he feel interrogated? Did he gain insight into what he plans to do? As for you, how did the experience feel? What do you think your questions revealed? What did they prevent from happening? How did this style impact your relationship?

As we proceed through the chapter, we will ask you to listen to the recorded conversation and note the kinds of questions you asked. We will also invite you to examine the timing of your questions, the manner in which you asked them, and the kinds of responses you received.

answer. They are typically used to obtain facts, to verify information, to close off lengthy explanations, or to control the flow of the interview (Sommers-Flanagan & Sommers-Flanagan, 2009). They may begin with such words as *do, is, are,* or *have.* Their form is best recognized by the implicit demand of the question to answer directly and briefly. Here are some examples of closed questions:

- Are you ready to proceed?
- Is this the book you were talking about?
- Do you agree?
- Are you interested?
- Do you want to continue talking about this?

## Open Questions

**Open questions** invite exploration and conversation; they help create clarity and generate new learning. An open question may direct the client to a theme of discussion, yet it allows ample latitude to explore thoughts and feelings. A reflection of content or feeling is more likely to follow an open question than a closed question. When you ask open questions, you may receive lengthy responses that you may choose to paraphrase or summarize

to ensure understanding. Open questions may begin with words such as *how, what, would, could,* or *why.* Some examples of open questions include the following:

- How has your program been going lately?
- What kinds of activities interest you most?
- What specific outcomes are you hoping to attain through this coaching relationship?
- What have you learned thus far?
- Why is this an ideal week for you?

## Indirect Questions

**Indirect questions** are statements that imply a need for response. They are a less intrusive way of seeking information and can often unlock unconscious understandings of issues (Groth-Marnat, 2009). Especially when the coach has been asking many questions, the use of indirect questions may break the pattern and ease the pressure of questioning for the client. Here are some examples of indirect questions:

- It would help me to understand your perspective if you said more about this.
- I am curious to hear how you reacted.
- It seems you have something else on your mind today.
- I don't know exactly what you mean by that last statement.

# PROBLEMATIC QUESTIONS

The structure of a question affects both the answer you receive and the quality of the relationship you want to nurture. Most experts in the communication and helping fields believe that a lengthy questioning process diminishes rapport in addition to reinforcing unproductive power and dependency dynamics in the relationship (Ivey et al., 2010; Kottler, 2008; Shebib, 2010; Young, 2009). The following discussion addresses aspects of problematic questioning.

## Leading Questions

A question is said to be leading when the way it is phrased most likely influences the response. Often these questions are phrased as negations, making it difficult for the client to disagree with or deny something. Here are some examples:

- Wouldn't you like to try this?
- Isn't it a lovely day?
- Is this so difficult that you won't even try it?
- Don't you think it would be a good idea to have your brother join you?

## Loaded Questions

This type of ill-formed question has a built-in assumption that may be erroneous. In order to provide an answer, the respondent has to embrace the assumption as if it is a reality. Typically, loaded questions elicit defensiveness. Examples of loaded questions include the following:

- Why is this always so hard for you to do?
- What is the matter with you?
- What has to happen for you to stop making excuses?
- Why are you so resistant to me?

## Limited-Option Questions

A question of this sort not only contains embedded assumptions but also limits responses to the options provided, even though these options may not include all the possibilities. In some forms, it is a forced choice in which all answers are potentially incorrect. Examples include the following:

- Would you rather have a green shirt or a red shirt?
- Are you going to run tonight or tomorrow night?
- Do you want to meet Tuesday, Wednesday, or Thursday?
- Which of these activities will you commit yourself to doing this week: running, swimming, or biking?

## Stacked Questions

This form of question is not so much leading or biased as it is confusing. The coach asks several questions at the same time, even though they may be unrelated to one another. The client may not know which question to answer first, or she may answer one and get so involved in her answer that the second question gets lost. Some examples include the following:

- Why do you think you need a coach, and what have you tried in the past to reach your goal?
- What are your main goals, and how long do you imagine we will work together?
- What I'd like to know from you is what motivates you most, what turns you off, what's the longest you've ever exercised regularly, and what is your vision for the future?

## *Why* Questions

For many people, *why* questions come in the context of a perceived interrogation. Parents ask their children, "Why did you do that?" Teachers frequently use *why* questions in trying to get to the bottom of things. By the time we become adults, we may be overly sensitive to *why* questions and react defensively, even though the intent of the questioner may be to help. For this reason, we need to remain aware of the possible effects of this type of question. Defensiveness in response to a *why* question may reflect the rapport between coach and client as much as it does to the type of question. Nonetheless, a safer approach is to use an alternative phrasing. Here are some examples of *why* questions and possible alternatives:

- Why do you want to lose weight? Alternative: What do you imagine the benefits of losing weight would be for you?
- Why do you want to work with me? Alternative: Help me understand your reasons for wanting to work with me.
- Why did you say that? Alternative: I'd like to understand what brought you to say what you just did.

No matter how well you phrase your questions, clients often answer with things they have on their minds, even though these replies may be unrelated to what you have asked. No doubt you have had exchanges similar to the following, in which the question requires a simple answer but the respondent uses the question as an opportunity to tell you something completely different.

**PERSON A:** Where were you last night?

**PERSON B:** Oh, I've been having a rough time in general. Things simply haven't been going well. Last week, I tried to . . .

Here's another example:

**PERSON A:** What time is it?

**PERSON B:** I think it's late. I'd better get moving. I have an appointment at 3.

Some communication theorists (Grinder & Bandler, 1976) propose that the meaning of your communication—or question, in this case—can be discovered in the response you receive from the other person. You may ask about someone's health, and he may tell you all about his family history. When clients are highly motivated to discuss certain things, the question you ask them is almost irrelevant. They will somehow find a way to turn your question into a means of expressing what they want to say.

Careful structuring of questions is essential for effective coaching. If you ask a confusing question and the person gives a seemingly irrelevant reply, you cannot be sure whether the response results from your poorly constructed question or something unique about the client. By contrast, if a client responds with a tangential remark to a well-formed question, the coach will have gained significant, though unexpected, information.

---

**REFLECTION 8.2**

Now would be a good time to listen to the recorded conversation from reflection 8.1. Can you identify the types of questions you asked? Which ones were well-formed questions? Did you use any of the problematic questions we discussed? How else might you have phrased these questions? Did the answers you received correspond to the questions you asked? Were there any types of questions that seemed to create defensiveness? Were there any that increased rapport and flow of information?

---

# STEPS IN QUESTIONING

Guidelines for asking questions may seem obvious. Nonetheless, let us review some steps that you might wish to consider (Cormier et al., 2009):

1. **Understand the purpose of your question.** You may ask questions out of curiosity as long as what you are curious about has a direct link to the client's agenda. Another aspect of this step applies to instances where you ask a question when you already suspect the answer. Using a question to influence a client to make public significant commitments, feelings, or ideas can be important to the coaching process. For instance, a client who schedules an appointment and shows great interest throughout the first session might nonetheless be asked the following question to confirm her commitment to the process.

**COACH:** What I have gathered from your remarks today is that you're committed to working with me for the next six months on the issues that we outlined. Am I correct?

**CLIENT:** Absolutely. I really want to work on this, starting right now!

2. **Determine which type of question best serves your purpose.** Recognizing the various purposes of questioning, do you want to moderate the pace of the session, refocus the conversation, explore an issue, confirm your perception, or look for a simple answer about something? Asking an open question will likely facilitate client expression. If this is what you want to achieve, then you have chosen the right type of question. Asking a closed question will likely provide a specific detail or answer. For instance, let's say your purpose is to have your client dig deeper into an issue and you ask, "Can you tell me more about this?" The question is formed as a closed question, so the answer may be "Yes." This may not be very problematic; it does, however, interrupt the flow of the dialogue. Instead you might ask, "What other things come to your mind in thinking about this issue?"

3. **When possible, embed the question in reflections.** Asking a series of questions without reflecting content or feeling can be intimidating or create distance. Framing the question at the end of a paraphrase or reflection rather than asking question after question is often a wiser strategy to promote comfort and trust. An example of this step would be "You mentioned that you want to add to your program and seem excited about this. I would like to hear what you have in mind."

4. **Evaluate the effects of your question.** Nonverbal cues may provide some appreciation for how people are receiving your questions. Verbally, the response you observe will either meet your intentions or yield new information. When clients use

your question to present information about other topics, you have a choice to either assess through additional questioning whether they understood the question or pursue the topics that they seem energized to discuss. All answers are helpful, even when they do not correspond to the specific questions that you asked.

People have different responses to being questioned, and we need to be sensitive to the timing of client responses. A client may pause for what seems an eternity before answering. If the coach is not in touch with the client's need to reflect, she may forge ahead by asking another question or simply repeating the original question, thereby confusing or pressuring the person. As a general rule, ask the question and pause patiently—a perfect use of silence—until you get a response. Note also that paralinguistic qualities of the client's reply may tell you as much as verbal responses. If the person normally answers quickly but responds only after a long pause to a particular question, you may want to reflect on the potential meaning of this pause.

Another point to bear in mind in the steps of questioning is that clients who have a preference for introversion will likely have a slower response rate than those who are extroverted (Quenck, 2009). Your reaction to these patterns will depend on your own style, that is, introverted or extroverted. Those who tend more toward introversion generally like to reflect and engage in internal self-talk before expressing their opinions; in this respect, their answers to probing questions may come after lengthy pauses. Those who are more extroverted, on the other hand, are likely to respond quickly while thinking aloud. Their responses will probably seem far more spontaneous. If you are extroverted, you may occasionally need to slow down the questioning process. Your own tendency to think aloud and to speak without extensive reflection could run counter to the needs of your clients. If you are introverted, you may have a pattern of reflecting internally on what the person has said before you ask the next question. When working with extroverts, however, you may need to process your thoughts out loud so that these clients can experience continuous engagement in the coaching process.

# UPSIDE OF QUESTIONING

The application of questioning in helping relationships has been widely explored (Anderson & Kil-

lenberg, 2009; Groth-Marnat, 2009; Kenny, Alvarez, Donohue, & Winick, 2008; Sommers-Flanagan & Sommers-Flanagan, 2009; Weiner & Bornstein, 2009). Let us consider the most common uses of questions and the benefits of questioning in coaching.

## Initiating the Relationship

Clients expect coaches to ask them questions about relevant background factors, needs, goals, and preferences. Implicitly, they may have a framework for determining whether a question is within bounds or whether it is probing beyond the legitimate domain of the relationship. For instance, if you ask, "How much money do you make?" the client may respond defensively rather than with a direct answer, because she may consider such information to be peripheral at best to her coaching topic.

## Encouraging Client Communication

In conjunction with active listening, questioning promotes communication. In the early stages of coaching, clients may need direction. They may arrive at the first meeting, smile, and then await your questions. A cycle of communication occurs in most coaching sessions wherein the coach intersperses questions with active listening to engage clients in relevant discussions about their agendas.

## Assessing Client Issues

Questions are invaluable to understanding and assessing issues. Coaches ask questions to explore topics, create new understandings, move clients toward action, and examine perceived limitations. Questions may focus on matters of who, what, where, when, why, and how related to various issues. As you might imagine, a client may be more or less open to questions, depending on the degree of rapport he experiences with his coach. Asking questions that are too pointed or abrupt may affect the quality of the client's responses and the coaching relationship itself.

## Testing Assumptions

Grinder and Bandler (1976) use the term *complex equivalent* to refer to cases in which the same word or phrase has different meanings for people. When someone says, "I was upset," we might assume that we know exactly what that person means because we have been upset at times. Of course, as coaches, we need to check our assumptions and verify the meanings of words and phrases used by the client. Often this process relies on the elicitation of concrete examples: "When you were feeling upset, what exactly did you do?" "What would I have seen had I been observing you in the moment when you were upset?" "How strong was this upset feeling? What would you compare it to?" You would not necessarily ask all these questions, but you would certainly want to pursue a clearer definition of the client's experience in order to obtain a deeper understanding of her communication.

## Expressing Interest

Asking questions can make the coach's keen interest in the client more evident. As noted in the steps in reflecting or summarizing (chapter 7), the last part of the coach's message is usually a question to check accuracy or request elaboration. Questions can be invitations to explore matters mutually (e.g., "Would you be willing to explore some of these issues in greater detail?") or to work together in a process (e.g., "How might I best assist you in your efforts to achieve your goals?"). These types of questions are likely to feel supportive and facilitate progress.

## Discovering Meaning

Questions can be used to probe for deeper meanings. As we discuss in chapter 9, skillful questioning enables clients to go beneath surface understanding to discover concerns that may motivate and direct behavior. A possible exchange in such a discovery process might sound as follows.

**COACH:** You've mentioned that you want to lose 20 pounds and reduce your body fat to 18% during the next six months. These seem to be highly important goals for you. What are you imagining these changes will bring to your life?

**CLIENT:** I'm not sure. I just thought I would look better and probably feel better. But now that you ask, I think part of what this is about for me is that I feel like I don't belong. Most of my friends are fit and athletic and I'm a bit of an oddball in the group . . . you know, the one

who finishes last or does the cooking for the group while they go out for a run.

**COACH:** So, these body-change goals are also about fitting in? Being part of the group rather than being an outsider? Is that what you're saying?

Seeking deeper understanding without implying that anything is wrong, the coach probes through questioning and discovers client needs that can serve either to modify his goals or create energy for his achievement.

## Creating Focus

Questions can be used to focus a client on specific issues. The coach can do this covertly or overtly. By reflecting selected parts of a client's comments and asking questions that draw her into the desired arena of conversation, a coach can covertly shift the focus of the session from broad topics to particular interests that the client might have. A more overt way of using questioning to shift focus involves an explicit announcement by the coach. This might sound as follows.

**COACH:** So far, we have been talking about fitness activities that you've done in the past. I'd like to shift our focus to the future, if that's okay with you. (*Pauses for verbal or nonverbal response.*) If you can imagine yourself one year from now, what activities might you hope to be doing then?

## Controlling the Process

Sometimes clients provide too much information about topics or use the session as a sounding board for a variety of concerns. Coaches can guide them back to the agreed-upon agenda by asking questions. There is a directive quality to this application of questioning (i.e., it represents influencing rather than attending), yet it is fully justified in terms of moving clients efficiently toward their goals. The following intervention is an example of bringing the discussion back into focus without disregarding the content of a digression by the client.

**COACH:** Would you help me understand how these things you have been mentioning in the past few minutes can be applied to the goals you want to achieve in your work with me?

# DOWNSIDE OF QUESTIONING

Questions give life to the coaching process. They engage the client in critical explorations. They generate insights and actions. They provide guidance for the journey. As necessary as questions are, however, coaches must use them judiciously. Caring and supportive questioning has a positive effect on clients, yet no matter how good the questions are, there are limits. Let us review some of the more problematic aspects of questioning.

1. **Overloading with questions.** Clients may be highly compliant in coaching sessions and continue to answer questions even though they experience increasing discomfort. Attention to nonverbal cues is important when asking questions. As mentioned in our discussion of reflection in the previous chapter, we suggest a varied approach to gathering information. Indirect questions may be less intrusive. Moreover, reflection skills may encourage clients to explore issues without your ever asking a question.

2. **Reducing autonomy.** When questioning is one-sided, people are likely to perceive that the person asking the questions is in a position of greater power. When clients are repeatedly on the receiving end of a questioning process, they may eventually abdicate responsibility in the relationship and come to believe that you have all the solutions. In so doing, the client becomes more dependent on you as the coach. A powerful question that returns control to the client might be the following.

**COACH:** I've been asking a lot of questions, and I'm not sure that what I'm asking is as useful as it could be. So, may I approach it this way? What questions would be most helpful for me to ask so that I can best help you achieve your goals?

3. **Privileging the positive.** Coaching is not therapy. It is not problem-focused; yet clients do have issues. If questions are slanted in such a way that only the bright side of the story is sought, clients may come to believe that they always have to shine luminously. Those who might see you as having it all together may be reluctant to share their true feelings, especially when the feelings differ from what they imagine you want to hear. A number of strategies are available if you sense that clients are presenting overly positive, socially acceptable

answers to your questions. As we discuss in chapter 9, self-disclosure or engaging the client in a here-and-now conversation can help ground the relationship in reality rather than in fantasy.

4. **Reinforcing vulnerability.** When two parties disproportionately share information, the person who has shared the most may feel more vulnerable than the other. In friendships, self-disclosures tend to be cyclical in an ever-deepening way; one person's self-disclosure induces the other person to open up (Johnson, 2009). Because of the nature of the relationship, coaches reveal far less of their personal values, beliefs, needs, and history than clients. Predictably, clients may feel vulnerable having exposed so much of their inner stories. Although this feeling of exposure may be inevitable with some people, you need to remain sensitive to the responsibility attached to obtaining extensive information about clients. Clients may need to be reassured that what they have shared with you is acceptable. On occasion, you may wish to level the field through relevant and timely self-disclosures done in the service of forwarding the clients' agenda.

A final caveat concerns levels of intervention. Given that information needs only to be gathered as required for the contracted coaching work, it is best to avoid probing in ways that extend beyond the client's needs and intentions. Though it may seem that the more you know, the more effective your work will be, the philosophy of coaching emphasizes action far more than it does diagnosis and reflection. Put another way, coaching focuses more on the present and future than it does on the past. The future is something that the coach and client cocreate through the coaching relationship. Smith (2007) and Williams and Davis (2007) offer sage advice

> ### REFLECTION 8.3
>
> Return now to the recorded conversation from reflection 8.1. Based on what you have learned from the discussion of the upside and downside of questioning, what can you see more clearly about your questioning strategy? How would you describe the purposes of the questions you asked? What did you intend to explore or discover? Were there any pitfalls in your approach to questioning? What other ways might you have gathered information?

for those who might want to explore deeper levels of the client's world. According to them, effective and ethical helpers gather necessary information to inform their actions with clients while guarding against pursuing deeper understanding for its own sake or for speculative reasons.

# POWERFUL QUESTIONS

As suggested by the title of this ICF core competency, coaches need to not only learn how to ask questions, they also need to master the art of asking powerful questions. The task may seem daunting at first: What is a powerful question? How and when do you ask it? This may come as a surprise, but a powerful question could sound as simple as "How will you do that?" or "What do you want to do?" Isolated from the rich texture of the coaching conversation, such questions seem anything but powerful. However, within the weave of words, the precise timing and sensitive delivery of a simple question can send shockwaves through carefully constructed walls of denial or seemingly hopeless scenarios.

When you listen deeply to what your client is saying and connect all the information, you gain a commanding appreciation of this person's world. Add your own intuition and knowledge to the mix and you have a strong basis for generating powerful questions. When someone tells you he is happy with his life yet continues to express regret about things he feels incapable of doing, it's easy to imagine a question that confronts this apparent contradiction. What would make the question powerful, however, is asking it in a timely fashion and framing it with respect and support. An essential point about powerful questioning is that it is highly dependent on the quality of your listening and the degree to which you have built trust and intimacy in the relationship (see Examples of Powerful Questions).

You are probably still wondering how to acquire the skill of asking powerful questions. Certain forms of questions can create compelling awareness, understanding, and forward movement. Let's take a quick look at seven types of powerful questions (de Jong & Berg, 2002; de Shazer, 1988; Kimsey-House, Kimsey-House, & Snadahl, 2011):

1. Miracle questions
2. Exception questions
3. *What else* questions
4. Scaling questions
5. Resourcefulness questions
6. Relationship questions
7. Presumptive questions

## Miracle Questions

Sometimes people get stuck in their thinking and can't see a way out. If you ask them what they can

## Examples of Powerful Questions

What deeply matters to you?

Where are you going?

When can you do that?

Who's there *just* for you?

What are you passionate about?

What do you think your purpose is in this precious life of yours?

What's your biggest learning from this?

How did you make that happen?

How can you make this happen?

What makes sense to you about this?

What's stopping you from getting what you want?

How are you feeling right now?

What keeps you going?

How can you set that boundary?

How can you let that go?

How are *you* taking care of *you*?

How might you deal with that feeling of_____?

How can you ask for this?

do to move forward, they repeatedly blank out or offer options they know will not work. The miracle question is a way to get beyond this impasse by making a grand assumption that the obstacle has magically dissolved or disappeared. It jettisons the client from her current state into her desired future where she has reached her goal. Miracle questions focus clients not on the road ahead but on an imagined road they have unknowingly taken. This question is shaped in the form of a dreamlike journey with a question such as this: "Imagine that while you were sleeping, a miracle happened and magically removed all barriers and obstacles, and because you were sleeping, you were unaware of what happened. When you woke up, you realized that you made the leap and reached your goal. Your world is different. Be there now. What do you notice that you are doing differently?"

As the client begins to describe her altered reality, she will likely see glimmers of how she got to that place. Projecting her forward gives her a new vantage point from which to observe the obstacles that she currently perceives as being in her way. As you continue to explore with her, she may gain a heightened capacity to look back over her journey to this new reality and appreciate what she needs to do to get there.

## Exception Questions

When we hear the words *never* or *always*, we are likely to think, "What's the exception to that pattern or belief?" There always seems to be an exception to the rule. A client says, "I've never been able to stick with a diet." You reply, "Never?" She pauses and adds, "Well, there was this one time . . ." When clients describe what they have tried in the past to achieve their goals, there is often a sense of inevitability and incapacity. Nothing has ever worked, no matter how hard they tried. Exception questions bring into focus the times when something did in fact work!

Clients may perceive themselves as incapable of doing certain things. "I could never stand up in front of a group and speak my mind," says Jane. The coach asks, "Has there ever been a time when you were with a group of people and you talked to them about your ideas?" And Jane answers, "Well, if you put it that way, of course I've done that! Just last week . . . ." It is true that we do some things better than others and that our talents are not equally distributed. Yet, this is not the same as saying we have

zero capacity in certain areas. You may not have run a marathon, but that doesn't mean you can't.

## *What Else* Questions

The first answer to a question that someone offers may be as far as he has gone in thinking through his options. "Well, I tried meditating to help reduce my blood pressure, and that didn't work!" So, you ask, "What else could you do?" Even when the person produces a lengthy list of alternatives, you may continue to stimulate creativity: "What else comes to mind?" The first answer isn't always the best, and the most promising answer may never emerge if the client stops generating ideas too early in the process.

Sometimes clients wear blinders when it comes to explanations for events in their lives. Over time, they tell the same stories about their experiences and why things happened as they did. This becomes their personal mythology. They lost out on the big job and as a result, things went wildly off in the wrong direction. Or, someone said something about what they were doing and it sounded so critical that they never tried again. Well, what if their interpretation was wrong? They might have to revamp their entire story about their lives. Asking questions such as "What else could have explained that happening?" or "What else could you have done?" may break open locked-in self-beliefs to the degree that clients start experiencing hopefulness and competency for the first time in a particular area.

A special use of the *what else* question can be found in brainstorming, which can be useful as a creative problem-solving method. Brainstorming is a technique that can help individuals or groups generate novel ideas and produce new methods to answer a question or address important issues (see Examples of Brainstorming). A few rules govern the technique of brainstorming:

- Define the question and the time frame; sometimes people are asked to complete a sentence stem to aid in generating new ideas (e.g., I would be happier if . . . ).
- Generate as many answers and ideas as possible in the given time frame.
- Welcome all ideas and record them (no matter how unusual or seemingly unrelated).
- Withhold all comments that imply evaluation or judgment.

## Examples of Brainstorming

Bryan wants to find new motivations to exercise every day. Both he and his coach engage in a brainstorming activity with the coach asking *what else* questions.

**Coach:** Bryan, without taking too much time to think about it, I want you to complete the following sentence stem:"I would want to exercise if . . ."

**Bryan:** I would want to exercise if . . . I had a friend to go with me.

I would want to exercise if . . . my partner came with me.

I would want to exercise if . . . I could see it as time just for me.

I would want to exercise if . . . I got results.

**Coach:** What else?

**Bryan:** I would want to exercise if . . . I had great exercise gear.

I would want to exercise if . . . I could go on a weekend away as a reward.

I would want to exercise if . . . I could do it at lunch.

I would want to exercise if . . . I had a little more time in the morning.

I would want to exercise if . . . my days weren't so stressful.

**Coach:** What else?

**Bryan:** I would want to exercise if . . . my supper were ready when I came back.

I would want to exercise if . . . I had a trainer.

I would want to exercise if . . . I could join that new gym.

I would want to exercise if . . . I had fun doing it.

**Coach:** What else?

This exercise could go on until Bryan completely runs out of new options. Any of the responses to the brainstorm could then be explored and put into action if Bryan thought that he would find motivation in the element he identified.

For further reading on brainstorming, see www.mindtools.com/brainstm.html.

---

- When there are no new ideas or the time is over, look back at all the ideas and combine them to provide a variety of answers to the brainstorming question.

## Scaling Questions

Most of us are accustomed to asking or being asked a question that begins with the words "On a scale of 1 to 10 . . ." In coaching, it is important to appreciate the relative strength of clients' beliefs and experiences. One special application of a scaling question is likely to arise at the end of a session: "On a scale of 1 to 10, how committed are you to successfully completing your action plan this week with 1 being 'absolutely not committed—will not do it' and 10 representing 'I'm gung-ho—I can't wait to get out of here to start'?" Of course, there are other types of scales. You can ask whether your clients strongly agree, strongly disagree, or believe something in

the middle. You can ask where they would place themselves on an undefined scale between the words *competitive* and *noncompetitive*.

Over a series of sessions, if you ask the same scaling question, you can develop a progress chart. Here is an example: "On a scale of 1 to 10, how satisfied are you with what you've accomplished in our session today, with 1 being totally dissatisfied and 10 being extremely satisfied?"

## Resourcefulness Questions

As people, we are often our own worst critics. Some clients may have a bias toward perceiving where they weren't so successful rather than acknowledging the strengths and capacities represented even in failed efforts. A woman tells a story of perseverance against insurmountable odds and focuses on her lack of success. You ask, "What enabled you to continue putting effort into doing this time and time again?" She feels a bit stunned and stammers, "Well, I guess, I, uh. . . ." Coaching empowers people to move forward partly by surfacing unrecognized assets and resources. Asking questions such as the following allows clients to see their deep capacities in spite of the undesired outcomes of their efforts:

- How did you keep going despite all the opposition you were facing from your friends and family?
- What did you do that prevented this situation from getting so much worse than it did?
- How in the world do you manage to cope with all that's on your plate?

## Relationship Questions

When a client is being hard on himself, it can be helpful to ask what others in his world would say about his situation or behavior. Coaches learn over time what their clients' social networks look like and where there is reliable support for the change process. They develop impressions of how others would see their clients in action and can call upon these voices to help them through tough moments. For instance, you might ask, "What do you think your brother would say about your progress to date?" Even when clients hang on tightly to beliefs about their limitations, they are likely to acknowledge that others in their world may have a more objective or fair-minded assessment of the situation. In some cases, you might bring yourself into the picture as the observer. A question such as the following might be asked: "If I had been a fly on the wall while you were learning how to tango, what do you think I would have seen?"

## Presumptive Questions

It is reasonable to assume that after a few sessions, you will have mapped your client's belief system to a degree where you can anticipate how she will respond to certain questions. For instance, you are likely to know whether she has an optimistic or pessimistic bias toward herself and her capacities. A presumptive question bears some similarity to a resourcefulness question, except that it consistently skips a step in order to project the client beyond her limiting beliefs. A woman may habitually describe ways in which she doesn't live up to her own standards. Yet, as her coach, you readily see all the ways in which she generates positive outcomes in

her life. So, you ask, "What's your personal success formula?" The question presumes—without making the presumption explicit—that she has been successful. A variation of this question might be "What personal qualities have enabled you to recommit yourself time after time?" Here, the coach presumes not only that the client has some specific assets but also that she perseveres no matter what. Of course, the use of presumptive questioning requires careful consideration. If you can predict that the person will challenge any assertion that she is better than she thinks she is, you may need to use another approach.

# COMMENTARY

As you pursue your coaching career, you will continue to discover unique ways to access pivotal aspects of clients' stories that will be insight provoking and empowering. What we have reviewed in this chapter and the previous are some enduring ways of helping people to overcome self-limiting perceptions and other blockages to growth. We have focused on fundamental coaching competencies that facilitate client openness and exploration while providing necessary support and guidance. As experienced professionals, we might occasionally assume that we accurately understand what a client is saying because we think we hear his words and because we have so much background against which to appreciate his remarks. In the previous chapter we discussed how active listening allows the coach to verify information through the use of reflections; we not only hear the client's words, we feed them back for a kind of validity check. Yet, active listening doesn't always get to the point as quickly as needed. From this perspective, questions are essential.

A blend of inquiry and reflection stimulates imagination and momentum throughout the coaching process. A key principle to bear in mind is that listening and questioning become detrimental to progress when they are used mechanically or without full awareness of their effects. In this respect, these competencies rely heavily on your coaching presence for their power. When you are fully engaged—mind, body, and spirit—your reflections and questions will feed disclosure, build intimacy and trust, and inform the path forward.

# 9

# DIRECT COMMUNICATION

## *I*n this chapter, you will learn how…

- feedback enables clients to reorient themselves and pursue their path forward with greater intelligence and awareness;

- confrontations sound severe, yet they actually represent compassionate ways of bringing clients toward greater commitment and self-appreciation;

- self-disclosure has many forms, all of which are strategically intended rather than personally motivated;

- immediacy as a coaching skill is a potent method for connecting with the client in the here and now; and

- information, instructions, and advice may seem simple and obvious, yet they can influence clients in unpredictable ways.

> Why would we resist the powerful visions and futures that emerge when we come together to cocreate the world?
>
> —*Margaret Wheatley*

Listening actively to clients' stories is essential. Yet the magic of coaching arises from the synergy of two people cocreating a new and more desirable future from old stories that might no longer be useful. The client comes into the coaching relationship with a strong desire to change and the coach acts as a catalyst in this process of transformation. A rich chemistry emerges when both willingly combine their energies in service of the client's agenda.

Unlike some other processes of helping, coaches neither dominate nor disappear in a coaching relationship. They do not unilaterally dictate actions or interventions, nor do they passively observe their clients fumbling through the darkness. Coaches have their own histories, wisdom, and personal insights that are different from those of their clients. In this chapter, we move into a more challenging domain where the coach becomes more visible. Direct communication is the final competency listed under the ICF theme of communicating effectively. It requires that coaches voice their ideas, perceptions, and insights. In contrast to active listening and powerful questioning, the coach's character and style take the foreground in dialogues where direct communication occurs. The underlying assumption is that clients are strong enough to accept or reject the perspectives the coach offers.

According to the ICF (2011c), the seventh core coaching competency of direct communication is the ability to communicate effectively during coaching sessions and to use language that has the greatest positive impact on the client. A coach who uses this skill effectively

- is clear, articulate, and direct in sharing and providing feedback;
- reframes and articulates to help the client understand from another perspective what she wants or is uncertain about;
- clearly states coaching objectives, meeting agenda, purpose of techniques, or exercises;
- uses language appropriate and respectful to the client (e.g., nonsexist, nonracist, nontechnical, nonjargon); and
- uses metaphor and analogy to help to illustrate a point or paint a verbal picture.

International Coach Federation 2011

In the lexicon of the helping professions, direct communication moves unequivocally into what has been traditionally known as the realm of influencing skills (Cormier et al., 2009; Ivey et al., 2010). A distinguishing characteristic of direct communication is that messages are conveyed by the coach; they potentially reveal as much about him as they do about the client. Direct communication implies that you speak directly to issues arising in clients' stories from a stance that is well thought out, personal, and tailored to the client's language. There is a quality of telling or informing clients about something with the intention of moving them toward their stated objectives. Coaching is a partnership, so there is nothing dictatorial about direct communication. There is, however, a shift in the relationship when you as the coach offer an opinion or observation that represents far more than mirroring what the client has said. In fact, you might be quite challenging to your clients in what you say through direct communication.

This chapter explores coaching interventions that intentionally deconstruct old views and perceptions of reality in order to create the foundation for a more viable and satisfying future. For lifestyle wellness coaches, this form of communication requires skillful application since it may prove rather automatic for some health, wellness, and fitness professionals to offer their expertise without reflection. As is true of all coaching processes, direct communication relies on your capacity to use language that is respectful of clients, their unique personalities, their cultural heritage, and their coaching agendas.

In discussing direct communication, we will first address the process of giving feedback. We will then explore the matter of confrontation and how it can motivate change. We will also take time to review self-disclosure, where coaches reveal aspects of their stories in service of clients' topics. We will then move to a discussion of immediacy, or here-and-now dialogue, that focuses on what is happening in the moment within the coaching relationship. Finally, we will consider direct input that can take the forms of advice, suggestions, and information.

# FEEDBACK

**Feedback** is an effective way of increasing clients' awareness of their behaviors and motivating them toward desired change. It is a process of providing people with specific data on how you see and experience them.

## Purposes of Feedback

The term *feedback* is associated with the field of cybernetics, where information is fed into a system to ensure the correction of processes directed toward achieving certain outcomes (Fradkov, 2007). With the advance of technology, most systems have built-in autoregulating devices so that when undesirable deviations from ideal performance occur, a feedback-initiated, self-correcting process begins. In the realm of human behavior (Carver & Scheier, 2010), feedback is a useful tool to bring something to a client's attention so that he might become aware of an area of needed change. It is also valuable to reinforce a behavior that is producing effective results. Unfortunately, feedback may occur only sporadically and be poorly done. Consider job performance evaluations. A manager may ignore important behaviors for a long time before suddenly confronting an employee with overwhelming evidence of ineffective performance and placing the person on probation or firing him. The need for timely and effective feedback processes is critical to success in most endeavors.

# Guidelines for Giving Feedback

There is strong consensus regarding guidelines for feedback in helping relationships (Brammer & MacDonald, 2003; DeForest, Largent, & Steinberg, 2005; Trotzer, 2006; Young, 2009). We will explore these guidelines with the perspective of coaching in mind. Some guidelines are discussed separately in this section, and others are integrated into the next section on steps in providing feedback.

1. **Feedback is about the behavior, not the person.** Most important, giving feedback in coaching is about highlighting behaviors that hinder clients from achieving their desired goals; it is never about the person or her character. Character assessments, such as "You just don't seem motivated," are inappropriate, poorly constructed, and potentially damaging; they do not constitute appropriate feedback. Clients might present patterns that are not advantageous to realizing their dreams (e.g., a shy executive has great difficulty making presentations to groups). In some instances, certain character attributes might push your buttons (e.g., a client consistently demonstrates a negative attitude to the world in general). If you say someone is smart or lazy or kind or generous or wild, you usually have inferred these character assessments from actions or verbal behaviors. Someone may overeat in certain situations or even most of the time, but this does not mean that he is a glutton.

Giving feedback to clients must not only focus on their behavior, it must also be offered when, and only when, it can be linked to their coaching agenda. For example, feedback to the shy client might sound like "I have noticed that you frequently speak in a barely audible voice and don't look at me as you are talking. I wonder how these patterns might show up when you are speaking to groups in your organization." Feedback to the pessimistic client might sound like "You keep saying that the whole world is going to hell in a handbasket . . . I wonder how this expression fits into your intention to be a source of positive energy for others."

2. **Feedback is most effective when the client asks for it or, at a minimum, consents to it.** When someone asks for feedback, she is more likely to accept responsibility for what she hears, even though she may not entirely agree with it. In coaching, feedback must never be imposed without consent even though it might have been part of the initial agreement as a way of working together. Cli-

ents who are surprised by the delivery of feedback in a session may feel emotionally unprepared and consequently resist your messages even when they are valid. Practically speaking, you are not always able to await clients' invitations to offer feedback. For this reason, you need to remind clients about their contract concerning feedback, and check for their continuing agreement.

3. **Feedback needs to focus on what clients can control.** There are things we can change and things we can't. Feedback must address issues that the client perceives as being under his control, that is, matters that are changeable and relevant to his goals. A person may be able to alter his response to a stressor, but he cannot change the fact that someone he loves is ill. He may be able to modify his lifestyle, but he cannot reverse his genetic composition.

4. **Feedback must not convey judgment.** When offering feedback, you might sometimes be motivated by a certain disappointment with your clients. Indeed, when you invest yourself heavily in your coaching relationships, you might take client behaviors personally. When emotions become caught up in the feedback, words and nonverbal messages can convey disapproval or rejection. This kind of feedback is inappropriate. Although at times it may be difficult, words that are evaluative, such as *good*, *bad*, *right*, or *wrong*, must be avoided. When you cannot easily contain your feelings and judgments, you may wish to seek supervision or speak with colleagues who can help defuse your excess emotional charge through compassionate and empathic listening.

5. **Feedback takes time.** Giving someone praise does not take much time. These joyful expressions are not what most of these guidelines concern. Feedback involving behavior that has deviated from its intended path or interactions that weaken the working relationship will likely take more time. Thus, feedback must be scheduled so that it does not occur at the end of a session, unless it is highly contained and unlikely to evoke defensiveness or emotional reactivity.

# Steps in Giving Feedback

The guidelines just discussed provide general parameters for giving feedback. The following steps will steer you through the process.

1. **Frame the feedback in small, clear units.** Even with praise, human beings seem to have a

limited capacity to absorb feedback effectively. For this reason, you need to organize your feedback to address the most critical issues in a timely manner and offer it in proportions that the client can digest. Feedback must be offered in small, coherent doses; it must be specific and focused. Often in feedback discussions, one of the parties may try to capitalize on the conversation by broadening the agenda, saying, "Well, since I'm telling you about this, I might as well tell you about that." Alternatively, the person receiving the feedback may use this opening in a defensive manner as a channel for voicing previously unexpressed complaints. Making a clear contract for the boundaries of feedback can control reactions that could easily snowball into an all-out defensive argument. In agreeing to a feedback dialogue, you and your client need to delineate terms so that you will address only an identified agenda—a specific issue—and thoroughly debrief it. You may acknowledge other topics arising during the feedback and schedule them for a future time.

2. **Collaboratively agree on the time and scope of the feedback.** Coaches and clients might initially agree to periodic feedback discussions in which identified topics frame the discussions and for which both parties come prepared with observations and data. When emergent or unanticipated issues surface, the client must be fully in accord with the decision to partake in a feedback discussion. To make this decision intelligently, he needs to know the exact parameters of the feedback, including the nature of the topic to be covered. Furthermore, he needs to understand that although this feedback may bring to mind issues he might have with you as his coach, he needs to contain the discussion to the agreed-upon agenda. As previously noted, you and your client can set up a date for further feedback that arises from this agenda.

3. **Target the behavior, not the person.** Coaches need to express their messages in a supportive manner with humility and nonattachment. A cardinal rule of feedback is that it represents the giver's interpretation of the receiver's behavior, not an unarguable truth. Therefore, it does not have to be accepted by the person receiving it. Feedback must be concrete and offered in a manner that can readily be validated; otherwise it may provoke reactivity and defensiveness. Specificity as to time, place, and circumstances increases the effectiveness of the feedback (see Examples of Feedback Mes-

## Examples of Feedback Messages

Compare the examples of poorly phrased feedback with those of well-phrased feedback to appreciate the effective use of this skill.

| Poorly phrased feedback | Well-phrased feedback |
|---|---|
| You're always late for our sessions. | I've noted that in each of our last four meetings you have been 10 to 20 minutes late. I'd like to discuss this with you. |
| I think you're fantastic. You've improved so much! | As you said you would, you went to bed at a regular time 6 days this past week—between 11:00 and 11:15 p.m. You are now getting an average of 7 hours sleep every night. |
| I know you're trying hard, but you're just not doing enough to reach your goals. | I can see by your record that you wrote every day. What concerns me, though, is the amount of time you spend writing—between 15 and 20 minutes. Would you be open to discussing this? |
| I can tell that you're going to succeed. You show every indication of being a success story. | I feel so hopeful for you. Here's what tells me you're likely to reach your goals: You've met or exceeded every target we've set for your nutritional intake. You have followed the walking schedule exactly as we agreed last month, and . . . |

sages). When you keep records of times or behaviors relevant to feedback discussions, you can produce these for your clients to review and consider.

This step also implies that clients' accomplishments, strengths, or assets will be equally acknowledged, especially when the feedback points to unproductive patterns. Clients may try, try, try, and never succeed. Or they may have excuses for every occasion when they did not reach the target. In the mix of problematic behaviors and good intentions, clients' strong points must be highlighted. Sometimes just showing up for the session is the strength, even when agreed-upon actions were neglected.

4. **Express feedback in the client's frame of reference.** Especially when providing technical feedback, remarks must be worded in a language that the client will readily comprehend. Moreover, when working with people from diverse backgrounds, you need to be sensitive to the norms for feedback within clients' cultural heritages or value structures.

5. **Relate feedback to the agreed-upon coaching agenda.** Feedback needs to serve clients' agendas. Even when clients engage in behaviors that are mildly annoying, their idiosyncrasies can only serve as the basis for feedback if they are related to the contracted agenda. For instance, someone may have an annoying pattern of giggling at periodic intervals. This behavior may suggest some personal issues that he may want to address in future work, but it may not be part of the agreed-upon coaching contract. Whatever feedback you provide must be linked to the coaching agenda. Even when you assume that the client will understand how feedback is pertinent, you need to verify if this is the case.

6. **Create opportunities for clarifications.** Some feedback may lead to emotional reactions. Though emotions can motivate us to pay closer attention, they can also cause us to distort messages, overemphasize certain themes, or misconstrue meanings intended by the speaker. A good practice to incorporate in feedback discussions is asking the client to paraphrase your feedback before discussing it. If this does not occur, the ensuing conversation may be skewed and contentious because the client may have thought he heard something that you either did not say or did not intend in the way he interpreted it. A secondary advantage of paraphrasing here is that in the process of paraphrasing, the client may release some of the emotional charge that could have been building during the feedback. Essentially, this practice slows things down.

Some clients may resist when you ask them to paraphrase your feedback. When that happens, such paraphrasing is more likely to be essential. One interpretation of this resistance is that some part of the feedback has triggered the client emotionally, causing him to have a distorted understanding of the communication. Both coach and client can use paraphrasing or a combination of reflection of content and reflection of feeling to avoid misunderstandings and prevent the discussion from spiraling into an argument.

7. **Request client response to feedback.** Once you are sure that the client has received the intended feedback message, encourage her to offer thoughts, feelings, or behavioral evidence relevant to the matter. Create ample opportunity for clients to describe any reactions related to the feedback and even to reject entirely what you have offered. Following their response, you might paraphrase the client's messages before offering any new input.

8. **Bring feedback to closure through mutual agreement.** The discussion ends when both parties believe they have said what they needed to say. The optimal results of feedback are that both you and your client have reached new understandings about how you can work together more effectively and how the client can better direct action toward his agenda.

## Upside of Providing Feedback

Feedback is essential to effective coaching. In this section, we review its contributions to the coaching relationship.

### Feedback Motivates Behavior

As Skinner (1938) demonstrated, giving people positive reinforcement for specific behaviors increases the chances that they will continue to perform those behaviors. Praise, compliments, awards, prizes, public recognition, and meeting personally defined targets are all examples of feedback. Certain benchmarks for behavior are needed to provide feedback. When clients are working toward goals through reliable adherence to a program, intermittent feedback about their successes can be highly motivating. For instance, although someone may ultimately wish to lose 30 pounds, significant weight reduction is unlikely to occur in the initial weeks of a weight management program. Giving this client feedback about adhering to agreements and actions may motivate him to continue in lieu of the direct evidence (weight loss) that he is seeking.

## Feedback Minimizes Errors

On some highways, rumble strips on the shoulders vibrate the wheels of vehicles, making a loud noise when drivers inadvertently veer out of lane. This kind of feedback is an effective mechanism for error correction, causing the driver to steer back into her lane and pay better attention to her driving. When clients engage in a coaching relationship, they often need feedback about how well they are doing in relation to their stated objectives. Some feedback can be codetermined so that you as the coach do not take the role of judge or police, reporting infractions back to your clients.

## Feedback Stimulates Joint Problem Solving

When goals are unclear or experimental methods are used to achieve objectives, feedback may center on the fact that the goal was not reached or that the process was ineffective. For instance, a client might be using a nicotine patch to quit smoking. The person may religiously apply the patch, yet this process alone doesn't produce the desired result. Feedback discussions can help clarify reasons for success or failure and provide guidance toward more productive solutions. In this respect, you and your clients assume the role of investigators endeavoring to unravel a particular obstacle to success; it is a collaborative rather than an antagonistic relationship.

## Feedback Promotes Understanding and Learning

Sometimes you won't know what hinders you from goal attainment until you take action and encounter the emerging obstacles. Actions planned in some coaching sessions may be designed as much to produce information and experience as they are to achieve specific results. Predicting the future is hard; it is difficult to see around the corners of change processes when they take you to places you have never been before. Clients' reaching their goals is not just about results. It is also about their learning and incorporating new skills that can have multiple applications in their lives. An encounter with what clients might interpret as failure may simply represent the discovery of something they needed to learn. Like Thomas Edison, who viewed each failure to invent a functioning light bulb as the successful discovery of yet another way not to do it,

you can help clients view failure as an exciting way to learn. Such an approach allows them to zigzag along uncharted routes where learning adventures abound and where the goal, although getting ever closer, is no more valuable than learning and growth on the path of progress.

# Downside of Giving Feedback

As essential as quality feedback is to promoting client progress, coaches may occasionally misuse feedback. Examining problematic aspects of feedback might produce deeper understanding of its appropriate design and application.

1. **Feedback as subterfuge for complaint.** Feedback must be carefully formulated within the parameters of the coaching relationship and its legitimate agendas. When you feel irritated by a client, when personality clashes occur, or when countertransference arises in unconscious ways, you may erroneously use feedback to criticize or to vent feelings. Being clear about your reasons for giving feedback and following the steps for providing it will help keep you on solid professional ground.

2. **Feedback that promotes client dependency.** One of the problems with the use of punishment (Skinner, 1938) as a behavior control strategy is that the recipient often has difficulty separating the punishment from the punisher. Similarly, when you reward someone, especially with praise and compliments, the recipient might have difficulty distinguishing the feedback from you, the person providing it. In this regard, clients may come to value the source of praise and then try to please you in order to experience new rewards. When they have few sources of praise in their lives, they may become highly reliant on you and your generosity in providing compliments. Ultimately, clients need to become capable of appropriately assessing their behaviors and being generous with self-rewards. The more factual and data-based your feedback is, the more likely it is that your clients will experience it as justified and originating in their own behaviors rather than resulting from your subjective feelings.

3. **Feedback in the face of counterdependency.** Sometimes clients need to experience their own trial-and-error process, and they may be resistant to the voice of one who suggests what to do. In fact, a client may have an ingrained pattern of resisting anyone who tries to suggest changes in his behavior. In the lingo of social science, the client may

be **counterdependent** (Bennis & Shepard, 1956), meaning that he becomes oppositional when others, especially those in perceived roles of authority, try to influence him. You can become trapped with a client in a vicious cycle of offering and rejecting ideas for change. The client may experience your feedback as an attempt to control him. Ironically, although the client is paying you to tell him what you see, this embedded pattern of resistance may emerge whenever you do so. Should this pattern continue to emerge, the viability of the coaching relationship may come into question.

## REFLECTION 9.1

To practice the skill of feedback, we invite you to engage in this two-part experiment:

1. Ask two people, a friend and a work colleague, if they would be willing to provide feedback on your behavior—separately, of course. You need to clearly specify the behavior you are seeking feedback about (e.g., "Please give me feedback about the way I greet people I have never met before"). The behavior needs to be the same for both observers. Remember that your friend and colleague may not have been trained in the art of providing feedback, so once the feedback has occurred, the only appropriate response is to thank them for their help in this task. Now, answer these questions: How did you feel when you received the feedback? What impact did it have on you? What did you like about it? What did you not like about it? What style of communication was evident in the feedback? How did it conform to the guidelines for providing feedback? What were the differences you experienced in receiving feedback from a friend versus a colleague? What implications can you draw from this experience?

2. The second part is to ask another friend or colleague if you can provide (positive) feedback on a specific behavior of theirs. Frame your feedback according to the guidelines and steps described previously. How did you choose the object of your feedback? What was its purpose? How was it received? What might you have done differently? What did you learn from this experience? How might positive feedback influence your coaching clients?

# CONFRONTATION

The term **confrontation** may sound harsh, as if it involves conflict and emotionally charged encounters. For some, it suggests hostility. Indeed, these elements are possible, but they are not the predominant meaning of confrontation as a coaching skill. The essence of confrontation is bringing discrepancies in a client's messages to the client's awareness. Such messages require delicacy and extreme sensitivity to the client's readiness to address incongruities. Confrontation has been referred to as *articulating* in some of the coaching literature (Kimsey-House et al., 2011), with the suggestion that the coach may need to present the hard truth in responding to the client's verbal and nonverbal messages.

Another expression that has been used as a substitute for confrontation is *challenging* (Schneider, 2008). The coach challenges certain aspects of the client's communications and thought patterns. Challenges in coaching are different than what is often implied in the health, wellness, and fitness fields, where challenging a person is more likely to be associated with efforts to motivate, raise the bar, or engage the individual in a competitive venture. One way in which confrontation and challenging have more congruent meanings is in the case where a coach challenges a client positively by noting the discrepancy between her potential and actual behavior. In so doing, this challenging confrontation may motivate the person to perform at higher levels (Gladding, 2009).

## Purposes of Confrontation

Confrontation may be one of the more difficult competencies to master in coaching. Effective confrontation is based on keen observation of client messages and behaviors over time. When important discrepancies or inconsistencies are observed, coaches may choose to use confrontation in order to explore aspects of thinking, emotions, or behavior that clients might otherwise overlook (Adler & Myerson, 1991). Confrontations can build trust rather than breach rapport (James & Gilliland, 2003); indeed, confronting issues is often necessary to foster forward movement. However, this must be done with care and empathy and in a manner that steers clear of judgment.

Confrontation needs to be aligned with the goals of the relationship. Evidence suggests that confrontation can help people "see more clearly what is happening, what the consequences are, and how they can assume responsibility for taking action to change in ways that can lead to a more effective life and better and fairer relationships with others" (Tamminen & Smaby, 1981, p. 42). Failing to confront clients on important issues may inhibit their success.

Confrontation enables clients to see themselves differently and come to greater self-acceptance (Kottler, 2010; Prochaska & Norcross, 2010). Egan (2010) associates this purpose with helping people gain greater awareness of blind spots. Clients may be missing certain pieces of information about their behavior or thought processes, and through a confrontation they may become more cognizant of their way of being in the world. For example, clients with body-image issues may choose goals based on distorted perceptions of themselves. Other clients may have inaccurate views of their commitment; they may overestimate their efforts and consequently feel disappointed with their results.

Most theorists (Chang, Scott, & Decker, 2009; Gladding, 2009; Kottler & Shepard, 2011) consider the identification of discrepancies as paramount in confrontation. Clients may show inconsistencies in words and actions; their words may differ either from their actions or from other words they express. Studies of human behavior (Argyris, 1970; Argyris & Schön, 1974) suggest that people tend to be inconsistent partly because of lack of feedback. Argyris and Schön describe this as differences between our **espoused theory of action** (what we say we do) and our **theory in use** (what we actually do). We have certain beliefs and values, yet our actions may fail to match what we believe. According to this perspective, healthy people respond appropriately to evidence that confronts them with their inconsistencies. They take action to bring behaviors in line with their values and beliefs. Coaching relationships are premised on the assumption that people who seek coaching are both able and willing to function in mature, responsible, and mentally healthy ways. Confronting coaching clients with incongruities, discrepancies, distortions, or other forms of inconsistency may be difficult, but when done skillfuly, confrontations will most likely yield positive results.

## Types of Confrontation

There are many forms of mismatched messages. To understand confrontation better, it may help to examine various types of mixed messages and how these can be addressed through the skill of confrontation (Fitzpatrick, Moye, Hoste, Lock, & Le Grang, 2010; Hackney & Cormier, 2009).

### Inconsistent Verbal and Nonverbal Messages

The person describes certain reactions or feelings, yet nonverbal communications suggest other meanings.

**CLIENT EXAMPLE:** A client describes his job as challenging and fun, yet the more he talks about it, the more he bites his lips, furrows his brow, and clenches his fists—all signs of discomfort and anxiety.

**COACH'S CONFRONTATION:** "You say your job is fun and challenging, and the more you talk about it, the more I see tightness in your face and your fists clenching."

### Inconsistencies Between Two or More Verbal Messages

The client makes one statement at one time and a contradictory statement at another.

**CLIENT EXAMPLE:** In the first session, the client says that his family totally supports his new commitment to be healthy, but in the third session, he mentions that his partner has been complaining about the time he spends at the gym.

**COACH'S CONFRONTATION:** "When we began our work, I remember you saying that your family totally supported your training, and now I'm hearing that your partner is complaining about the time you spend at the gym. Would you be willing to explore this with me?"

### Inconsistencies Between What the Client Describes and Circumstances

A client voices certain thoughts, wishes, or aspirations, yet her circumstances represent either insurmountable obstacles or conditions that contradict her words.

**CLIENT EXAMPLE:** A client who is planning to make a big leap into self-employment says that she is going to buy a new car in anticipation of her future success. You know that the job transition will involve at least a temporary reduction in earnings and that she currently has little discretionary income and only modest savings.

**COACH'S CONFRONTATION:** "I hear your excitement about your future and the idea of buying a new car. Based on other things you've said, I am wondering how the new car idea fits into your present financial state and the projected decline in your earnings as you make this job transition."

### Inconsistencies Between Words and Actions

What the client says differs significantly from how he acts.

**CLIENT EXAMPLE:** A client says he simply doesn't have time to cook the meals he agreed to prepare, yet he keeps talking about all the sports he watches on TV every night.

**COACH'S CONFRONTATION:** "May I check out something that I've heard? (*Pauses for agreement.*) You just told me that you don't have enough time to prepare the meals you agreed to cook for yourself, yet each day you said you watch about 3 hours of TV. Can you help me understand how these statements fit together?"

### Inconsistencies Between Two or More Nonverbal Messages

The client exhibits two contradictory or opposite nonverbal communications.

**CLIENT EXAMPLE:** A client massages a previously injured calf muscle while grinning at her coach after a tough training session.

**COACH'S CONFRONTATION:** "I'm aware of you smiling at me and I also see you rubbing that calf muscle you injured a while back. Is there something happening that I should know about?"

## Steps in Confrontation

Pointing out discrepancies to clients is no doubt easier when evidence shows they are doing far better than they say. Such confrontations may build client self-efficacy and increase rapport. For instance, indicating that a person's program adherence is much better than she perceives is likely to generate positive feelings and renewed commitment. In some of the examples just described, however, confrontation could create tension in the relationship. More optimistically, even when they concern difficult matters, confrontations can make the relationship more genuine.

People may do better when they discover their own inconsistencies rather than having them repeatedly identified by others. When they hear themselves verbalizing inconsistent thoughts or feelings, chances are that they will catch themselves delivering discrepant messages. The active listening skills reviewed in chapter 7 offer nonconfrontational ways of aiding clients in hearing themselves. In many respects, a delicately delivered confrontation might sound like a simple reflection of content or a summarizing response, and clients may not even realize that they have been confronted. Instead, they get to discover, through the coach's paraphrasing, the incongruity of their messages..

When applying the skill of confrontation, you may wish to follow the structure suggested here. These steps have been modified from a number of sources for the role of lifestyle wellness coach (Cormier et al., 2009; Ivey et al., 2010; Kottler, 2008; Shebib, 2010).

1. **Gather information.** The role of coach requires awareness and sensitivity. Although coaches are not responsible for keeping extensive data related to all of a client's actions, they may keep pertinent records of sessions that include information regarding client commitments and progress.

2. **Assess relevancy and timing.** When inconsistencies or incongruities relevant to the coaching agenda occur, a confrontation might be useful. It is important to ensure that the relationship has been sufficiently well established. In some of the examples provided earlier, confrontation was immediate. However, this is not always appropriate. The coach may gather information and wait to surface issues either when the inconsistency recurs or when it seems timely to do so.

3. **Formulate a nonjudgmental message with specific data.** Messages about inconsistencies may be difficult for clients to digest. To ease the process, your wording must in no way imply judgment or blame. Moreover, the more objective, factual, and nonemotional the message, the easier it will be for clients to hear it. You may have noted in some of the earlier examples that the coach simply stated the discrepant information without a conclusion and then invited the client into a discussion.

4. **Request client permission.** Coaches may assume that they have chosen a good time to offer a confrontational message, yet they cannot be certain. In addition, clients may be aware of their own inconsistencies

and simply not want to address them. Just as when delivering feedback, enlisting the client's permission to discuss the topic is crucial. When clients accept responsibility for the discussion, they are less likely to close it down abruptly. You may want to headline the topic so that the client has a clear idea about the matter to which she is agreeing.

5. **Encourage client discussion.** Similar to feedback, confrontation takes time. In some instances, the client may only need to acknowledge the discrepancy and integrate this awareness in a continuing dialogue. For instance, when someone says her experience was positive but looks pained in describing it, she may simply hear the confrontation, acknowledge it, and express more fully her feelings about the experience. When a confrontation runs counter to the client's strongly voiced desires, such as the case where the client wants to buy a new car in the face of impending income reductions, the coach may need to encourage further discussion while making sure to handle defensive reactions

constructively. Coaching dialogue 9.1 offers an example of a confrontational exchange.

6. **Connect the confrontation to the client's agenda.** If the client is unclear about the reasons why certain discrepancies are being pointed out, the coach will need to highlight their relevance. Of course, if the client denies, discredits, or refuses to address the matter, another approach will probably be necessary. In these instances, you will have the challenging task of dealing with the client's readiness to be coached on this topic.

7. **Codetermine implications for the future.** When the issues addressed in the confrontation warrant it, the concluding segment of the discussion should concern not only implications for the current coaching goals but also how this information might affect future ways of working together. For instance, if a client falsely reports information about program adherence and the coach confronts him with this fact, what will need to occur in order to reestablish trust?

---

## COACHING DIALOGUE 9.1
# CONFRONTATION AS VALUE CLARIFICATION

Clients sometimes make requests that if taken at face value might deprive them of the opportunity to dig below the surface and uncover damaging patterns. As coaches, we are committed to forwarding the client's agenda through the effective use of skills meant to uncover limiting beliefs and assumptions. In the following example, the coach uses confrontation to uncover a client's underlying motivations.

### Background Information

Laura is a 46-year-old woman who has been involved in a coaching process for four months. Her original goals were to work on her body image, self-esteem, and energy levels through regular daily activities: self-affirmations, journaling, and yoga exercises. In discussions with her coach, she determined that improving her body image through the exercises she had chosen would probably make her feel better about herself. At the beginning of this session, she mentions to her coach that she wants to reduce her coaching sessions for financial reasons. A while later in the session, she mentions that she has started going for weekly massages; she also notes that she has scheduled some elective cosmetic surgery.

### Coaching Dialogue

**Coach:** Laura, I've been hearing some things from you today that I believe would be important for us to discuss further. Would that be okay with you?

**Laura:** I guess. What do you mean?

**Coach:** It's hard to headline it without getting into it. It pertains to some of the decisions you've announced today. I imagine it will take about 10 minutes for both of us to look at the issues. This would help me to know what direction we're heading in.

**Laura:** Okay, go ahead.

**Coach:** I want you to feel as much in charge of this discussion as I am, so let's take it step by step. You can let me know if you're still okay with it as we go along.

**Laura:** Yeah, great.

**Coach:** You mentioned that you found our work together to be really important, yet you want to cut back our sessions to once every three weeks because of the cost.

**Laura:** Yeah, that's right. I simply can't afford it every week anymore.

**Coach:** I can understand the economics of coaching. Doing this work is a financial investment. I appreciate your commitment to the sessions and the activities we codesigned.

**Laura:** Thanks, it's really good . . . although doing yoga is still hard for me.

**Coach:** I realize that and I've also seen steady improvement in your energy levels.

**Laura:** That's true. I do feel better physically and I feel better about myself.

**Coach:** Great! (*Pauses*) You also mentioned going for weekly massages starting a couple weeks ago and that you want to schedule some optional surgery, which you said will be expensive.

**Laura:** (*Slightly defensive*) What are you getting at?

**Coach:** I'm trying to understand the choices you just described in relation to how important you say this coaching experience is for you. From my side, I'm not sure at this time whether a coaching session every three weeks would support you very well in your goals.

**Laura:** Well, I like getting a regular massage. It feels good, especially with the stressful job I have.

**Coach:** I couldn't agree with you more. A good massage can be important in reducing stress.

**Laura:** Yeah, well, I know that it costs money, too, but I need it.

**Coach:** No doubt that's why you've decided to do it. Makes sense to me.

**Laura:** Okay, so this surgery thing is definitely going to cost a lot of money, and I need to budget for that.

**Coach:** Uh-huh. Elective surgery is expensive.

**Laura:** (*Defensively*) Why do you say "elective"? I really need to do this.

**Coach:** So, you believe you need to do this, and my saying "elective" didn't land well?

**Laura:** No, it didn't. Daily affirmations, journaling, and yoga have helped, but I need something that's guaranteed to make me feel better about myself—right now!

**Coach:** So, the activities are helping but you're not getting to feel better about yourself fast enough—and you think surgery will give you a guaranteed, fast change. Is this it?

**Laura:** Yes, well, maybe. . . . I'm not entirely sure, but I think so. (*Pauses*) Maybe I'm just doing my old thing.

**Coach:** What "old thing" is that?

**Laura:** You know. I talked about it at the beginning. If I don't see results right away, I look for a quick fix. (*Pauses*) I think I'm doing that again.

**Coach:** So, surgery may be a quick fix?

**Laura:** Yeah, I think so. . . . Maybe I shouldn't act so impulsively. Maybe I need to think this through some more.

**Coach:** Well, you seem to be slowing it down right now and thinking about it. I'd like to add that whatever you do is entirely up to you. You're in charge. From my point of view, I needed to understand better what was happening, and I needed to let you know that a reduction in coaching could affect your results.

**Laura:** You had every right to ask, and I thank you for bringing it up.

**Coach:** You're welcome, and I thank you for allowing the space for our discussion. We've spent about 10 minutes, as I thought we might, so I'd like to ask you how you'd like to continue the session from here.

# UPSIDE AND DOWNSIDE OF CONFRONTATION

Relationships will stall interminably unless pivotal issues are confronted. We all have experienced the elephant in the room that no one wants to talk about and that blocks any progress. Yet, with all of the benefits it can provide, confrontation is not always warranted. It can backfire even when the coach's intention is to improve the climate of the relationship and facilitate goal attainment. Some clients may prefer to avoid the truth, hide out, and attempt to engage the coach in a process of collusion. As in the story of the emperor's new clothes, some clients may find it easier to have the coach pretend along with them rather than live in reality. Let's explore some problematic applications of confrontation.

1. **Confronting peripheral matters.** What is the client's topic? You may be highly skillful and have evidence that is entirely accurate, yet unless issues relate to the coaching contract, confronting them is likely to be out of bounds. When the coach implicitly

broadens the agreed-upon agenda by confronting matters that have only indirect relevance to the stated goals, there is reason for concern.

2. **Unsubstantiated confrontations.** Some approaches to coaching recommend speaking spontaneously from your intuition, or, as the technique is described, *blurting* whatever you authentically believe to be happening in the moment (Whitworth et al., 2007). Indeed, a coach may speak from hunches and the effect can be entirely beneficial. However, when speaking from intuition, it is important to be aware of the data that formed your impressions. You may have had an experience of a person saying something similar to the following to you: "I have a real sense about you. I just know that you are feeling [fill in the blank]." When queried about this sense, the speaker may be unable to produce any validating data, even as he continues to assert that his sense is correct. In coaching, undocumented confrontations are troublesome. They increase the mysterious powers of the coach and may either distance the client or, conversely, deepen dependency. Coaching is not a guessing game. Whenever coaches confront clients, they must be able to back up their impressions, and in doing so, trust the client to confirm or disconfirm the information.

3. **Piggybacked confrontations.** Usually, the process of confronting discrepant messages involves some emotional charge and people may be defensive. If the coach offers one confrontation after another, the client may rightfully feel attacked. You need to be aware of clients' need to save face. As a result, it will be important for you to do whatever possible to support clients' confidence and self-esteem. If confrontations begin to erode clients' sense of self-efficacy, switch tracks—quickly! Failure to do so may have negative consequences for all involved.

4. **Confronting as a control strategy.** When coaches jump on discrepant messages through confrontations with the intention of proving their expertise, they may be expressing a need for control. They might simply want to demonstrate their power by seeming to have extraordinary awareness of thoughts, feelings, and actions. This will likely backfire in the long run. Although some clients might become dependent on the coach, others will recognize the strategy for what it is. In either case, the coach will have failed to promote autonomy.

5. **Confronting too deeply.** Coaches may be aware of deeper issues that, if confronted, could help clients achieve fundamental changes. Never-

theless, the possibility also exists that through such confrontations, clients will have far more to deal with than they had originally contracted for. It is unlikely that coaches will have sufficient justification for deep interventions that go beyond contracted agendas. However, when a coach believes she has ample reason to use confrontation to bring important issues to the client's awareness, she might consider opening a discussion to renegotiate the original agreement.

# SELF-DISCLOSURE

Transparency and authentic behavior are linked to positive well-being and health (Kernis & Goldman, 2005; Palmer, 2000; Sheldon & Kasser, 1995). Such behaviors entail showing up in a genuine way, unafraid to be seen for who you are. Raines (1996) has noted that clients sometimes need to know their coaches in order to see them as real people. Clients are likely to feel a greater sense of hope and connection through the shared experience that self-disclosures afford (Mathews, 1988). Yet, client curiosity has to be considered carefully. What information can you share? What wouldn't you talk about? More important, why would you, the coach, say anything about yourself during coaching sessions?

Johnson (2009) provides a useful analysis of **self-disclosure** within an interpersonal, nonprofessional context. He defines it as "revealing to another person how you perceive and are reacting to the present situation and giving any information about yourself and your past that is relevant to an understanding of your perceptions and reactions to the present" (p. 48). In this definition, self-disclosure supports interpersonal relationships. Johnson emphasizes that in order to be most beneficial, self-disclosure should be structured to (1) focus on present reality rather than history, (2) include references to feelings as well as facts, (3) cover a wide range of topics, (4) have depth in terms of personal revelations, and (5) be reciprocal, especially in the formative stages of a relationship.

These specifications for appropriate self-disclosure in everyday life stand in sharp contrast to the emerging wisdom about self-disclosure as a skill in professional helping relationships. For the most part, self-disclosure in a professional context refers to "a conscious, intentional technique by which the helper strategically shares personal information in order to achieve a specific benefit to the relationship or for the client" (Simone, McCarthy, & Skay, 1998, p. 174). Varying from advice to counselors and psychotherapists, the coaching profession takes a more favorable view of self-disclosure, no doubt because of the assumption that coaching clients are presumably stable and emotionally healthy (Martin, 2001; Whitworth et al., 2007; Williams & Davis, 2007).

Regardless of its benefits, using self-disclosure in any professional relationship requires a high degree of self-awareness. Coaches need to understand their own needs and issues and how they might relate to the client in the moment. Effective self-disclosure also relies on a strong sense of self-acceptance. Coaches who take the risk of exposing their vulnerabilities need to have accepted their own behaviors and imperfections, particularly as these are portrayed in the stories they tell. If clients react negatively, a coach's expectations of acceptance or approval might result in defensive or critical reactions. Predictably, these responses would be counterproductive to the coaching relationship and the attainment of the client's agenda.

## Types of Self-Disclosure

Not all self-disclosures carry the same weight or meaning. We offer some important distinctions among four types of self-disclosure.

1. **Professional information.** Clients need to know that their coaches are qualified to provide the services for which they have been hired. It is therefore necessary for coaches to disclose the nature of their training and credentialing. This information can be shared in a straightforward manner through a brief professional résumé.

2. **Personal information.** It has been pointed out (Pedersen, Crethar, & Carlson, 2008) that each culture has norms about sharing information. For some cultural groups, coaches would not be expected to reveal personal information such as age, relationship status, number of children, and so on. However, people from other groups might expect them to share some of these details. Moreover, coaches need to be aware of the potential meanings that certain biographical information may have for clients. A person who asks about the coach's age may be asking, in an indirect manner, whether he can trust her because he equates age with wisdom.

3. **Content-congruent stories.** Think of social conversations in which a person uses some aspect of the speaker's remarks to launch into a personal revelation. People share stories and disclose personal

---

**REFLECTION 9.3**

The more you explore ways you have used self-disclosure in the past, the more insight you will gain about its appropriateness and applications to professional work as a coach. Recall some recent experiences where you told a detailed story of a life experience to someone with whom you have a personal relationship. What was your intention in telling this story? What effect did it have on the other person? How did you feel after telling your story?

Now, recall another experience in a professional or work context when you told someone a story about your life, knowing that you wanted to make a particular point with the story. What was your intention? What effect did it have on the other person? How did you feel after telling your story? You may also recall experiences where you were the client and a professional shared personal details or disclosures with you. How did that work out?

You may recall other occasions when you disclosed details of your life to others and the outcomes were mixed or problematic. What was it about these instances that seemed to trouble you? Was it how the other person reacted? Was it your concern about how the person seemed to perceive you? Did anything change in your relationship as a result?

information to pass time and establish a sense of commonality. When coaches have stories that have similar content to those of their clients, they may choose to share them intentionally and strategically, assuming that these stories will enhance their clients' capacities to address goals successfully.

4. **Thematic stories.** Embedded in each story is a theme—one of victory or defeat, of hope or despair, of love or loss. Coaches are unlikely to always have stories with content that corresponds well to their clients' stories, yet they may have had experiences with similar themes. For instance, if someone tells a story about being discouraged and not being able to find the resolve to overcome obstacles confronting her, the coach may choose to speak about a personal experience containing the same themes or dynamics to help the person move forward.

## Steps in Self-Disclosure

The steps outlined in this section apply primarily to the stories coaches tell (content-congruent or thematic stories) rather than to professional or personal information they share with their clients.

1. **Evaluate the purpose.** It's better not to chime in too often with self-disclosures of personal success in response to clients' stories of victory. Self-disclosure is more appropriate when clients' stories contain messages of confusion, uncertainty, defeat, or even despair. In such instances, a personal experience might be shared as a means of instilling hope or clarity, or perhaps as a way of encouraging the person to develop new perspectives about certain dilemmas (Egan, 2010). If the goal of your self-disclosure is to increase trust, build rapport, provide new perspectives, or increase self-acceptance, you need to assess whether you have sufficient reason to believe that a specific self-disclosure will accomplish one or more of these purposes. Your story must be true and have sufficient content and process overlap with the client's story so that he can recognize his own experience in another light. Your intention must never be to match experiences to show identification with the client or to compete with him.

2. **Assess client readiness.** How ready is the client to receive the coach's personal stories? Simone and colleagues (1998) provide some evaluative questions that can help in determining client readiness:

- Will your story take the focus away from the client's experiences?
- Will the boundaries of the coaching relationship remain intact?

- Might your seeming vulnerability disturb the client?
- Will the client see you as less capable because of the self-disclosure?

3. **Ensure proper timing.** If the intent of the self-disclosure is to provoke discussion, there needs to be enough time in the session for the client to respond to and integrate the message. On the other hand, if the self-disclosure is meant as a takeaway reflection to be mulled over during the interval between sessions, the timing is less crucial.

4. **Formulate the story.** How the story is told is pivotal. Its details must clearly match either the themes or the content of the client's experiences. Moreover, there must be a strong likelihood that the client will construe your embedded messages in a manner that is congruent with her intentions. The story must be told succinctly and delivered with sensitivity in terms of how it is received.

5. **Disclose with awareness.** Your self-disclosure must occur with awareness of the here and now. Nonverbal cues often reveal whether the client is receiving the self-disclosure in a positive, neutral, or negative way. Commitment to telling the story must never supersede refocusing the session on the client if her reaction warrants immediate attention. For instance, your client tells a story without fully experiencing her own emotions, and as you start telling a similar tale, she begins to cry. Most likely, the appropriate response is to pause and inquire about the client's immediate experience.

6. **Refocus on the client.** At the conclusion of the self-disclosure, you return the focus to the client. Although the client may probe for additional details about your experience, providing such information is appropriate only insofar as the requested details continue to serve the coaching agenda. Otherwise, you might frame a question to the client such as "I wanted to share this story with you because I hoped that in some way it would be helpful. Does my story create any new awareness about your own experiences?"

## Upside of Self-Disclosure

What justifies self-disclosure in the coaching process? Here are some suggestions.

### Modeling Behavior

For coaching to advance, clients must reveal essential details of their histories and experiences. When done with intentionality, you may engage in appropriate self-disclosures to model styles of disclosure and thereby support your clients in sharing relevant information (Bitter & Byrd, 2011).

### Increasing Trust

Because roles differ considerably in the coaching relationship, clients may feel threatened by perceived status differences or the unidirectional nature of questioning and disclosures. When you share appropriate details and information, clients may come to see you as more human, less distant, more trustworthy, and more authentic (Egan, 2010; Helms & Cook, 1999).

### Developing New Perspectives

In friendships, one person may describe a particular kind of experience and the other joins in with a similar report. The purpose is connection, demonstration of similarity, and perhaps identification; it is not intentionally helpful or therapeutic. The purpose of sharing in coaching is to motivate or to help clients achieve new awareness.

### Increasing Self-Acceptance

Clients may think that they are the only ones confronting particular issues. Coaches may strategically share some of their own disappointments, failures, or other unsettling life events as a way of helping them be more self-accepting. Through appropriately matched self-disclosures, you can communicate that you also experience difficulties and have strong feelings about issues (Hackney & Cormier, 2009).

## Downside of Self-Disclosure

Human experience has many commonalities, yet when professionals attempt to match their self-disclosures to a client's framework, there is much room for error (Abend, 1995). For this reason, self-disclosure is thought to be a risky strategy (Hill & Knox, 2002; Watkins, 1990). Professional relationships normally do not include much self-disclosure in the earliest stages because the helper knows so little about the client (Farrell, 2001). It can also be precarious to disclose too much personal information to clients who are poorly suited to the coaching process.

In many instances, clients may perceive self-disclosing coaches as more caring than those who disclose little (Capuzzi & Gross, 2009). To broach inappropriate subjects or self-disclose in order to gain approval, however, can offend clients and harm the relationship (Myers & Hayes, 2006; Wells,

1994). Moreover, too much self-disclosure may result in the coach consuming valuable air time in the session, which in turn leaves the client confused or alienated (Myers & Hayes, 2006). It is also problematic to share experiences without a clear purpose and without assessing the client's readiness.

To better capture the problematic aspects of self-disclosure by coaches, three points deserve reiterating (Young, 2009):

1. **Incompatible themes or content.** As discussed earlier, you must know enough about the client and her experiences to predict with reasonable accuracy that she will perceive your story as meaningful. Sharing a story simply because it has some content connections may be unsuccessful and could lead to the impression that you are acting like a friend rather than a professional.

2. **Inappropriate deepening of the relationship.** As social creatures, we are likely to match the depth of another person's story. If someone describes a frivolous, superficial happening, we might do the same. However, if you tell emotionally significant stories to lead clients along the same path without clear justification and agreement, you may be operating inappropriately and unethically.

3. **Overexposure.** Self-disclosure must be done sparingly, especially when the stories being told are detailed and involved. There are other means, such as immediacy (see the following section) and feedback (see earlier in the chapter), to increase transparency and a sense of authenticity without telling extensive stories.

## IMMEDIACY

**Immediacy** has been described both as a skill (Egan, 2010; Hill & O'Brien, 2003) and as a component of empathy (Ivey et al., 2010). Immediacy involves the coach's sensitivity to the present situation within the relationship. It requires comprehension of what is happening in the moment and willingness to openly and directly explore the here and now (Capuzzi & Gross, 2009; Egan, 2010). Immediacy may also involve expressions of the coach's desires, needs, or wants in the moment (Turock, 1980).

Immediacy may seem similar to the processes of confrontation and self-disclosure. What merits its separate consideration is that this skill represents a special case of self-disclosure or confrontation. Immediacy can be challenging because it often requires that you as the coach discuss your own feelings and reactions (Capuzzi & Gross, 2009; Turock,

1980). It involves a heightened, moment-by-moment awareness of the subtle shifts and communications during coaching sessions. That is, you may see or feel something in the moment and then comment on it. There is no hiding out in immediacy; the client is likely to feel seen and you will also be quite visible.

Immediacy isn't always about major moments in coaching. Sometimes an immediate response reflects something simple and direct. Here are a few examples:

- I see you smiling broadly and I imagine that you are feeling pretty good about yourself right now.
- I heard that deep sigh when you finished that story. I wonder what that means.
- I, too, feel excited about all the great results you've been getting from your efforts.

Associating immediacy with any particular stage of coaching is difficult because it may be applied at various points depending on what needs to occur to foster client progress. As Shebib (2010) comments, immediacy is a tool for exploring, evaluating, and deepening the relationship. We include it under the ICF core competency of direct communication since it derives from the coach's perceptions. However, it could also be considered under the competency of creating awareness, which is presented in the next chapter.

## Types of Immediacy

Immediacy is always about what is happening right here, right now with the coach, with the client, or in the relationship (Cormier et al., 2009). One instance occurs when a coach consciously chooses to express her own thoughts and feelings. Another happens when she decides to direct a comment to something happening in the present moment related to the client. A third occurrence is when something pops up in the relationship that provokes an immediate response.

### Immediacy Related to the Coach

Immediacy is involved whenever you express thoughts or feelings reflecting your in-the-moment experiences. Expressions of this nature may range from simple statements of welcome to admissions of personal feelings. Some examples are as follows.

**COACH:** I feel flattered by your feedback.

**COACH:** I am excited by the work we're doing.

**COACH:** I have a headache and I can't seem to focus.

One way of differentiating immediacy and self-disclosure involves the purpose of the intervention. When you intend to focus on the relationship per se, it is more likely that you will be using immediacy.

### Client-Related Immediacy

This form of immediacy is akin to giving feedback. It involves sharing your perceptions about your client as they occur in the moment. In this form, immediacy may serve multiple purposes, including increasing client self-awareness, acknowledging the client, or pursuing an issue. Examples include the following.

**COACH:** Seems like you're struggling to understand what I'm saying. Your brow looks furrowed, and you're looking very intently at me.

**COACH:** I imagine you're feeling happy for discovering that fact. What a wonderful, big smile you have.

**COACH:** I wonder if you're upset with yourself. I see you wringing your hands and shaking your head from side to side.

### Relationship Immediacy

What is the climate of the working relationship? How well are coach and client functioning together? Shebib (2010) writes of relationship immediacy as focusing on the way the relationship is developing rather than on a specific incident or here-and-now occurrence. He offers that a helper could use immediacy to explore his and the client's feelings, hopes, or annoyances as a way of assessing the strengths and weaknesses of the coaching relationship. Relationship immediacy might be called for when difficult feelings and resistance to coaching are adversely affecting progress. This application of immediacy is a means for enhancing the working relationship between you and your client (Cormier et al., 2009). Coaching dialogue 9.2 provides some background and a simulated conversation representing an expression of relationship immediacy.

## Steps in Using Immediacy

The effective use of immediacy relies on the relational foundation of trust and rapport between coach and client (Gazda, Asbury, Balzer, Childers, Phelps, & Walters, 1999). Especially in a health, wellness, and fitness context, some people may not be

# AN EXAMPLE OF RELATIONSHIP IMMEDIACY

Read the following dialogue to understand how immediacy can be used to address emergent concerns in the coaching relationship.

## Background Information

The coach and Jack, the client, have been working together for six months, meeting at a regular time each week. Although Jack seemed highly motivated at first, over the past month he has been showing up late for appointments. Whenever the coach asks for information about his progress, Jack seems reticent to provide details. Should obstacles to progress be identified in a session, he rejects any ideas that his coach puts forward.

## Dialogue

**Coach:** I'm noticing some things about how we are working together lately that might be worth discussing. Would you be willing to talk with me about how coaching seems to be going? I can't be sure how much time it'll take, but we can set an initial time limit of 10 minutes and then reassess at that point. After 10 minutes, we'll talk about the specific agenda you're bringing today or continue on this subject. I'll leave the decision to you. Does this work for you?

**Jack:** Yeah, 10 minutes would be okay.

**Coach:** I've noticed a few changes over the past month in our relationship. Before last month, you were always on time. . . .

**Jack:** (*Defensively interrupting*) Yeah, well, I've been real busy this month so if that's it, then let's not bother discussing it because I can't control my boss, and that's why I've been late.

**Coach:** So, you're telling me you've been late entirely because of work reasons, so we needn't go any further in this discussion?

**Jack:** Well, not entirely . . . please continue.

**Coach:** Sure, because the lateness is only part of what I want to discuss. The other parts are about how we seem to connect in these sessions.

**Jack:** (*Again interjecting defensively*) Connect? What do you mean? I don't see anything different. I come here, we talk, we decide what I'm going to do, I try to do it, and then I give my report the following week.

**Coach:** (*Noticing that the conversation is being redirected, yet also aware that what the client is saying may be related to the perceived difficulties*) That's helpful to know. You're saying you haven't been aware of any changes in our relationship.

**Jack:** Well, maybe a little.

**Coach:** Maybe if you told me about the "little" changes you notice, we could accomplish the same objective. Would you be willing to do that?

**Jack:** (*Looking energized and leaning toward the coach*) Yeah, sure. It's no big deal, but it feels to me like this is all about business these days. When I first started, you used to ask me all kinds of questions about my life, my work, my family, my friends, my interests—you name it, you asked me about it. And now it seems all you want to know about is whether I did what I said I would do.

**Coach:** I am so sorry that I'm coming across this way. I can see that the way you see us relating upsets you.

**Jack:** (*Minimizing the importance of what he has just said*) Well, I said it was no big deal.

**Coach:** I guess, then, it's just a big deal to me. I was wondering what had changed, and now you've given me a picture of how I'm coming across to you. Thanks. I believe we can deal with this. I am so appreciative of the fact that you told me how you were feeling. I've been concerned about this for some time.

willing to address conflicts, differences, or feedback about behaviors that they define as irrelevant to their topics. In this regard, initial discussions need to establish clear parameters for the working relationship. If a potential client indicates an unwillingness to consider any input other than performance and adherence reports, then the coaching process itself may not be viable for this individual. If she understands that feedback may be broader than what might occur in a more expert-driven, advice-oriented process, the question of timing remains. Timing concerns when it might be appropriate to use immediacy as a strategy, both within an individual session and within the larger context of the coaching relationship.

These cautionary words refer, of course, to situations where the coach's use of immediacy raises significant and potentially sensitive issues. An expression such as "I am so happy to see you today" is a form of immediacy that is far simpler in its dynamics.

The following material describes steps in using immediacy. The steps are based on the works of Egan (2010), Hepworth and colleagues (2010), and Cormier and colleagues (2009). They have been modified for applications in coaching.

1. **Practice awareness.** The use of immediacy begins with an awareness that something is happening in the relationship that pertains to the coaching agenda. You might sense that something significant is going on that hasn't been addressed. Ideally, mindfulness and self-awareness entail not projecting your own issues on the client and not using the relationship to meet your own needs. Stated more positively, awareness requires ongoing monitoring of the relationship, of nonverbal messages as they relate to the client's verbal expressions, and of your internal state and intuition. It also requires analysis of how all this relates to the coaching agenda.

2. **Consider the potential effects and meanings of your observations.** What are the potential effects of what you are observing or noticing? Are they important enough to address? Are they related to the coaching agenda? What do you imagine is going on? Do you have a hypothesis about what the client's behaviors mean? Are there alternative explanations? Have you thought through all the ways of seeing or interpreting these actions? Sometimes you need to sit with the observations and reflect until a comprehensive appreciation of all the possible meanings and implications emerges. This would especially be the case where you intend to speak to certain relationship dynamics. Of course,

some behaviors require immediate comment. For instance, if the client acts in a denigrating, critical fashion, this circumstance alone may be important to discuss. Verbal abuse must never be tolerated even when clients are successfully addressing their agendas. When someone speaks in a way that you experience as disrespectful, the behavior must be addressed immediately (see Judgmental Versus Nonjudgmental Examples of Immediacy).

3. **Determine what you want to achieve.** Sometimes we get triggered when someone hits a sensitive area with a comment or behavior. Clients are likely to push your buttons at various times, intentionally or not. Part of being a professional is referencing all your interventions to the goals of the relationship and the values that you wish to represent in your actions. If an immediate response will serve little purpose other than getting something off your chest, it may not be justified. There needs to be a well-articulated reason for using the skill of immediacy, and this reason must serve the relationship and its objectives.

4. **Time your statement.** In emotionally laden uses of immediacy, timing is of utmost importance. Raising issues toward the end of a session or when a client seems highly motivated to pursue something else may be unwise. Additionally, if someone comes into a session with a passionate interest in discussing a particular topic, rarely would you sideline the desired agenda to address matters that he may be unwilling, unmotivated, or resistant to consider.

5. **Be open to a variety of responses.** Some clients may lack awareness of their impact on others. Consequently, the use of immediacy could serve as a significant wake-up call for them. They may begin to make connections between what just transpired in coaching and similar issues in other relationships. They may need space for reflection. Of course, another potential client response to immediacy may be defensiveness or denial. Rather than attempt to prove the correctness of your observations or perceptions, you may simply want to recognize this impasse and consider it in determining how best to proceed.

6. **Emphasize the relevance of immediacy to the goals of coaching.** If the meaning of the immediacy intervention is not entirely clear to the client, you may wish to review why the information was brought up and how it relates to his goals. This step would occur after your observations have been adequately discussed. A learning moment in the coaching relationship might take place when the rationale for using immediacy is clearly stated.

# Judgmental Versus Nonjudgmental Examples of Immediacy

The coach has noted the following pattern: The client seeks advice about how to handle various situations, yet when she provides suggestions, the client invariably rejects them by finding fault with some aspect of the suggestions. Later in the session, the client suddenly discovers a solution, almost always something that the coach had suggested earlier, and congratulates himself on answering his own dilemma. At the same time, he wonders aloud why the coach couldn't be as creative.

## Judgmental, Evaluative, or Critical Immediacy

1. I am feeling a bit frustrated here. I don't think I'm being given due credit. The solution you just came up with was something I told you earlier, yet you're acting as if you never heard it before!

2. Can we talk about something? I've been noticing a pattern that you need to be the smart one here. It always has to be your idea, even though the fact is that every idea you've discovered is something I told you about previously. Your ego always has to win.

## Neutral, Factual, and Nonjudgmental Immediacy

1. I would like to discuss something with you. Would you be willing to take a few minutes with me now? (*Pauses for agreement*) I'm not sure what this is about, so I really need your help. When you just came up with an answer to the problem you shared earlier, I felt glad for you and I hope it will work. My puzzlement is that earlier in the session I said what I thought was the same thing, and in your words, you replied, "That's crazy. That will never work." Do you remember this happening? Do you have any thoughts about what I've just said?

2. Can we take a minute to look at something that may be happening between us? (*Pauses for agreement*) I have been noticing what I think is a pattern, and because it just seemed to happen again, I wanted to get your thoughts about it. You just came up with what you described as a great solution to your problem, and I agree with you that it seems to be a good one. Yet, I remember saying the same thing to you 10 minutes ago, and you told me the idea was crazy and wouldn't work. Do you remember this? Am I describing this accurately in your view? (*Pauses for agreement*) It seems like a pattern, and I sure would appreciate your help in figuring it out.

# Upside of Immediacy

Immediacy may be used for a number of reasons. To highlight some of these, let's review the potential values represented in expressions of immediacy (Cormier et al., 2009; Shebib, 2010).

## Fostering Awareness

A coach might experience a dynamic in the coaching relationship that resembles how the client ineffectively manages other relationships. For example, a woman wants to get her life in order and aims, among other things, to acquire time management skills. She remarks that people in her network often complain about her being late for appointments. You have observed that she usually makes it to coaching sessions in the nick of time and out of breath. Because the coaching relationship can be a microcosm of how the client acts with other people (Teyber & McClure, 2011), you may decide to talk about how you are personally experiencing this behavior.

## Demythologizing Clients' Impressions

A client may make a number of flattering comments that convey the impression that you have it all together. For instance, in describing how he messed up one time, he says, "I know you'd never do anything that ridiculous." You decide to demythologize this characterization by using self-disclosure and immediacy. In so doing, you will not only confront the mistaken beliefs, you may also share some of your own shortcomings.

### Sharing Immediate Observations

Some of your clients' behavioral patterns may interfere with how they engage with others who are crucial to their goal attainment. Immediacy can be a powerful intervention when you experience these patterns in sessions. For instance, a client frequently interrupts you when you are speaking, sometimes causing you to lose your train of thought. On a particular occasion when this occurs, you mention it to your client and ask what she thinks this is about for her.

## Downside of Immediacy

The power of immediacy for moving the relationship toward more productive dialogue cannot be underestimated. Conversations framed in the here and now can be quite potent. They capture the spirit of both coach and client, and these moments can promote stronger relationships and the discovery of deeper meanings. Applications of immediacy may require great courage and equanimity. And developing the capacity to be mindful of relationship dynamics can be demanding. Let us review problematic uses of immediacy, some of which we have touched on in earlier discussions.

1. **Immediacy as an end in itself.** Immediacy is not something that is done for its own sake (Egan, 2010). In intimate relationships, people may talk about their mutual feelings and the dynamics of their relationship quite regularly. This deepens the relationship, reduces misunderstandings, and avoids the potential buildup of negative feelings. Expressions of caring, concern, or affection play an important role in increasing interpersonal connection. How much of this will be crucial to a coaching relationship is questionable. Certainly, when misunderstandings affect the work, you might choose to focus on the relationship through the process of immediacy. Yet, the satisfaction that may result from increasing intimacy levels needs to be weighed against how central it is to the achievement of the client's goals—and what the long-range implications might be. Such an innocent expression as "I

was really looking forward to our session today" may represent a minor boundary crossing that could eventually cause your client to generate a problematic perception of your relationship.

2. **Immediacy as countertransference.** When coaches fail to engage in self-reflection concerning their coaching relationships, they may not observe how certain assumptions or even fantasies that derive from other pivotal relationships in their lives are shaping their experiences with certain clients. As previously noted, the tendency to see countertransference as pertaining to the more in-depth domain of counseling and psychotherapy needs to be deconstructed. These types of reactions are common to virtually all intense, ongoing professional relationships. Here are two simple manifestations of countertransference that might easily occur in coaching.

- **Situation A:** A male coach recently had an argument with his partner in which he was accused of not living up to his part of the bargain in the relationship. His partner criticized him for shirking responsibilities at home. While still in turmoil about this argument, he meets his first client of the day, who subtly shames him for forgetting to call her during the week as they had agreed. He angrily confronts the client and expresses displeasure with her.

- **Situation B:** The young client of a female coach physically resembles her son, who happens to be a bit of a sneak. The coach often finds out about her son's wayward behavior from neighbors or occasionally from authorities. In the present session, her client omits a particular detail about his action plan, which emerges later in the discussion. She asks somewhat accusingly, "Are you telling me *all* I need to know in order to do the very best with you?" The client feels put off by the question, especially because the coach has asked it more than once.

3. **Immediacy as fostering client dependency.** When coaches provide immediacy interventions based on feel-good experiences with the client (e.g., "You are such a joy to work with") or when they deepen the relationship through intimacy-creating dialogues, clients may be enticed to continue with coaching more for the emotional boost they get than for the contracted agendas. It is important to celebrate client successes and to be a source of support and praise. However, it is equally relevant to stay attuned to client responses, noticing whether a pattern of approval seeking is developing.

Generally speaking, becoming skillful in using immediacy will be important in your coaching. The more comfortable you feel being in the moment with your clients, the more ease you will convey about issues you choose to address through immediacy. Even so, clients don't always have to get it. They don't always need an epiphany or significant catharsis. You don't have to create an atmosphere of being buddies; simply use immediacy when it has a justifiable purpose within your clients' agendas.

# DIRECT INPUT

**Direct input** involves messages to clients that provide instructions, information, and advice based on the wisdom and expertise that coaches have gathered through education, training, and professional practice. When offered by a lifestyle wellness coach, these highly influential communications are likely to be perceived as legitimate, appropriate, and even expected. Just as someone walking into a nutritionist's office will anticipate that the professional will provide sound information rather than asking him to choose whatever he likes, clients working with lifestyle wellness coaches may expect some direction.

Before examining similarities and differences among instructions, information, and advice, we want to mention some special considerations about this category. When considering the concepts of giving people direction or attempting to control their behavior, certain questions may arise: Who can rightfully give direction or exert control? Who has legitimate expertise within the relationship? Looking at this in the context of health, wellness, and fitness professionals and their clients, we can define a direction and control continuum such as that depicted in figure 9.1. The role of lifestyle wellness coach would most likely occupy a place close to the center, that is, with client and coach providing more or less equal direction. Personal trainers, bodyworkers, and wellness consultants might be somewhat left of center, whereas athletic coaches, technicians, group fitness instructors, and expert advisors would fall to the far left of the continuum.

The emphasis of coaching is on collaborative, bidirectional processes that are embedded in its patterns of interaction. This can create dilemmas for coaches when they give instructions to clients because this type of communication is stylistically linked to unidirectional decision making and control. The degree to which instructions, information, and advice are present in coaching communications will determine the extent to which clients see themselves as responsible collaborators or passive recipients.

Let us examine the three skills in this category to understand ways in which they can best be used in coaching. We begin with brief descriptions

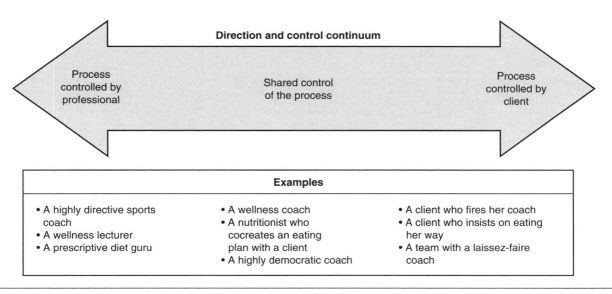

**Figure 9.1** Direction and control continuum of health, wellness, and fitness professionals.

and purposes for each and then consider steps for application and other matters for the three forms of direct input.

# Instructions

In matters of health, wellness, and fitness, clients often require **instruction**. They might not know what they need to do, or they might be unaware of the procedures. The level of instruction offered by a coach depends on the work contracted. Some coaches may serve in a variety of capacities, partly as guide, partly as support, partly as resource, and sometimes as expert. Others may work in a team approach whereby the coach monitors implementation of programs along with allied health professionals.

Instructions indicate to a client what he needs to do in terms of thoughts, feelings, or behaviors (Ivey et al., 2010). Examples of instructions include the following.

### Thoughts

Think about it this way.

Focus your mind on your breath.

Imagine your boss as someone who wants you to win.

### Feelings

Feel what's happening inside your body right now.

Sense the energy in your center radiating out through your arms and legs.

Smile inwardly just as you are about to speak.

### Actions

Do that again.

Lower your center and relax your breath.

Breathe in to a count of 4 and then slowly release your breath to a count of 4.

Instruction will take on different faces when coaches engage in dialogues with clients versus when they work with them in practical applications. In program implementation, instruction can take the form of verbal messages describing how to perform certain actions and perhaps also nonverbal messages, including hands-on postural corrections. Within coaching dialogues, instruction might take the form of mental imagery exercises, mental focus training, or clear reinforcements for action (e.g., "Continue doing exactly what you have been doing!"). Guided imagery may be used to help clients overcome anxieties related to performance or to facilitate envisioning positive futures toward which clients can direct action.

When clients engage experts in professional settings, they usually expect to receive clear instructions. However, when coaches communicate with clients, the permission to use instruction must be negotiated. The following example may clarify this latter case.

**COACH:** So, it seems that when you are in a competitive situation, you're not sure what happens, but you suddenly become aware of a shakiness in your knees and something like fear in your stomach. Is that what you're saying?

**CLIENT:** Exactly. But I don't know how I go from feeling so calm when I'm sitting on the bench to feeling so anxious when I'm out on the court.

**COACH:** Would you be willing to try something with me? (*Pauses for an answer*) Maybe we can get some more information about this. I'm going to ask you right now to close your eyes. (*Pauses until client closes eyes*) Now, imagine you are sitting on the bench about to go out on the court. Tell me how you're feeling.

This interaction, which relies heavily on instruction, is the beginning of a behavior rehearsal strategy (Suinn, 1986). It demonstrates how the coach enlists the client's permission and collaboration at the beginning of the process.

Providing instruction is appropriate under certain conditions (Shebib, 2010; Young, 2009). These conditions include the following:

- You have expert knowledge or training related to the client's agenda.
- You have extensive experience in helping clients with the specific approaches being used.
- You are fully aware of the limitations of the approach and appropriately advise the client about the potential benefits and liabilities.
- You have adequate understanding of the client's history, needs, capabilities, and limitations.
- You are able to adapt instructions to fit the client and the circumstances.

# Information

According to Young (2009), giving **information** means providing data that can help clients pursue their goals. Information might include ideas about how to accomplish something or to correct errone-ous notions. Young notes that information should be provided sparingly; too much information can overload clients and will likely be ignored.

Health, wellness, and fitness professionals rely heavily on using information as a strategy for guiding and motivating change. Clients may put themselves unnecessarily at risk out of igno-rance, and you can help them become aware of the consequences of actions by offering information. Conveying information may take a multitude of forms, from verbal descriptions to recommended readings, videos, or websites. As Cormier and col-leagues (2009) suggest, giving clients information is generally appropriate when it relates to their goals and well-being. These authors suggest that helpers determine whether to use information by asking and answering three questions: What does the client need to know? When does she need this information? How can I best deliver it to achieve optimal results?

Information is seldom unbiased or value free. When informing clients about options or activities, coaches often present their own knowledge about a topic or refer them to certain resources. None of these may be exhaustive, but they may be represen-tative of available knowledge. As you engage with an increasingly diverse clientele, you will need to be cognizant of various caveats based on the particular backgrounds, capabilities, limitations, needs, and interests of your clients. You can use information to persuade them to engage in certain actions, in which case it is wise to ensure that the data are accurate and credible.

## Advice

Of the three forms of direct input, giving **advice** or suggestions is the most problematic and likely the most widely used (Brammer & MacDonald, 2003). In relationships with friends and family, advice is one of the most common responses that people give each other (Johnson, 2009).

People from certain cultures may prefer direct advice from coaches because they consider them to be experts (Corey et al., 2011). Novice coaches may be especially vulnerable to the expectation that they should provide expert advice. Yet, as Kleinke (1994) notes about giving advice in therapy, "Clients can get all the advice they want from acquaintances, friends, and family members" (p. 9). If advice is what they want, they hardly need to pay a coach to tell them what to do. Steele (2011) offers an even stronger rebuttal to this type of approach. In his view, helpers who give advice are more concerned

about showing off their competency than support-ing their clients' own inner wisdom.

A more positive way of framing this issue comes from the work of Compton, Galaway, and Courn-oyer (2005), who conclude that the wisdom of helpers pertains less to what they know and more to their ability to facilitate client self-determination. Coaching is about supporting clients in generat-ing alternatives for themselves, making decisions among alternatives, and pursuing their choices. The bottom line seems to be that coaches need to focus more on helping clients think and decide than on providing them with answers. The question then becomes this: In which circumstances would giving advice be appropriate? Borrowing from arguments in the broader helping professions (Brammer & MacDonald, 2003; Shebib, 2010; Young, 2009), the following applications seem pertinent to coaching relationships:

- Offering suggestions so that clients become aware of unforeseen consequences of their actions

- Providing advice when clients may be at risk of harm or injury

- Recommending courses of action that the client may not know about or might have overlooked

- Making recommendations based on exten-sive experience, knowledge, research, or valid information

- Providing clients with strategies for dealing with issues instead of offering solutions

- Suggesting communication processes that might help clients deal more effectively with their agendas

### REFLECTION 9.4

The type of reflection we propose here might be coun-terintuitive. We invite you, when at all possible in the next 24 hours, to refrain from providing information, instructions, and advice, even if someone asks you for direct input. Instead, work with the person so that she will find a suitable answer. Then reflect on the following questions: How easy or difficult was this for you? How did people react? Did they come up with answers you would have provided? Or did they create something unexpected? Were their solutions or answers reason-able and safe? Or did you have to tell them something so they didn't get into difficulty? Were there any sur-prises in this process for you?

## Steps in Direct Input

Coaches must be intentional when it comes to giving instructions, information, or advice. The following steps (Cormier et al., 2009; Ivey et al., 2010; Shebib, 2010) pertain to instances for considering direct input.

1. **Assess the need.** What does the client need at this moment? Is it information? Is it your opinion? Is it instruction? Or is it a need to resolve her issues? Although you may optimistically believe that clients have all the resources they need to resolve their own difficulties (Martin, 2001; Whitworth et al., 2007; Williams & Davis, 2007), clients may not have all the necessary information or the requisite skills. At times, it is appropriate to provide instruction and information that is well aligned with their agendas.

2. **Determine the strategy.** Communication skills other than direct input may achieve the same results as giving information, instruction, or advice. When clients need to discover their own answers, active listening might have a more positive long-term effect on client self-efficacy and self-determination.

Shebib (2010) offers creative alternatives to advice. The following questions might draw out the client's intrinsic wisdom in lieu of giving advice:

- What are your ideas about this?
- How might you approach this situation?
- Have you had any thoughts that merit deeper exploration?
- If I were to give you advice, what do you think it would be?
- What might your best friend suggest to you?
- What do you think your options are?

When it is a matter of choosing among information, instruction, or advice, there may be good reason to prefer one over the other. Depending on the trust and rapport in the coaching relationship, you may decide to be highly influential by adding your own weight to clients' deliberations. This action would imply offering advice rather than giving information. Comparisons of these three approaches appear in the following coaching dialogue.

---

### COACHING DIALOGUE 9.3

# USE OF INSTRUCTION, INFORMATION, AND ADVICE

In this scenario, offers of instruction, information, and advice are contrasted. The risks and benefits accompanying each type of message can be estimated by imagining how the fictional client might respond to the type of input that the coach provides. You will recognize in some instances that the coach's input may have a low probability of success or may not match the implied needs of the client.

### Scenario

A 62-year-old man wants to better manage his stress. He defines himself as a rigid person and hopes that beginning to exercise regularly will help him loosen up a little in his personal life. Through coaching, he has determined to support his desired objectives with novel (for him) fitness classes.

**Client:** I think I'm way too stiff to do the exercises in some of these classes. Besides, I feel strange going into classes where there are mostly women. I feel awkward and embarrassed. What do you think I should do?

### Coaching Instruction

**Coach:** I want you to go to your fitness center and ask a staff member which classes men take a lot. Then, schedule yourself for one of these classes.

### Coaching Information

**Coach:** It's normal for people to feel a bit uncomfortable when they try new things. But as you continue, a level of comfort and familiarity will eventually develop. My experience is that it seems to take about six weeks of going to a new class for people to learn the ropes and start feeling more at home.

### Coaching Advice

**Coach:** My opinion is that it's a good idea for you to just keep doing it for a while longer. I believe your gains are going to far outweigh the discomfort you feel. And I think you need to do this to accomplish your goals.

3. **Formulate the message.** Though clients ultimately choose what to do, manipulative or highly persuasive ways of communicating must be avoided. The goal is not always to provoke immediate change; it might only be to stimulate thinking or to help clients reframe their situations. What would be most helpful to say or do in this situation with this client?

4. **Deliver the message.** Having a clear strategy in mind with awareness of its varying consequences, deliver the message while maintaining keen sensitivity to client responses. As always, if the person shows signs of discomfort or overt resistance, it is best to discontinue the delivery and ask about her immediate experiences.

5. **Invite a response.** At the conclusion of the message, clients may be invited to comment, reflect, or otherwise respond to what was said. Even if it takes a while for them to integrate the information, instruction, or advice, it is best to pause deliberately until they speak.

6. **Evaluate the impact.** If you are not clear how the message affected the client, ask directly. For example, "Now that we've talked about this, would you be willing to say what you're taking away from our discussion?" Using the skill of immediacy, you might also want to ask about the implications of the message for the coaching relationship: "You asked me for my opinion, and I willingly offered it. I'm wondering now if I could ask for your opinion about something. How do you think this discussion and the opinion I gave you might affect the way we work together?"

## Downside of Direct Input

When you use direct input in your sessions, ideally you are responding accurately and appropriately to your clients' needs. Advice and suggestions tend to be risky interventions, so they should probably be used as a last resort, except in emergencies or to steer clients clear of imminent danger. The following are some ways in which direct input might be used inappropriately in coaching.

1. **Input that is out of bounds.** Over time, clients may attribute to their coaches levels or kinds of knowledge unwarranted by their actual training and experiences. Seeing you as a wise, intelligent, and sensitive human being, clients may be inclined to ask you for advice on a wide range of topics unrelated to their coaching agenda. A red flag of caution in responding to someone's request for advice is when you hear "I know this isn't your area, but I wanted your opinion anyway." In this regard, even if you try to temporarily step out of role (e.g., "Well, this isn't my field, but in my experience . . ."), clients will most likely discount your disclaimers about expertise.

2. **Unsupported input.** Hesitation to make public your ignorance, especially when you believe that you *should* know the answer to a question, is quite normal. However, rather than stumbling through an ill-informed response, it may be better to tell clients that you will check into matters about which you are uncertain or simply confess ignorance.

3. **Input that increases client dependency.** Giving clients the tools to address their own issues empowers them to be self-determining. Instruction is often necessary in technical matters, but you will need to examine carefully the potential impact of being the go-to expert on client dependency and consider other ways to help them reach the same ends. Fortunately, simply encouraging clients to tap into their own strengths can reduce dependency even when direct input is provided (Young, Klosko, & Weishaar, 2003).

4. **Input as a means of control.** Giving information or instructions might be things the coach does well, and clients may value what they receive. Yet, over time you may become more intent on controlling a client's actions than on following a potentially slower path of fostering resourcefulness and autonomy. Power and control can be heady experiences; as such, these issues must be ongoing areas for reflection if you want to be an effective coach.

5. **Poorly timed input.** As with all coaching skills, timing is key. The core messages of information, instruction, or advice may be sound, but the delivery may be ill timed.

# COMMENTARY

As noted throughout the book thus far, coaching represents a weave of communications that emerges from the unique combination of who clients are, what they need, who you are, and what you are best able to provide. In an elegant coaching process, a natural flow of communication advances clients' agendas while nurturing and supporting their need for trustworthy connection.

Before concluding, we want to mention that in its list of the components of direct communication, the ICF includes the use of metaphors and analogies. Although we do see metaphors and analogies as forms of direct communication, we have chosen to discuss these applications under the core competency of creating awareness, which is addressed next.

We are acutely aware that the approaches reviewed in this chapter may take years of practice and reflection to master. You will need to thoroughly understand feedback, confronting, and self-disclosure not only for what they potentially offer clients but also for how they can adversely alter the working alliance. In looking forward to the ideas presented in the next chapter, we are excited to be able to explore with you other ways of generating opportunities for clients to fulfill their dreams.

# 10

# AWARENESS AND ACTION

**I**n this chapter, you will learn how…

- the Johari window guides the areas of awareness emphasized in coaching,

- focusing is a directive strategy that orients a client's attention to a specific area of goal pursuit,

- reflection of meaning provides clients with deep connections to their intentions and actions,

- interpretation is a delicate yet potent method for catapulting clients beyond barriers and obstacles, and

- the competency development model affords a holistic framework for ensuring robust action planning.

> You have to leave the city of your comfort and go into the wilderness of your intuition. What you'll discover will be wonderful. What you'll discover will be yourself.
>
> —*Alan Alda*

The adage "ignorance is bliss" stands to reason—occasionally, it's simply better not to know things. However, when clients seek coaching, they not only want to change patterns and behaviors, they might also want to gain awareness so they can have greater control in their lives. Historically, behavior change was thought to require insight and understanding. Current evidence veers in the direction that action feeds awareness and vice versa. We have stated previously that the hallmark of coaching is its focus on action. However, coaching also fully embraces the importance of insight and awareness, with the caveat that these must be in service of forward movement—or action! Coaching creates learning loops where clients experiment with action and then reflect on their learning. Rather than puzzle interminably over what to do, clients are encouraged to take the leap into action. Mostly, these actions are well designed and limited in scope at the outset. In this way, they don't rush off to do things that are ill considered, irreversible, or potentially disastrous.

In this chapter we address the ICF theme of facilitating learning and results. We discuss the interrelated eighth and ninth core coaching competencies of creating awareness and designing action. Combined, these two competencies provide a framework for learning in action. According to the ICF (2011c), creating awareness is the ability to integrate and accurately evaluate multiple sources of information, and to make interpretations that help the client to gain awareness and thereby achieve agreed-upon results. A coach who masters this competency

- goes beyond what is said in assessing the client's concerns, not getting hooked by the client's description;
- invokes inquiry for greater understanding, awareness, and clarity;
- identifies the client's underlying concerns, typical and fixed ways of perceiving herself and the world, differences between the facts and the interpretation, and disparities between thoughts, feelings, and action;
- helps clients to discover for themselves new thoughts, beliefs, perceptions, emotions, moods, and so on that strengthen their ability to take action and achieve what is important to them;
- communicates broader perspectives to clients and inspires commitment to shift their viewpoints and find new possibilities for action;
- helps clients to see the various interrelated factors that affect them and their behaviors (e.g., thoughts, emotions, body, background);
- expresses insights to clients in ways that are useful and meaningful for the client;
- identifies major strengths versus major areas for learning and growth as well as what is most important to address during coaching; and
- asks the client to distinguish between trivial and significant issues, situational versus recurring behaviors, when detecting a separation between what is being stated and what is being done.

International Coach Federation 2011

Coaching is less focused on looking over clients' histories than it is about creating new stories around which insights can be generated. Some clients come to coaching with clear goals and a reasonable approach to action. In such cases, the coach's work might be simply to sharpen the plan through a structured goal-setting approach and then to monitor implementation of action. That sounds pretty straightforward, perhaps so much so that we might wonder why the person needs coaching. However, more likely scenarios are ones where clients have a destination but most of the routes they have taken in the past haven't worked out particularly well for them (Hargrove, 2008). Creative solutions are needed—and these may require more than active listening or asking questions.

The beginning of this chapter emphasizes the creation of awareness. We examine the processes of focusing, reflection of meaning, and interpretation. We then present a developmental perspective of action wherein movement forward is based on the generation of building blocks to address all the relevant elements not only to begin but also to continue on the path to goal attainment.

# FOSTERING AWARENESS

At the outset of coaching relationships, you probably know little about your new clients. And though they may know a great deal about themselves, all of us have blind spots. Even when they are highly self-aware, how much clients are willing to share depends on a number of factors, including the nature of your relationship, their level of trust in you, personal values regarding intimacy, and even their ability to describe their internal states and processes.

In a simple yet enduring model of the relationships among self-disclosure, feedback, and self-awareness, Joe Luft and Harry Ingham (Luft, 1969) described a matrix of awareness or self-knowledge. This model, known as the **Johari window**, is helpful in conceptualizing knowledge about clients and thereby strategically investigating areas appropriate to their agendas (see table 10.1). The more you know about a client, the richer your strategies and the greater their chances of realizing their dreams.

## Public Self

What someone shares with her coach is part of the public self. She may not discuss this information with everyone, but by describing it to the coach, she makes these aspects of herself public. Coaches may use all forms of active listening, questioning, and other skills to broaden the dimensions of this quadrant of awareness for clients.

**Table 10.1    The Johari Window: An Awareness Model for Coaching**

|  | **Known to self** | **Unknown to self** |
|---|---|---|
| **Known to others** | **Public self**<br>What I know about myself and am willing to make public | **Blind self**<br>What I don't know about myself but others have observed about me |
| **Unknown to others** | **Private self**<br>What I choose to keep private | **Unconscious self**<br>What I don't know about myself and what is also unknown to others |

## Private Self

This area represents self-knowledge that clients have not yet disclosed. Because they need to share only what is necessary to assist coaches in their collaborative efforts, large areas of their lives may be off limits. Coaches may inquire about personal matters they deem important. However, if clients hold back, chances of success will diminish proportionately to the importance of the information to their stated agenda. If, for instance, a client has an eating disorder or a serious substance addiction and wants to work on achieving optimal levels of wellness, this information is likely to be important in order to proceed in the most appropriate manner or, in some cases, to determine whether the coaching relationship is viable.

## Blind Self

You often see things in others that they seemingly have little awareness of. In the coaching process, the task is to help clients become aware of relevant aspects of themselves that they manifest through actions or unconscious communications. Of course, you would not always disclose information of which clients are unaware. Timing is critical, as is a regard for the legitimate agenda of the relationship. If the information is pertinent to the coaching process, then, at an appropriate time, you may need to use various approaches to create client awareness. When the information is irrelevant to the coaching agenda, it may well be left unsaid.

## Unconscious Self

Much of the early work in psychoanalytic theory (Freud, 1949) was premised on the belief that we all have significant areas of unconscious experience, and this information remains virtually unknown to us or to anyone else until pivotal events surface

previously unconscious material. Freud (1953) thought dreams represented the "royal road to the unconscious" because a careful analysis of dream content brought to conscious awareness aspects of our previously unknown selves (p. 25). We know that painful memories of traumatic experiences are often repressed. Indeed, some people have little recollection of significant periods of their lives, typically in childhood and adolescence. One function of certain psychotherapies is to enable people to bring forth these memories so that they can resolve the presumed effects of these repressed experiences.

In considering the agenda of lifestyle wellness coaching, this unconscious domain is never the focus of direct intervention. As a coach, you are not attempting to unveil aspects of your client's unconscious. This does not mean, however, that the person's unconscious self is irrelevant to coaching. Any process that has a substantive effect on someone's functioning stands some chance of bringing to light memories or awareness that may not have been within the person's conscious mind and that the coach had not expected to emerge. This simple yet poignant story illustrates the point:

A client working with a health professional decided that, as part of her program, she wanted to commit to drinking at least eight glasses of water a day. Her work through all the processes of establishing a goal, planning action, preventing relapse, and creating social support brought no great awareness of any underlying issues related to this simple goal. She merely thought that drinking more water was important for her health.

While engaged in goal pursuit, the woman became aware of how frequently she would sit at her desk with a bottle of water within arm's reach and yet refuse to pause long enough to quench her thirst. A growing awareness of this blatant self-denial stunned her. The experience so profoundly affected her that she began recalling other instances of self-denial in her life. Eventually, she recalled critical messages from childhood. When this woman was a young girl, her mother repeatedly labeled her as selfish. Her mother's words came back to mind with resounding force: "Stop thinking about your own needs so much. You're so selfish." These messages became so ingrained over time that they formed a way of life. All this arose from a simple intention to drink more water!

The story is true. The likelihood that coaches will encounter these kinds of revelations is hard to estimate. In working with this woman, the professional only needed to be supportive. The client uncovered a major influence on her behavior of ignoring or denying her needs over a lifetime. She not only reached her goal of drinking a daily quota of water, she also set other goals for health improvement that she engaged thoughtfully and successfully during the following year. Should she have wished to discuss this particular matter further, a lifestyle wellness coach might have considered referring her to a competent counselor.

The Johari window (Luft, 1969) is a practical guide for reviewing the knowledge we have about clients vis-à-vis the information we believe necessary to work effectively. Here are some other reflections about the model and its relevance to coaching:

- When critical knowledge remains in the area of the client's blind self, effective coaching must generate awareness of this information in a sensitive manner that promotes trust and intimacy.

- Should the client be withholding information (private self), the coach needs to be skilled in creating comfort and safety for the client in discussing these personal matters.

- When the client talks extensively about life issues that are not related to the coaching agenda (public self), the coach needs to know how to help him define appropriate boundaries for self-disclosure.

- Should troubling memories be triggered in the client's unconscious self during coaching, strategies for addressing and managing these experiences need to be available as part of the coach's repertoire of interventions and referral sources.

Some methods are more potent than others for creating awareness. Even so, the fact remains that people sometimes gain awareness simply by telling their stories to an attentive and concerned coach. Coaching offers multiple lenses from which to appreciate clients' stories. Looking through these novel lenses at stories that clients have repeatedly told from unproductive perspectives can provoke moments of awareness. Coaches may **reframe** or interpret issues that their clients bring forth and then offer back these interpretations for their consideration. They may become aware of new meanings in what clients say and wonder out loud whether these perspectives resonate at all for them. Or, they may focus intentionally on particular aspects of communications because they suspect that there is special value in certain details. Let's explore three well-tested ways of creating awareness: focusing, reflection of meaning, and interpretation.

# FOCUSING

A popular interpretation of the skill of **focusing** is based on the work by Eugene Gendlin (1981), who represents it as a type of awareness enhancement. According to Gendlin, focusing allows clients to direct their attention toward a specific theme, or, at times, on their felt experience, almost as a meditative act. Within the realm of sport and competition, attentional focus, or concentration, has also been widely explored as a strategy for performance enhancement (Abernethy, 2001). The perspective of focusing represented here derives more from the work of Jean Baker Miller (Baker Miller, 1991; Baker Miller, Stiver, & Hooks, 1997) and interpretations of her work by Ivey and colleagues (Ivey, Ivey, & Simek-Morgan, 1997; Ivey et al., 2010). It allows the coach to take a number of specific angles for listening and responding to a client's messages. Let's see how this multiangled perspective offers a variety of ways to understand a client who is expressing difficulty in adhering to a stress management process to which he firmly committed in a previous coaching session.

**Client:** I'm simply not doing what I agreed to, and it's not just because of me . . . I don't mean to make excuses, but work has been rough . . . way too much traveling . . . and my kids have needs, too. I can't always expect my spouse to shuttle them around to all their sports and lessons. I'm disappointed nonetheless. Exercising and meditation require a lot of time and effort.

Maybe you should have come up with a more flexible plan for me.

A comprehensive paraphrase would reflect all elements of this client's message, yet if you had been working with this man for a while, you might have a hunch about the most productive lead to follow. You might choose one of the following perspectives for focus.

**Perspective A: Empathy.** You might believe that the client is simply having a rough time meeting all his objectives. You could choose to focus on his felt experience of disappointment, empathizing with the dilemma in which he finds himself. A focusing response of this nature might sound as follows.

COACH: Sounds like you've had a rough week with work, family, and no time for your program. I hear your disappointment and imagine it's hard to believe that things can get better—even though you really want to follow through on your commitment to yourself.

**Perspective B: Responsibility.** You might believe that the client is blaming others for not doing what he agreed to do. You could bring the focus on his responsibility for the contracted agreement and on his tendency to excuse his behavior. A response of this sort might sound as follows.

COACH: I hear you. You're feeling disappointed, and there are a number of reasons you're suggesting for why you didn't follow the plan. Would you be willing to explore with me what you might have been able to do this past week to deal with the problems you've identified? What could you have done differently to live up to your commitment to yourself?

**Perspective C: Planning.** Based on your knowledge of the person, you might choose to focus on planning. The client has a highly unpredictable job that requires him to continually adjust his agreed-upon actions. He may plan to train at his lunch hour but instead finds himself on the way to the airport. A response of this sort might sound as follows.

COACH: I can truly empathize with your disappointment. You planned to exercise and meditate according to the schedule we laid out and instead you ended up traveling. With the kind of last-minute business trips you take, it doesn't leave much time. What do you imagine would be possible for you to do when unplanned events take over your schedule?

Even if the client responds by saying that there is nothing he can do, the effect might be to reduce his disappointment. Along with you, he can then brainstorm contingency plans for the future.

**Perspective D: Offering new viewpoints.** You might believe that the client is feeling up against a wall with few options and not much hope. You could make a decision to inject new ideas or perspectives into the interaction by sharing personal experiences, providing information, or offering advice. A response of this sort might sound as follows.

COACH: Sorry to hear about your week and how disappointed you feel. Based on your experience this week, I have some ideas I would like to share with you. There are some things you might be able to do that will help you reach your goals even when you can't follow your plan to the letter. Would you be open to my offering a couple ideas?

The points of focus just described derive from the content of the client's story. In a more comprehensive way, Ivey and colleagues (Ivey et al., 2010; Ivey et al., 1997) have described seven global areas of focus that a helper can consider in formulating a response to a client's message. Briefly, these are as follows.

1. **Focus on the client's immediate experience.** Who is the client and what is he experiencing right now? What messages are you receiving in the present moment? You may be trying to absorb many details, but how does all this information coalesce into a useful image of the person before you?

2. **Focus on the problem.** Turn attention not so much on the client as on an aspect of her experience. Separating the person from the issues is not always easy, but by depersonalizing the client's messages and focusing on what needs to be resolved, you and your client may be able to dissect the matter with more objectivity.

3. **Focus on significant others.** When other people can affect a client's commitment, you may wish to draw out his awareness of these influences. The absence of significant others in a client's story does not necessarily mean that they do not exist or that social connections are unimportant. The lack of detail about relationships would potentially

justify an exploration of this area before drawing conclusions.

4. **Focus on family.** What are the client's family relationships and responsibilities that might affect goal setting or program implementation? What is the client's family history that might have bearing on beliefs, attitudes, or behaviors? The attitudes of family members toward a client's commitments can either hinder or help goal pursuit.

5. **Focus on the coaching relationship.** Sometimes it is valuable to bring the focus close to home, that is, to the relationship between you and your client. This focus might mean emphasizing expectations, attitudes, roles, or feelings. When you have indications that clients have strong expectations of you or when you sense that they are experiencing certain feelings that have implications for the working alliance, you may decide that it is timely to bring these matters into focus.

6. **Focus on the coach's world.** In listening carefully to client stories, you may hear distortions, fallacious beliefs, or seemingly irresolvable problems. Drawing on either professional knowledge or personal experience, you may have important points to add to clients' perspectives.

7. **Focus on contextual or background factors.** When trying to locate the client in a matrix of sociocultural, gender, geographical, occupational, and other contextual variables, you may become aware of certain influences on your client's attitudes, beliefs, and behaviors. Unless these influences are accounted for in strategies for working together and implementing action plans, they will continue to have an impact on the client and on the way she engages in goal pursuit. For example, a clinically obese woman with a negative body image may not do well in a mixed-gender fitness center. Clients with strong gender stereotypes may restrict themselves to pursuing certain kinds of activities involving only people of their own gender group. Ethnic and cultural backgrounds, sexual orientations, religious or spiritual associations, socioeconomic status, and other relevant contextual factors of diversity are all important elements that might influence clients' expectations of coaching, programming, and relationship dynamics.

Focusing is critical to the competency of creating awareness in that it acknowledges the multiple lenses through which clients might reexamine their agendas. It opens avenues for exploration that might not be at the forefront of their minds. It brings under the microscope key elements for creating commitment.

We have chosen not to dissect the approach of focusing in the way we have for other coaching processes (e.g., describing steps and upside and downside). In part, this is because focusing relies on skills we have already described, such as powerful questioning, active listening, and direct communication, among others. What is unique about focusing is how the coach shines a light on a specific aspect of the client's messages.

Focusing speaks to your internal process as a coach in your decision about how to respond to a client's messages. Multiple options for responding will always exist, and some will prove more productive than others. Knowing which to pursue derives from accurate knowledge of who the client is and what he needs, coupled with your self-awareness of agendas or biases that may drive your own behavior.

---

**REFLECTION 10.1**

As a coach, you have your own **worldview** (Senge, 2006), your personal values, beliefs, attitudes, and opinions about people and the reasons things are the way they are in the world. Your history has shaped you, and you have come to value certain things more than others. When applying focusing, it is critical to be aware of your worldview. You don't want to focus on an aspect of the client's communications because it is your preferred channel of inquiry. Your focus needs to serve the client's process and goal achievement. Embracing diversity requires that you hold onto your perspective lightly, at least while you are in sessions, in order to comprehend which focus will be most fruitful for your client's intentions.

In previous chapters, we asked you to reflect on your worldview and how your core values inform the work you do with clients. Reflecting again on your belief system, what are some of the topics that draw your attention in conversations? How might these areas of focus be valuable for your clients? How might they hinder you from fully listening to their stories?

---

# REFLECTION OF MEANING

Creating awareness is about helping clients gain clarity about their topics. It is about discovery and understanding. It involves the creation of a broad perspective that enables clients to uncover sources of strength and motivation they had never imagined. It is about deep meaning.

As a health, wellness, or fitness professional, you may be familiar with the following scenarios.

**Scenario A:** Julie, a 36-year-old woman, has been relatively inactive for most of her life. She just joined a running group and wants you to help her train for a 10K race.

**Scenario B:** Roger, a 50-year-old man, comes to you for stress management. He wants to find balance in his life. He smokes excessively and is currently in the process of a divorce. He has few friends and works at least 70 hours a week.

**Scenario C:** Maria, a 45-year-old recently widowed woman, wants to get back into life. She led a rather reclusive existence taking care of her ailing partner for the past five years and has lost contact with most of her old friends. She thinks that joining a book club at the nearby community center would contribute to feeling better about herself and help her develop new relationships.

Assuming that these clients are presenting their issues to you, would you begin to plan strategies to help them work toward their stated objectives, or would you want to know more about them and their goals? What thoughts come to mind when reflecting on their agendas? What information might you want to obtain? A recent survey of coaching clients (ICF, 2012) indicates that improvements in personal growth, interpersonal relationships, and self-confidence are among the most frequent topics addressed in coaching. As a lifestyle wellness coach, you are undoubtedly aware that if you help clients change one dimension of their health it will affect other areas as well.

Taken at face value, some of the clients' interests portrayed in the previous scenarios could be addressed through straightforward wellness programs. A diet might be prescribed for one and a smoking cessation program for another. Or, you may choose to go beneath the surface; in fact, it's probable that this is what the clients are asking for. Kimsey-House and colleagues (2011) note that clients' initial objectives are likely to be superficial, concrete, and object oriented. That is, they may want to practice meditation, breathe easier, build muscle, make friends, lose weight, test limits, or compete successfully. The magical thinking often incorporated in these objectives is that obtaining these ends will bring fulfillment. After the person has more friends, better sleep, bigger muscles, or less fat, life will be rosier, and he will feel fulfilled! Of course, in portraying the matter this way, you

are likely to agree that achieving goals does not necessarily make people happy; well-being is a state that a person must realize in each moment of her life.

Asking a man who is on the brink of a divorce and works 70 hours a week why he wants to focus on finding balance may seem pointless. Herein lies the dilemma: Although a goal may seem to have transparent value, as a coach you still want to inquire about the values your client associates with his desired state. Perhaps out of curiosity more than anything, a fitness adviser may want to discover what has suddenly inspired a 36-year-old woman to train for a road race. For a lifestyle wellness coach, understanding the motivation would be essential to working with this client. Similarly, when presented with the question of how to coach someone who wants to make friends while improving her self-regard, a coach would want to inquire about where this person is psychologically in her grieving process, what happened to all those old friends as she was going through the trauma of caretaking, and so forth. There are countless avenues that can be pursued to discover the deeper meanings of these clients' goals.

Human beings are meaning-making creatures (Frankl, 1969; Stringer, 2007). Others may not ask us the somewhat taboo *why* question, although we often ask it of ourselves. Why did I do that? Why is this so important to me? Why do I want to be with this person? Why does this continue to happen to me? Existential psychologists suggest that crisis and tragedy prompt people to search for meaning (Binswanger, 1963; Bugental, 1965; Frankl, 1969; May, 1996; Yalom, 1980). An obese client who decides to lose weight may be responding to self-perceptions or the judgments of others and may want to change those views. An entrepreneur who wants to slow down and enjoy life is likely to have experienced an important value shift that energized this redirection.

As Prochaska and Norcross (2010) comment in their description of existential theories, "We create meanings in our lives by the lives we create. We are not born with intrinsic meaning in our existence, but we are born with a creative self who can fashion intrinsic meaning from our existence" (p. 74).

Coaching involves appreciating the meaning clients are creating from their experiences and what new meanings they are yearning for. In the early stages of a coaching relationship, clients are encouraged to tell their stories. As coaches, we need to be attuned to the meanings that people attach to current experiences and future visions.

The search for meaning may run deep. We need to understand only enough to work with the client's more potent motivations and help ground her goals in reality. For instance, a person who wants to run a half marathon to overcome a sense of fear and self-doubt may need to find other supportive processes, such as reading, counseling, or human development workshops, to support his goal achievement. Alternatively, he might realize, through dialogue with a coach, that his reasons for focusing on this particular goal merit reexamination. Consequently, he may discover reasons for pursuing change that are not fear driven.

## Purposes of Reflecting Meaning

**Reflection of meaning** relies on other competencies such as active listening and powerful questioning. Through reflections of meaning, coaches help clients become more aware by discovering the personal significance of events, thoughts, needs, and objectives. Reflection of meaning serves purposes such as the following.

### Deepening Understanding

Perhaps the most straightforward purpose of reflection of meaning is simply to understand the client better. If someone says, "I want a new car and I'd love to have a summer cottage," you might immediately identify with those interests because you, too, would like to have those things. The trap arises from the fact that the same objective phenomenon, whether it is a car, a house, or a new job, can have substantially different meanings for different people. It can be problematic to assume that these objective things represent the same internal motivations. Using reflection of meaning allows you to discover what clients' experiences, desires, or goals mean to them. When someone tells you a story about certain life experiences, you may say things such as "I can certainly relate to that." But can you really? Remaining forever curious is key in coaching (Martin, 2001; Whitworth et al., 2007). You need to hear the client's story and you might also want to probe for the story behind the story. Only by doing so can you make sense of the whole person, not just one isolated dimension of her identity.

Although a client may be specific in identifying her intentions or goals for coaching, understanding what the goals mean to her is critical. Why does this goal matter so deeply? What will these intended changes allow her to do differently? How will the changes affect her life? What personal values does the goal represent?

### Confronting Myths and Fallacies

In listening to clients' stories, we sometimes hear assumptions about the world, about themselves, about the effect of their behaviors, or about what will happen in the future if certain things do not change. Some examples of client mythologies include the following:

> If I get a college degree, I'll lose a lot of my friends.
>
> If I have no energy to begin with, how can I possibly think of exercising?
>
> Going on an eating plan means I can never eat the foods I like.

Reflection of meaning is not about contradicting a person's erroneous beliefs. A client who believes that his spouse will love him more if he is more relaxed might be told point-blank that this assumption is not necessarily the case. Or, the coach could reflect this belief back to him in such a way that he becomes more likely to dissect his assumption and therefore find more personal, self-serving motives for his desired change. Imagine that this client based a stress management program on his stated motivation (to regain his wife's love and affection). No matter how much progress he makes, unless his intimate relationship changes, he will not feel that he has achieved his goal. Moreover, the coach would have no way of assessing the viability of this outcome or influencing it directly through coaching.

### Identifying Potent Motivations

Coaching is a strategy for helping clients become more self-directing and autonomous in addressing life's challenges and opportunities. As seen in coaching dialogue 10.1, the questioning that is involved in reflection of meaning assists clients in discovering the core values associated with their actions. By exploring dreams and desires through reflections of meaning, clients can find the energy and commitment to sustain engagement in their change processes.

### Discovering Options

When coach and client explore meaning in a coaching process, clients can better appreciate who they are, what they need, and the fullness of their agendas. They are able to target specific action strategies while also appreciating the big picture of

# DISCOVERING CORE MOTIVES THROUGH REFLECTION OF MEANING

The following dialogue demonstrates how a coach might discover a client's deeper meanings and the core values that will support efforts to achieve her goals. Through the coach's use of reflection of meaning, the client discovers the true reasons that will likely serve her better in attaining her objectives.

## Background Information

Jan, the client, is a 36-year-old single woman in a highly demanding executive position. She has exercised irregularly over the past 15 years and now wants to "get really fit and healthy." She smokes a pack of cigarettes a day and wants to quit. She eats reasonably well some of the time. At other times, she completely lets go and gains a few pounds, after which she starves herself until she sheds the extra weight.

## Dialogue

**Jan:** I want to be really fit. I want to be able to run 10K races without even having to think about it. I want to wear sleeveless shirts and have great arm muscles, and I want people to cringe with envy when they see my abs.

**Coach:** *(Using paraphrasing and questioning skills)* It sounds as if you want to be in peak form so that running a 10K would be easy and your body would be so fit that it would really make people notice. Are these your goals?

**Jan:** You've got it. That's what I want.

**Coach:** *(Probing for meaning)* Tell me this. If you were able to run a 10K race with ease, and if your body looked like the models in fitness magazines, what would this give you? What would it mean to you?

**Jan:** Well, it would mean that I look young and athletic . . . and people would look at me differently.

**Coach:** *(Probing further)* Okay, go on. You'd look young and athletic and people would see you differently. And what would that mean for you?

**Jan:** Well, I'm 36, you know . . . and I'm beginning to notice some changes in my skin and in how firm my body is.

**Coach:** *(Using reflection of feelings)* Am I hearing some concern about aging?

**Jan:** It's more than that. I used to take pride in my appearance. I counted on it. I guess my smoking doesn't help that, and neither does the way I eat.

**Coach:** *(Using reflection of meaning)* It sounds like your emphasis is on looking healthy by exercising regularly, yet you also seem to be aware that your eating and smoking may need to be modified.

**Jan:** Yes. I've been ducking this. I thought I'd get that great healthy glow from just exercising, but you're right, smoking doesn't do a lot for my complexion.

**Coach:** Uh-huh.

**Jan:** You know, now that you've said it, I want more than just looking healthy. I could have a perfectly sculpted body and still be unhealthy unless I'm willing to deal with the whole package.

**Coach:** *(Using reflection of meaning)* Are you saying that your deeper desire is to be healthy inside and out?

**Jan:** Yes, I am! I like the idea of looking young and fit and strong but I want it to be for real, not just an external show. I want to be that way from the inside out.

their desired future. Coaches can support clients in creating goals that are profoundly encompassing. They can also help them frame their expectations more realistically. As indicated in coaching dialogue 10.1, the 36-year-old client may choose to address her smoking and eating issues as part of her overall strategy for developing that strong, healthy glow. Alternatively, she may decide to proceed in a stepwise manner, dealing with her exercise involvement first. Then, having gained confidence and motivation from addressing that agenda, she could take on the challenges of quitting smoking and eating better.

## Steps in Reflecting Meaning

Reflections of meaning comprise four interrelated components: thoughts, feelings, behaviors, and, of course, meaning (Ivey et al., 2010). *Meaning* implies values, beliefs, deep-level motivations, and the significance that a person attributes to various facets of life and human action. Thoughts, feelings, and behaviors, however, do not provide perfect reflections of meaning. People must discover meaning through a process of inquiry, whether they do this privately or in dialogue with a coach.

Reflecting meaning relies on reflections of content and feeling, questioning, focusing, and even confronting, where discrepancies are highlighted in the dialogue. Whatever the stimulus for initiating a process of meaning reflection, the client must perceive such explorations as legitimate. A reflection of meaning reveals what lies beneath the surface, and although this method is generally appropriate for coaching relationships, clients who expect coaches to function more as technical experts may not welcome questions such as "What is it about this that so deeply matters to you?"

You might want to consider the following steps when using reflection of meaning:

1. **Determine need and timing.** This skill will be much more successful when appropriate boundaries for the coaching work and the methods of working together are clear. When clients tell their stories, they may volunteer the meanings beneath the surface, in which case there is little need to probe and explore further. More likely, they will offer only the surface information, which may have little potential for generating and sustaining meaningful change. Once the need to probe for meaning is evident, the next question is whether the timing is right. Reflection of meaning optimally occurs on the foundation of trust and rapport. Recognizing that clients may feel uncomfortable exposing sensitive personal information to someone who is a relative stranger, the deeper process of reflecting meaning might be postponed for a session or two until the relationship conditions (see chapter 6) have been sufficiently established.

2. **Formulate a theme.** Reflection of meaning needs a general direction. Inquiring out of general curiosity about the meaning a client attributes to life, relationships, or work is inappropriate. Such questioning may be perceived as quirky, unnecessarily philosophical, or simply out of bounds. When a man offers straightforward goals, such as "I want to learn how to eat well so I can feel more upbeat and energized throughout the day," a coach could easily offer support for this objective while at least wondering, "If you achieved this, what would it mean?" Moreover, the client may not fully understand some of his own words, such as *energized* and *upbeat*. So, at a minimum, the coach could explore the client's meaning of those words.

3. **Introduce the theme.** In simple reflections of meaning, a straightforward question such as "What does the word *upbeat* mean to you?" may suffice. However, when a theme has woven its way through a number of sentences or even sessions, it is likely that, first, it has significant bearing on the client's agenda, and, second, the client can benefit from an opportunity to explore these overlapping messages. The coach may begin a process of reflecting meaning by summarizing. Coaching dialogue 10.2 illustrates the initiation of a reflection.

4. **Blend approaches in the search for meaning.** When an issue is easily accessible to the client, only one or two questions might be necessary to discover the deeper meaning. In this case, the client knows the meaning, but the coach does not. Bringing this information into the public venue of their relationship will foster progress. More often, neither the coach nor the client fully understands the meaning of an issue, and therefore the process of discovery takes effort. If the client is barraged with probing questions, she might experience the process as a kind of interrogation. Defensiveness and emotional distance might result. A more effective strategy might rely on the considered use of a variety of approaches that pace the client in the process, that encourage openness, and that minimize defensive reactions (see coaching dialogue 10.2). The use of active listening may follow initial probes and may

# EXPLORING A MAJOR THEME THROUGH REFLECTING MEANING

The following dialogue weaves a number of coaching skills in the process of reflecting meaning. It exemplifies how a client can achieve clarity of his deeper motivations through the competent application of meaning reflections.

## Background Information

Phil, a 59-year-old man in relatively good health, has recently retired from a well-paid position as a research scientist. He believes that he has denied himself the opportunity to follow many of his dreams throughout life, but he now has the time and the financial security to pursue them. Many of these dreams involve high-risk pursuits. As a wise and cautious person, he wants to make sure that he's in the best condition to embark on these adventures. After three introductory meetings and some preliminary action planning, his coach chooses to address a theme that she has heard several times.

## Dialogue

**Coach:** *(Asking permission)* Phil, would you be willing to allow some time today for me to frame a theme I think I'm hearing from you—and for us to discuss it together?

**Phil:** Sure, sounds intriguing!

**Coach:** *(Using reflection of content)* The picture you have drawn of yourself is of a highly successful scientist who got where he did by being careful, being conservative, and never taking chances. Is this part accurate?

**Phil:** Yes, that certainly was the old me.

**Coach:** *(Using reflection of content)* Now I'm hearing that you want to engage in some pretty rugged and even dangerous activities because they have been your dream and you never took the time for them. This seems to be a kind of shift in the way you have lived your life. I'd like to understand more about what you are seeing in this new direction, especially when you contrast it with your previous patterns.

**Phil:** Frankly, I'm not 100% sure about this, but I think I lost an important part of me playing the scientist all these years, and I want to start having fun. I had fun discovering things but not like the fun I think I could have had sailing in the Bahamas. I've been a good scientist but I had to stuff a lot of my wilder side all these years.

**Coach:** *(Using reflection of meaning and questioning)* I hear you . . . and you imagine that sailing or something like that would allow you to get to know that wilder side better.

**Phil:** I think so. I want to go about this carefully, but I need to break out of that darn box that I've allowed myself to live in all these years.

**Coach:** *(Using reflection of feeling)* It sounds as if you have strong feelings about this.

**Phil:** I think so . . . even though I've had a good life, it's just time for a change. I'm still young enough and healthy enough to push it a bit, so why not?

**Coach:** *(Using powerful questioning)* So, why not?

**Phil:** Yeah, why not? I hope you can help me keep things in balance, because this isn't just about doing wild things, it's about me and how I see myself. I want to get reacquainted with that zany teenager I once was. I was a great student, but I also knew how to have fun.

**Coach:** *(Using a blend of skills)* This seems really important to you. I hear that all of this is about being your whole self, the way that you have always seen yourself but have not always allowed yourself to be. It's about bringing more excitement into your life in a careful way, even though it looks a lot riskier than what you've been like for the past 30 years.

**Phil:** Wow. What a great way of saying it! I'm going to think about this some more because having talked about it, I think I understand it better and I feel more in charge of it. Sometimes I just feel this urge to do it all, and now I have a better sense of where this is coming from.

lead to additional questions. Some powerful questions that have been suggested for accessing clients' meanings (Ivey et al., 2010) include the following:

Which of your values are best represented here?

What will this mean to you if you are able to achieve it?

What makes this so important to you?

Tell me how this makes sense to you.

If you were to put this all together, what would it represent to you?

Why do you want to do this?

Why this goal and not that one?

5. **Connect meaning to coaching goals.** Because the purpose of reflecting meaning needs to be practical more so than philosophical, the derived meanings must be connected to the client's goals. Some clients have moments of insight when they readily link their discoveries with the goals they have for coaching. In other cases, the connection may not be as evident, so the link needs to be made explicit.

## Upside and Downside of Reflecting Meaning

The upside of reflecting meaning was reviewed in our previous discussion of its purposes. Discovering clients' deeper meaning and values in their change objectives not only assists coaches in costructuring successful interventions but also generates ongoing motivation for action. If we think of the popular approach of having clients identify positive affirmations that, through constant repetition, direct and energize change (Goldman, 2001), then we can readily imagine how critical it is to find words and images that can reliably fuel action. Reflecting meaning enables clients to understand why they are choosing certain goals, why they want to change now, and what they desire from the coaching process. Yet, as with all other methods, certain uses of meaning reflections can become problematic. Here are some issues to bear in mind.

1. **Reflecting meaning as an end in itself.** Coaching contracts relate to agendas that clients deem important to pursue. Reflecting meaning can be rewarding in itself. Some clients may revel in processes of self-discovery, but because coaching is action oriented, such discovery processes must always help advance action and goal attainment.

2. **Steering the agenda.** Imagine a client who states certain objectives that you, for personal reasons, disagree with. For instance, a client may want to do whatever it takes to become an elite amateur bodybuilder and you may privately disapprove of this agenda. By using reflection of meaning, you could lead the client to question her own values and goals. Implicitly, you may convey disapproval of the client's agenda by the way in which you ask, "Why exactly do you want to do this?" The discovery process may continue until you redefine the client's agenda. Unfortunately, she is likely to feel shamed and demoralized if her important goals have somehow been discredited through a biased reflective process.

3. **Probing too deeply.** As noted throughout this section, reflecting meaning gets beneath the surface. How deep it needs to go depends on the agenda and agreements about how coach and client will work together. Coaches need to estimate how much information they need in order to formulate strategies. More is not always better. In fact, with some clients, minimal meaning reflections will suffice. Going deeper may cause them to spin in indecision and uncertainty. The process may unduly broaden the agenda or produce too many options to consider. Bringing up the bottom, that is, unearthing profound questions and concerns, is not always a great strategy. Some clients may have struggled to find the motivation to engage a coach to help them with their work, and they may live with barely concealed dissatisfaction about a number of other issues. Asking too many questions about their

---

**REFLECTION 10.2**

Reflection of meaning promotes self-awareness and mindfulness. We invite you to take a few minutes and sit back to think about why you do what you do.

When you think about the things you do, particularly your deep passions, what meanings can you find in your pursuit of these agendas or practices? Why did you choose these and not other things? Particularly, when you find yourself struggling with something for a long time yet continuing despite the hardships, what do you think this is all about for you? What purposes are being served in your life? What are the bigger values that are represented in these actions?

reasons for wanting to achieve certain health goals may reawaken self-rejecting thoughts and feelings that cancel out their positive motivations.

# INTERPRETATION

**Interpretation** is one of the oldest approaches in the helping professions (Clark, 1995) and one of the most widely misunderstood. Interpretation is often associated with the highly complex and esoteric works of psychoanalysis (Freud, 1964). However, according to Frank and Frank (1993), virtually all professional helpers interpret their clients' behaviors according to the theoretical frameworks in which they were educated. In coaching, the term *interpretation* continues to be widely used (Kimsey-House et al., 2011; Neenan & Dryden, 2002; Williams & Davis, 2007), although it is often associated with concepts such as reframing and the use of metaphors.

Ivey and colleagues (1997) describe interpretation as "the renaming of client experience from an alternative frame of reference or worldview" (p. 248). The client tells the coach a story; the coach puts the client's words into his own language and feeds that back to the client with the intention of creating greater awareness or behavior change (Brammer & MacDonald, 2003).

Whitworth and colleagues (2007) refer to interpretation, or reframing, as a hunch or intuition that a coach has about the client's situation. In this view, interpretation is not a judgment or even something definite. Coaches develop a sense about what is going on, and in their own words, they try to communicate their hunches to their clients. Borrowing more from the concept of reframing, Williams and Davis (2007) indicate that what coaches do is "find other words or descriptors for something that appears to be a challenge, problem or deficiency in the client's view. You place the behavior or perception, as articulated by the client, in a new context or frame. This allows the client to see whatever the situation or concern is in a new way. Rather than viewing the problem as a weakness, it can be seen as an opportunity for learning" (pp. 107-108).

## Types of Interpretation

Examining different types of interpretation might remove any remaining beliefs that this skill belongs more to counseling and psychotherapy than to coaching. To some degree, the following types might be seen as occurring along a continuum of depth. (See coaching dialogue 10.3 for examples of the types of interpretation.)

### Interpretations That Add Implied Messages

Interpretations can be seen as a form of additive empathy (see chapter 6). The coach includes aspects of the client's message that she seemed to imply through nonverbal or verbal cues but did not state directly (Egan, 2010). A woman may look sad or elated when describing an experience but never label her feelings. If the coach were to reflect the content of the client's messages and add the unspoken element of feelings, this would be a kind of interpretation. It nonetheless represents an interpretation because the coach rather than the client brings in the unstated meaning; it had to be interpreted from nonverbal indicators.

### Interpretations That Connect Messages and Add Implications or Conclusions

We noted in chapter 7 that summarizing involves bringing together various messages that a client has delivered over time. When a coach summarizes a number of client messages and then adds something that may be implied or even something that he infers (a hunch) from the information, this process is more accurately described as interpretation. It may seem like splitting hairs, but the distinction between reflecting actual messages and adding something that has been unspoken can have major consequences for the relationship and the client. Coaches may think that what they are sensing in a situation must be obvious to the client as well. Possibly it is, yet making the implicit explicit can be important. When it is not evident to the client, the coach will have brought to awareness something in the individual's blind self that may foster positive movement.

### Interpretations That Reframe the Client's Issue

This form of interpretation has sometimes been described as looking on the bright side of things (Whitworth et al., 2007), but it is much more than that. When clients are struggling with issues, they may be unaware of the strengths that they are exhibiting or the potential in their dilemmas. Walking

## Common Metaphors in Everyday Speech

I feel blue today; I feel on top of the world; I feel flighty; I feel inside out.

She's cute as a button; she has a heart of gold; she's a witch; she's a money magnet; she's an angel; she's a devil.

Life's a beach; life's a bowl of cherries; life's a roller coaster; life's just a dream; life's a hard road to travel; life's a gift.

He's cold as ice; he's a rock (a snake, a pig, a knight in shining armor, a diamond in the rough).

Time is money; a stitch in time saves nine; don't cry over spilled milk; make hay while the sun shines; a bird in the hand is better than two in the bush; a penny saved is a penny earned.

in a fog, we may not realize what lies just beyond our range of vision. To the person involved, a situation may seem hopeless, whereas to someone less involved, possibilities may abound. Reframing is a way of taking what people are describing and presenting a more adaptive view for them to consider as an alternative. As noted, reframing generally provides perspectives with greater potentiality and hopefulness, although not always. A reframe could also present the dangers or negative implications of a scenario with the intention of alerting the person to unforeseen consequences so that he might avoid them.

### Metaphors

Metaphors may be simple or complex (Lakoff & Johnson, 1980; Lawley & Tompkins, 2000). "You seem to be *rising above* it all now and seeing it for what it truly is" is a metaphorical expression implying that the client is extricating herself from a situation to gain perspective. This simple metaphor captures in visual imagery some aspect of an experience; however, the description comes from the coach rather than from the client. Metaphors that are more complex may take the form of stories that illuminate certain dynamics of what the client has been expressing. Fables and fairy tales are elegant metaphors from which coaches hope their clients are able to draw a useful moral. See Common Metaphors in Everyday Speech for examples of metaphors frequently used in everyday speech.

### Theory-Based Interpretations

When a particular theory informs a coach's work, interpreting a client's thoughts, feelings, or behaviors within this framework can provide an entirely new way of understanding. Chapter 3 describes

the TTM. When clients' behaviors are described through such a framework, coaches are using a theoretical interpretation. Similarly, if they use certain inventories or profiling tests and communicate meanings extracted from these measures, they are using a theoretical interpretation.

## Purposes of Interpretation

Interpretation serves a number of purposes that are similar to those of other coaching methods, including reflection of meaning, summarizing, and immediacy. What distinguishes it from some of these other methods is that the coach is explicit about the meaning she is adding to the dialogue. In reflecting meaning, she may ask, "What sense do you make of this?" whereas in interpretation, she is more likely to say something to the effect of "Here's the meaning I see in this." Interpretations serve several purposes, including the following.

### Developing Insight and New Perspectives

When coaches reframe clients' experiences, reflect unspoken messages, or describe their stories in metaphorical ways, clients hopefully gain insight into the reasons for their behavior or come to see themselves in a new light. Such insights and perspectives are not ends in themselves; they serve to propel movement toward the person's desired future.

### Revealing Resources

In the last quarter of the 20th century, when women returned to work after raising their families, they often confronted the difficult task of putting

# TYPES OF INTERPRETATION

The following dialogue depicts the different types of interpretations that can be derived from a client's statements. You will find some more potent than others, though all have the ultimate goal of moving the client forward.

## Background Information

Jenna, a 27-year-old financial analyst, has been working with a coach for more than six months on a multifaceted program to build confidence and compete successfully in an amateur tennis association. She performs well in practice but invariably makes errors in competition that she almost never does in practice sessions. The coach has worked with her using mental imagery along with guiding other aspects of a cross-training program and adherence to sleep and nutrition commitments determined through consultations with a doctor and a nutritionist. In recent sessions, Jenna has made these remarks, which the coach has noted carefully.

**Comment 1:** Even at work I seem to clutch whenever I feel someone is watching. I don't like people looking over my shoulder.

**Comment 2:** I want to win so bad that I make stupid mistakes because I'm trying too hard.

**Comment 3:** I hate competition.

In this session, the client is upset about a recent loss against an opponent whom she always defeats in practice.

**Comment 4:** I can't believe it. I threw the game away. She can't play anywhere near my level of tennis, yet she trounced me yesterday. I'm such a loser.

## Types of Interpretation
### Adding Implied Messages

**Coach:** Jenna, it sounds as if you're feeling frustrated with yourself, like someone who's determined to defeat herself.

### Connecting Messages and Adding Implications or Conclusions

**Coach:** Jenna, I can really hear how disappointed you feel with yourself, and I sense from other things you've said—like about work and about trying too hard—that when the spotlight shines on you in competition, you "clutch" and "make stupid mistakes." There seems to be something in this about not being able to perform well when it counts the most.

### Reframing

**Coach:** Jenna, I hear you . . . how disappointed you feel with yourself . . . like you set yourself up for failure. Yet, maybe there's another message in this. I remember you telling me one time that you hate competition. Perhaps some part of you is trying to get through to you that how you are engaging in this game doesn't work for you. You do well in practice because you're having fun. As soon as you define the situation as competition, the fun exits—and this overaggressive, angry competitor that you don't want to be comes roaring out.

### Metaphorical Interpretation

**Coach:** Ouch . . . it seems like you're really hurting and upset about this. I have this image of you tying your shoes before you go out on the tennis court and saying to everyone watching, "Look at me. I'm going to make it as difficult as I can for myself to win. It reminds me of that children's story *The Little Engine That Could*, except you're saying, "I know I can't, I know I can't, I know I can't."

### Theory-Based Interpretation

**Coach:** Jenna, I can see how upset you are and how you're blaming yourself for all this. Things you've said to me over the past few weeks make me wonder whether this all might be about a *fear of success*. You know that your inherent skills are far better than what you demonstrate when you're competing, and you've also said that you hate competition, yet you continue to place yourself in the limelight at these kinds of events. So you do what you don't like or even hate under conditions that you normally find upsetting, that is, having people watch you. Then, no surprise, you fail, almost as if you set it up to happen that way. I guess the unknown in this little theory of mine is what it would mean to you if you were to be successful at something that you wanted so badly.

together a credible résumé of skills and experiences. Not having held a salaried position for many years, they tended to view themselves as unskilled and therefore unemployable. Only through reframing the tasks they engaged in while raising children and managing homes were they able to understand the extensive talents they had been nurturing and perfecting over many years of unpaid employment. The skill of interpretation opens windows for clients on experiences they have had so that they can appreciate latent talents, uncover opportunities and resources, and imagine new pathways. Interpretation feeds development by breaking through self-defined limitations and restrictive worldviews.

### Generating Energy

When clients awaken to a new vision of themselves as a result of an interpretation, they typically discover new reserves of energy that they can use to foster their chosen agendas. As the lights go on, clients seem to wake up and feel motivated to act.

### Building the Relationship

Although interpretation involves a degree of risk, when it is successful, clients are likely to express more trust and feel more comfortable in exploring other issues that may be impeding progress toward their desired goals. At the very least, the coaching relationship can be strengthened; potentially, clients will want to bring their new awareness to others for further exploration and connection.

## Steps in Interpretation

Interpretation relies on having sufficient rapport to permit coaches to influence clients and to manage potential negative effects of its misguided use. Simple interpretations can be drafted and offered without complication, whereas deep-level interpretations need to be constructed and implemented with great sensitivity. The following steps have been suggested in discussions of interpretation in the helping professions (Brammer & MacDonald, 2003; Cormier et al., 2009; Ivey et al., 2010). They are reframed here for coaching roles.

1. **Ensure rapport and trust.** Significant themes in a client's messages are usually repeated numerous times. When carefully noted, these themes can inform interpretations. However, to estimate the likelihood of successful interpretation, you must appreciate the way in which your client responds to situations, her openness to new ideas, and her receptivity to your comments in general. All of this relies on the prior establishment of a trusting relationship.

2. **Structure interpretations.** As seen in dialogue 10.3, a number of interpretations can be used, from simple images to complex metaphors. The varying depths of different types of interpretations must be carefully considered. Coaches will need to structure their interpretations according to clients' capacities to absorb the ideas presented.

3. **Time the interpretation.** In long-term relationships, the amount of information that you have about your client and the degree of rapport established will likely allow for the repeated use of certain interpretive messages in order to highlight some of the client's patterns. For instance, someone who seems to be walking on eggshells in all realms of life might benefit from a reminder whenever the pattern emerges. When a deep interpretation is delivered for the first time, however, clients must be ready and sufficient time allowed to process the client's responses.

4. **Deliver the interpretation.** For straightforward and simple interpretations, you may blend the message with an image, metaphor, or observation amid reflections or feedback. When the interpretation is more involved, you may want to ask for the client's agreement before proceeding.

5. **Appreciate the impact.** When delivering an interpretation, your awareness remains on the client. If your interpretation is lengthy (e.g., telling a story), you may need to suspend delivery of your message if there are indications of resistance or discomfort. Following the interpretation, you will want to work with your client to appreciate meanings drawn from the interpretation.

6. **Explore the client's associations.** When interpretations are complex, clients may be encouraged to connect the relevant aspects of the interpretation to as many domains of their thoughts, feelings, and behaviors as justified within the parameters of the coaching relationship. Bearing in mind that people exhibit certain degrees of consistency across areas of their lives, you need to guard the boundaries by helping clients shape implications of interpretations within the legitimate realm of the contract.

## Upside and Downside of Interpretation

We have discussed how interpretations can foster understanding, develop new perspectives, lead to the pursuit of new directions, and enhance the working alliance. We also have acknowledged that because you are offering something that is unspoken by the client and framed in your own worldview, a degree of risk accompanies this strategy. The following points highlight problematic aspects of interpretations.

1. **Expanding the agenda.** A client may manifest certain behaviors or even attitudes that could interfere with some realms of his functioning; if the coaching contract does not extend to these domains, however, you must either renegotiate the scope of the contract or allow these matters to go without comment.

2. **Shooting from the lip.** Some schools of coaching encourage coaches to freely express their hunches and intuitions (Whitworth et al., 2007). The more experience and knowledge a coach has, the more likely it is that this can happen effectively. However, it remains a risky approach. Clients may not be ready—and you could be dead wrong. It's hard to erase what has been said, and given the power that you hold as a coach, clients may be

strongly affected by a poorly conceived interpretation.

3. **Poor timing.** Well-formed interpretations are generally based on sound evidence gathered over time. Even when core themes are identified early in the coaching process, an opportune moment must arise to offer interpretations. Brown and Srebalus (2003) argue that interpretation is most likely to be appropriate after the initial tasks of relationship building and contracting have been accomplished.

4. **Interpretations as ends.** Interpretation as a coaching skill is never an isolated event; it must be framed within the purposes of the relationship. You may have exquisite intuition and create impressive images of how your clients function, or you may have wonderful stories carrying inspirational messages. As long as they relate to the agreed-upon agenda, they are appropriate.

5. **Irrefutable interpretations.** You can be right about your interpretations, but if the client resists strongly, it is unwise to argue the point. Trying to convince clients of the accuracy of your interpretations, especially by presenting supposedly irrefutable evidence, can be detrimental to the relationship.

6. **Mysterious interpretations.** Offering clients interpretations is not about being psychic. A hunch, an intuition, or some visual image comes from somewhere. You need to be able to articulate the bases of your interpretations rather than imply that clients should simply trust your inner wisdom.

Clients tell their stories from a personal perspective, emphasizing some elements and ignoring others. Stories are rarely complete representations of one's realities; in fact, some may be quite impoverished. Some people may focus on what's wrong, what's missing, or all the reasons why they can't do something. Interpretations are used to promote positive change, yet as a coach you are not a cheerleader. You are not there to reframe lemons into lemonade. And your intention is not to offer fairy tales. Creating awareness is often necessary and powerful—and it is always in service of change.

## DESIGNING ACTION

We now move to the ninth ICF core competency of designing action within the more encompassing theme of facilitating learning and results. In chapter 4 we described our flow model of coaching, which was divided into the two phases of engagement and goal pursuit. The core competency of designing

---

**REFLECTION 10.3**

Simple and complex metaphors are potent interpretations in that they leave space for people to derive implications and personal meanings. As you work with clients or even as you interact informally with others around you, we invite you to do the following:

1. Become aware of when you are using metaphors to express messages, thoughts, or feelings. How might others be interpreting your metaphors? How do they respond? Do your metaphors add clarity, or are they too ambiguous? Do they open up the conversation?

2. Think about some of your clients or people you know who are experiencing significant changes. Imagine a metaphor that might describe how each person seems to be amid the changes they are pursuing. Especially when they are struggling with the change process, what metaphors might best capture them in their experiences? If something clearly connects for you and you can safely and appropriately offer the metaphor, try it out with humility and a willingness to explore.

actions is strongly aligned with the goal-pursuit phase of this model.

Designing action is, according to the ICF (2011c), the ability to create with the client opportunities for ongoing learning, during coaching and in work–life situations, and for taking new actions that will most effectively lead to agreed-upon coaching results. A coach who clearly evidences this competency

- brainstorms and assists the client to define actions that will enable the client to demonstrate, practice, and deepen new learning;
- helps the client to focus on and systematically explore specific concerns and opportunities that are central to agreed-upon coaching goals;
- engages the client to explore alternative ideas and solutions, to evaluate options, and to make related decisions;
- promotes active experimentation and self-discovery, where the client applies what has been discussed and learned during sessions immediately afterward in his work or life setting;
- celebrates client successes and capabilities for future growth;
- challenges the client's assumptions and perspectives to provoke new ideas and find new possibilities for action;
- advocates or brings forward points of view that are aligned with client goals and, without attachment, engages the client to consider them;
- helps the client "do it now" during the coaching session, providing immediate support; and
- encourages, stretches, and challenges but also offers a comfortable pace of learning.

International Coach Federation 2011

As mentioned earlier, action and insight are intricately related; each informs the other. Imagine that a woman approaches you with a desire to become a wellness consultant working with groups and organizations. Assuming that you have expertise related to this agenda, you take on the challenge. What is the starting point? What has she done? What does she know? What are her skills? How well does she relate to people? These are just a few of the questions that immediately cross your mind. In your initial session, you discover that this client is quite talented—and that she still has a lot to learn. Where do you start designing action? What do you emphasize first? How do you go about exploring her background to further define her skill set? What learning would help most as she goes about building her career? The more complex the client's agenda, the more facets you will need to consider. Yet, even when working with seemingly straightforward agendas, there are social elements, financial components, personal habits, knowledge pieces, work issues, and maybe even moral matters to consider. Designing action in these less complex agendas is still more than doing just one thing; it is multidimensional.

Designing action relates to the question of what to emphasize at this point to connect clients' awakened understanding of their agenda to a well-structured and organized process of forward movement. It is about discovering what the options are and identifying avenues of action that are likely to be more productive than others. It is about locating and removing obstacles. It concerns finding the client's preferred pace of movement and her capacity to manage multiple efforts in addressing the dimensions essential to creating her desired future.

# THE COMPETENCY DEVELOPMENT MODEL

What kind of framework can we use for appreciating the multidimensional nature of any client's agenda for change? Let's begin to answer that by considering the following scenario:

A highly stressed manager goes to his doctor for a checkup. The doctor says, "You have mild hypertension. I want you to take this prescription. Come back and see me in six months." The man complies. He goes to the pharmacy and takes a pill every day for the next six months. What has changed? You might say, "Very little." Think again. Is this now the same man who walked into the doctor's office? Mostly yes, but he knows something about himself that he didn't know before. That knowledge may change his self-definition from "I am a healthy man" to "I am a man with heart disease." Does he behave the same way? Well, maybe. But he may also think more about what's causing his hypertension, and he may try to do something about it.

Imagine he's married with kids. Is his social world the same? Unlikely. His partner may be concerned and scrutinize his actions and diet. He may talk to friends and find himself relating more to guys who also are taking similar pills every day. Will anything change financially? He may look at his life insurance policy a bit more closely, but if he wants to increase his coverage, he may have to pay an extra premium now. And on it goes.

Clients don't come to coaching with an expectation of getting a magic solution to their issues—or if they do, they will be quickly dissuaded from this illusion. Let's imagine now that the man with hypertension described in the previous scenario is your client. He's tired of popping pills. He doesn't think this is the best answer for him. If your background is in fitness, maybe your first thoughts will be about exercise programs. If you are trained in nutrition, you might leap to dietary adjustments. If your area of expertise is in stress management, you might look at ways this man can engage in a mindfulness-based stress reduction practice. However, jumping to any one avenue rather than looking at the whole picture can be highly problematic and limited in effectiveness. It is also true that taking in the whole picture will have challenges. Maybe your client hired you because he thought you were going to work with him on only exercise or nutrition or meditation.

You may be wondering, "Can I really address the whole person if he just wants an exercise program or a nutrition program?" Before answering this question, let's consider two ways in which your client might state his interest in a coaching relationship:

**Option A:** The client says, "I want to deal with my hypertension by exercising regularly. I need your help in designing and sticking to a heart-healthy exercise program."

**Option B:** The client says, "I have hypertension and I'm quite stressed. I want to give up my meds and live in a way that keeps my blood pressure within normal parameters."

Clearly, option B is going to be more about the whole person, but guess what. Option A is as well! You may have more latitude for the ways in which you work with this person with option B, but even with option A, you must appreciate all the relevant dimensions of this man's life. To help someone change just one aspect of his life, you need to con-

sider the whole person and all the ramifications of this one change. No matter how you define your coaching practice, any potential challenges to continuity must be addressed for change to be robust and long lasting.

In this section, we offer a perspective for designing actions that address the whole person, even when coaching agendas are narrow in scope. As a core competency, designing action speaks to the coach's ability to ask powerful questions, to listen supportively, to create new awareness, and to maintain the client's forward focus. Skill components related to this competency have been covered in previous chapters. Rather than reiterating these skills, we offer a whole-person framework for competency development as a powerful new perspective about structuring change initiatives.

The **competency development model** derives from the seminal work of Howard Gardner (1983, 2006) on multiple intelligences. Gardner originally described seven areas of human intelligence. Later theorists expanded these areas into other frameworks (Armstrong, 2003; Ellison, 2001; Wilber, 2000c). We prefer the term *competency* to that of *intelligence* because it implies the possibility of development more readily than does the construct of intelligence, which might suggest something fixed and innate.

In the world of coaching, competency development can be seen in the integral coaching approach of Joanne Hunt (2009) and Laura Divine (2009), which exquisitely articulates a philosophy and methodology for addressing the wholeness of clients. Sourced by the work of Ken Wilber (2000a, 2000b, 2000c) and his integral theory, Hunt and Divine propose that the client's agenda be apprehended in the complex nature of who the client is and his ways of being in the world. Within this framework, the client's agenda is approached through multiple lenses of his strengths, lifestyle, habits, personality, thought patterns, feelings, and relationships.

When considering what a client needs to do to move forward, Hunt and Divine propose that we consider six lines of development: cognitive, emotional, somatic, interpersonal, moral, and spiritual. These lines of development are analogous to what we describe as the clients' competencies pertaining to the goals they want to achieve. Coaching is sometimes a matter of clients' mobilizing capacities they already have; at other times, clients need to master new competencies that are critical to the steps required to move forward. The following example will help contextualize this idea.

> A woman wishes to live a long and healthy life, yet she currently has a strongly ingrained pattern of unhealthy behaviors. At a physical level, she may need to learn new skills to engage in physical activities; moreover, she may need to develop the capacity to sense how her body is feeling in the moment. She may need to practice stress management, which could involve the interpersonal skill of asserting herself in order to say no to demands on her time and the cognitive skill of retraining her thought processes. She may have certain emotional triggers that cause her to pick up a cigarette or to eat beyond satiation. Morally, she may struggle with her definition of fairness as she rearranges her time commitments to work and family. As the example indicates, it would be naive to assume that this person currently has all these capacities necessary for the design of actions. Equally, it would be unrealistic to propose action plans that require her to "just do it." She needs to build these specific capacities over time. This is the essence of the competency development model.

To assist clients in moving forward, a series of actions are usually planned to accomplish certain things at certain times. Some actions may be about building new competencies, while others may focus on tapping into and reinforcing existing strengths. As the coaching relationship progresses, clients are likely to engage in overlapping actions that occur both simultaneously and sequentially.

Achieving goals such as completing a marathon, losing a certain amount of weight, quitting smoking, or maintaining blood pressure at normal levels takes a master plan. That plan can be roughly sketched in the first few sessions, though modifications are likely to occur due to new information and learning along the way. Neither coach nor client will have a fully developed strategic plan at the beginning. Much needs to be discovered. As time goes on and with the results of actions that clients engage, evidence emerges about where they are strong and where they need to develop other competencies.

Coaching rarely looks like a monolithic effort to do just one thing over a number of months. Rather, a series of interrelated initiatives will begin at various points in the relationship. After months of persistent effort, tangible effects can be seen and a critical mass of progress accumulates. New competencies have been developed, and old ones have been strengthened. As a result, clients feel sturdier in facing the challenges of their new ways of living. There are multiple celebrations for achievements and the acknowledgment of milestones that have been met and surpassed. Clients have been engaged in concerted efforts that shift interrelated dimensions of their lives.

In discussing the competency development model, we outline six competencies that are most pertinent to a holistic view of a person engaged in a coaching relationship. These are general knowledge, self-knowledge, and emotional, somatic, interpersonal, and moral competencies. We will describe each before applying them systematically to coaching situations.

## General Knowledge Competency

What does the client know about the issues related to her agenda? Here we are considering information and data as well as scientific evidence and opinion. Beyond this, we would want to know her degree of competency in translating knowledge into action strategies. How capable is she of applying relevant knowledge to her agenda? In working with someone whose goal is to reduce stress, we might inquire what the person knows about stress, its causes, and strategies for managing it. For this client to be autonomous and self-directing in the future, what knowledge does she need to learn? Where can she find reliable information? Once the lacunae in her general knowledge pertaining to stress have been identified through the coaching dialogue, actions to address these gaps can be constructed and initiated.

## Self-Knowledge Competency

How accurately does the client know herself in relation to her agenda? How knowledgeable is she about her personal style as it relates to her agenda? If her goal is stress management, how well does she understand how she generates and manages stress in her life? Does she recognize her triggers and sensitivities? Does she know about her optimal stress levels for performance? What is her mental model of stress? How readily can she translate self-knowledge into behavioral prescriptions for what she needs to do regarding stress? The difference between self-knowledge and general knowledge can be illustrated as follows: Knowing about your specific triggers for stress reactions is self-knowledge, whereas understanding that the process of stress typically involves triggering situations or stimuli is general knowledge. If this client needs to develop self-knowledge, then actions to increase her mental framework for understanding what stress is for her and what she knows about herself in stressful encounters might be an avenue to pursue.

## Emotional Competency

What are the client's emotional capacities related to her agenda? Is she able to identify emotional experiences—her own as well as others'—with a high degree of accuracy? Can she differentiate among levels of emotional experience, especially as they arise in the context of her coaching topic? This competency is comparable to Goleman's (1995) proposal of emotional intelligence. If the desired goal is smoking cessation, for example, how attuned is she to her emotional world as it relates to this behavior? What are her competencies in emotional self-management in general? How does she deal with her emotions other than through smoking? What feelings arise in regard to her self-concept pertaining to her agenda (e.g., "I feel embarrassed to be a smoker")? Do these feelings overwhelm her, or does she have perspective about them? What are her strengths in appreciating and managing her emotional world? Action planning for developing emotional competency in this instance would concern actions that this client most needs to do (e.g., expressing emotions, managing feelings, journaling) in order to make progress toward her goal.

## Somatic Competency

What is the client's body knowledge related to her agenda? What competencies does she have at a physical level to move forward? If her topic is increasing her exercise levels, what physical capacities does she possess? What body knowledge does she have? How sensitive is she to somatic messages of well-being or impending illness? How does she regard her body? Does she see it as an instrument that is somewhat separate from her? Or does she inhabit her body comfortably, experiencing strong mind–body connections? Is she aware of which somatic practices would help her most in moving forward? Which ones would give her greatest satisfaction? Which ones would challenge her yet offer long-lasting benefits? What area of her physical

being does she need to work on right now to set the foundation for future development?

## Interpersonal Competency

Similar to Goleman's (2006) concept of social intelligence, this competency addresses the client's competencies in relationships with others. Does she have an accurate and useful social map of her world related to her agenda for coaching? How do others influence her (e.g., "I smoke more whenever I am upset with someone")? How does she influence others? What is the quality of her relationships with those around her? Can she successfully engage with friends, colleagues, family, and strangers in matters essential to forward movement? If her goal is developing greater self-confidence, how do others play into her experience and self-presentation? How aware is she of these interpersonal influences? How able is she to deal with them effectively to achieve desired outcomes? What actions does she need to take to develop her interpersonal competence?

## Moral Competency

Borrowing from Kohlberg's (1981) propositions regarding moral development, this competency examines the client's judgment process related to her agenda. How capable is she of understanding her goals and the path toward these objectives in a way that is fair and compassionate toward herself and others? What is her competency in minimizing blame, shame, and guilt and transforming such judgmental experiences into more empowering perceptions? If her agenda concerns body image and weight, how compassionate and nonjudgmental is she toward herself and others? Is she able to transcend a self-negating view of her body and appreciate herself in more adaptive perspectives? What might she need to do to reduce judgmental tendencies and generate greater acceptance?

Each of the competencies is framed in the perspective of the client's agenda rather than in a global view of the client's life. For instance, concerning general knowledge, the coach does not consider how much a client knows about the world but rather how much knowledge she has pertinent to her topic and how capable she is of manipulating that knowledge base to formulate intelligent goal-related actions. As a coach, you will be interested in creating awareness pertinent to each of these six competencies in order to codetermine what is available to your clients and what they yet need to grow.

Let's come back to our client dealing with hypertension. Imagine he states his agenda in a broad fashion as wanting to live in a way that keeps him in the normal range for blood pressure with reduced stress levels. Should you choose to work toward creating a multilayered program of exercise, nutrition, work–life balance, and meditation, you would need to examine his competencies for each component of his program. He may know a lot about nutrition but little about exercise. He may have good interpersonal competencies for fitness engagement but come up short on being able to say no to stress-producing work assignments. He may feel anxious going to novel fitness classes but be competent in managing other emotional reactions within fitness settings. When he travels, he may experience a high degree of emotionally driven eating but show greater control at home.

Some clients may be sufficiently self-aware to know what their competency levels are in each of the six areas as related to their agenda, whereas others may have relatively little insight. Coaches might need to create client awareness of the strengths and resources they have and those they need to develop in order to motivate action. By asking questions and checking for understanding, they come to know whether clients would be self-sufficient in doing things such as beginning an exercise program without supervision.

One of the priceless gifts of the competency development model in relation to designing actions is that it focuses on growth over time. The six areas in the competency development model provide structure for organizing what clients might need to address to sustain positive change in their lives. The model provides a practical framework with which to inquire and formulate practices that clients can systematically and continuously engage in. The relative importance of each competency needs to be assessed in the context of what clients most desire and how they most efficiently learn. Determining which competency people need to address first will always involve a degree of judgment about its centrality to change and the degree to which progress will feed motivation. Of course, it is likely that designed actions can influence learning on more than one competency. For instance, an action plan wherein a client writes down her inner dialogue during stressful moments can feed self-knowledge, emotional, and moral competencies.

As implied earlier, there is an essential and reciprocal relationship between competency development and goal achievement. A client's goal refers to what she wants to achieve, whereas competencies pertain to the methodology, or *how* she will succeed. The client may want to live a healthy and balanced life or complete an Olympic-distance triathlon. These are goals she wants to achieve. It will take an in-depth coaching conversation to understand what she might need in order to reach her objective. In the process she will discover capacities, resources, behavioral patterns, values, motivations, and other dreams she may have. Some of what will be uncovered will pertain to specific competencies she needs to develop. Completing a triathlon, for instance, requires competencies in running, biking, and swimming along with sufficient endurance to go the distance. She may need to master emotional concerns about falling off her bike or neglecting other life responsibilities as she trains for the big event. She will probably need to understand the technicalities of completing a triathlon (general knowledge) as well as knowing how she is going to cope with the mind noise that she hears whenever she does tough things (self-knowledge and emotional competency). These issues represent parts of the *how*, and they pertain to competencies that she will need in order to live her dream.

# COMMENTARY

Beyond the learning and doing related to achieving goals and dreams are the realities that clients create along the path of change. As weeks of coaching and action pass, clients know that the lights have gone on. Not only has their new awareness shown the way, but they have a growing sense that they can keep these lights shining. That is, they have awakened to an ever-changing and increasingly satisfying new world. Awareness continues to feed action, and action in turn stimulates new awareness. That is the cycle. Though at times it may seem never ending, there are plateaus or resting places. There are zones of experience where clients simply take in all that they have created for themselves, inside and out. Ideally, we are all lifelong learners. As coaches, our work generates awareness and forward movement. Yet, as noted in the elements of the ICF's core competency of designing actions, coaches wisely make space to celebrate progress and acknowledge milestones, and perhaps they even create reflective occasions where clients pause without intention and without the need to move further or faster. They signal to their clients that it is okay to stop and savor the new realities generated through intelligent and dedicated engagement.

The subject matter of this chapter speaks to heady moments in the coaching process. There is much excitement in seeing clients grow in awareness, self-appreciation, competency, and achievement. It is stimulating when, through our collaborative work, clients' impossible dreams are embraced more and more as emerging realities. In short-term coaching relationships, there may be a continual sense of rushing to the finish line, whereas in long-term projects and change initiatives, clients need to find balance between doing and being. Pacing progress and allowing time for action and reflection can be as pivotal to success as the powerful methods we use to forward the action.

# BUILDING ENDURING FUTURES

*In this chapter, you will learn how…*

- each component of action planning needs to be articulated to maximize clients' chances of success;

- SuPeRSMART elements apply to outcome, performance, and process goals;

- the competency development model applies to both phases of the coaching flow model;

- the ending of coaching represents a process rather than a static event; and

- management of endings will ideally promote client autonomy, self-efficacy, and the transfer of learning.

> If you want to identify me, ask me not
> where I live, or what I like to eat, or how I comb
> my hair, but ask me what I am living for, in detail,
> ask me what I think is keeping me from living
> fully for the thing I want to live for.
>
> —*Thomas Merton*

Many clients enter coaching relationships after a number of unsatisfactory attempts to change. They may have lost and regained weight, quit smoking dozens of times, begun a meditation practice every few months, or tried repeatedly to create work–life balance, all without enduring success. It seems far less difficult for people to initiate change than to stick with it over the long term. In the TTM (chapter 3), the action stage is transcended only after six months of sustained commitment. Then comes the maintenance stage, which technically can last a lifetime, though clients are thought to be on relatively solid ground after another six months or so.

Novice coaches often wonder what experienced coaches do after the first few months. Coaching in the early stages can be stimulating and highly challenging. Coaches get to discover the inner worlds of new clients. They successfully engage them toward lasting change. They plan and experiment. They uncover new resources and opportunities. Insight and awareness abound. Then, the client has it—she has articulated a way forward that she believes she can maintain. Do coaches then babysit their clients for the next six to nine months? Will clients continue to pay for that? Will coaches find meaning in this kind of work?

There are clients who get it quickly and whose continuing commitment is unquestionable; they are not the majority. There are others whose goals are tangible and time limited, such as training for a marathon. A lot will depend on the clientele you choose to attract. What if your coaching niche is working with adults who have long-standing health issues or characteristics that put them at risk of disease or even premature death? How long do you think it will take for those who have had a lifetime of poor eating habits, substance abuse, chronic stress, or unhealthy patterns to get it for good? Well, maybe a lifetime, but how long will you be able to work with them in meaningful ways that are challenging and productive for them and responsible and engaging for you?

Many coaches like to frame the initial commitment with their clients somewhere around 3 months. Data from the ICF's survey of practices (2012) show that, in North America, 14% of clients engage in a coaching relationship for 3 months or less, 47% for 4 to 6 months, and 26% for 7 to 12 months. Only about 8% remain in coaching for over a year. These findings suggest that a large number of clients are on their own during a time when changed patterns are stabilizing but not necessarily set as lifelong habits.

The gift of coaching that will enable clients to continue on their own long after the coaching relationship has ended has much to do with the robustness of action planning and comprehensive strategies for change that coaches encompass in their work. We referred to this in the previous chapter while discussing designing actions. In this chapter, we want to take this topic further. When coaches are engaged with their full range of sensitivities and skills, clients remain in the fire of a change process for the duration of the coaching relationship. To realize this, the work must have continuing intensity once the goal and action plan have been defined.

As mentioned before, change is rarely linear. As the client engages in action toward attaining her initial goal, evidence and patterns continue to emerge about who this person is and how she goes about fulfilling her commitments. With unwavering focus on the client and her agenda, the coach can recognize early warnings that she might be slipping before she is even aware of it. As a result of this intense work, clients learn to identify their own patterns. They come to perceive their covert exit routines and amass sufficient strategy and skill to put themselves back into action should they slip even slightly.

In this chapter, we consider goals and their ideal structures. The competency development model discussed in chapter 10 assumes that the outcome of coaching is the accumulated learning and development generated by multiple actions toward interrelated goals pertaining to the client's overall agenda. Therefore, we examine the staging of actions in order to achieve an overarching goal. We also discuss what happens in that transitional zone when clients are no longer in their old realities and have not yet arrived at their desired futures. To help us in this effort, we address the final two core coaching competencies within the ICF theme of facilitating learning and results. These are planning and goal setting and managing progress and accountability.

The 10th ICF (2011c) core competency of planning and goal setting is the ability to develop and maintain an effective coaching plan with the client. The coach who masters this competency is one who

- consolidates collected information and establishes a coaching plan and development goals with the client that address concerns and major areas for learning and development;
- creates a plan with results that are attainable, measurable, and specific and have target dates;
- makes plan adjustments as warranted by the coaching process and by changes in the situation;
- helps the client identify and access resources for learning (e.g., books, other professionals); and
- identifies and targets early successes that are important to the client.

International Coach Federation 2011

The 11th ICF (2011c) core competency of managing progress and **accountability** has been described as the ability to hold attention on what is important for the client and to leave responsibility with the client to take action. A coach who excels in this competency

- clearly requests of the client actions that will move the client toward her stated goals;
- demonstrates follow-through by asking the client about those actions that the client committed to during the previous sessions;
- acknowledges the client for what he has done, not done, learned, or become aware of since the previous coaching session;
- effectively prepares, organizes, and reviews with client information obtained during sessions;
- keeps the client on track between sessions by holding attention on the coaching plan and outcomes, agreed-upon courses of action, and topics for future sessions;
- focuses on the coaching plan but is also open to adjusting behaviors and actions based on the coaching process and shifts in direction during sessions;
- is able to move back and forth between the big picture of where the client is heading, setting a context for what is being discussed, and where the client wishes to go;
- promotes the client's self-discipline and holds the client accountable for what she says she is going to do, for the results of an intended action, or for a specific plan with related time frames;
- develops the client's ability to make decisions, address key concerns, and develop himself (to get feedback, to determine priorities and set the pace of learning, to reflect on and learn from experiences); and
- positively confronts the client with the fact that she did not take agreed-upon actions.

International Coach Federation, 2011

These competencies differ from those covered in previous chapters in that they speak to the focus of dialogue once clients have become clear about what they are fully committed to doing. The coaching competencies of planning and goal setting and managing progress and accountability rely mainly on skills of active listening, powerful questioning, direct communication, and designing action. We will begin with the topic of goal setting and proceed to consideration of the big plan and all its potential elements.

# GOALS AND GOAL SETTING

Coaching is goal focused; it is about promoting action in relation to a particular goal. Some goals are more important than others and some goals can be subdivided into steps or stages. If we subsume all of the terms we have used in the previous chapters (*topic, agenda, dream, vision*) under the framework of goals, we might be able to move toward clarity by examining the literature on goals and goal setting.

In the field of exercise and sport psychology, three categories of goals have been identified: outcome, performance, and process (Weinberg & Gould, 2011). All three types can play important roles in the change process (Tenenbaum & Eklund, 2007). **Outcome goals** typically focus on the end of some engagement, such as a final result or a target behavior. One client may aim to win a prize, while another intends to lose a certain amount of weight. Both are outcome goals. **Performance goals** represent the achievement of certain standards of behavior, irrespective of others' actions. A client may have a performance goal of eating according to a specific regimen, whereas another may want to get seven hours of sleep every night. Finally, **process goals** emphasize the qualities that one wishes to experience in her behavior. One client may have a process goal of enjoying a hobby, while another may have a process goal of feeling balanced in his daily life.

A slightly different take on outcome and process goals is framed within the context of helping relationships (Shebib, 2010). For coaches, this would concern what a client wants as a result of engagement in goal pursuit (outcome) and what means he is willing to commit to in order to attain these outcomes (process). Process goals can be further subdivided into actions codetermined by the coach and the client and aspects of the coaching relationship itself. How often will coach and client meet? What are the terms of the relationship? What responsibilities do clients and coaches bear for activities between sessions?

An important differentiation among types of goals can be found in the works of Kimsey-House and colleagues (2011). These authors have presented three goal types—fulfillment, balance, and process—as a kind of progressive focus in long-term coaching relationships. When people first contract for coaching, they often have a specific objective in mind, such as completing a certification, losing a certain number of pounds, or adopting a meditation practice; these are known as fulfillment goals. After experiencing a number of successes in reaching these fulfillment goals, people may shift interest toward balance goals. Here, the emphasis is on creating a well-rounded life pattern of work, play, learning, and relationships. Finally, in what seems to be a more evolved focus, clients express a desire to alter their ways of being in the world so that they might find harmony and peace. This is a process goal where the way they live moment to moment is what matters.

Regardless of the type of goal clients propose, clarity is essential. Goals provide direction (Senge, 2006) and thereby guide actions. Goal statements can also clarify the boundaries of the coaching relationship—what is being deliberately pursued and what is off limits. In this regard, Cormier and colleagues (2009) suggest that clear goals permit helpers to determine whether they have the skills, experiences, and credentials to effectively address clients' agendas. Having clear goals also directs coaches to use particular strategies and interventions appropriate to clients' goal attainment. Finally, clear goals enable coaches to create concrete frameworks for evaluation and assessment of progress (Smith, 2007; Stober, 2006).

In health, wellness, and fitness, whether clients are focused on an objective *outcome* of completion or an ongoing *process* of maintenance will influence the nature of the coaching relationship and perhaps its duration. Outcome goals suggest that once the client has obtained the prize, the relationship has served its purpose and may be ended. Process goals may benefit from coaching relationships that endure over several years with the frequency of meetings waxing and waning according to client needs and development.

## Seven Qualities of Effective Goals

Much of the work on goals and goal setting derives from the pioneering efforts of Edwin Locke and his followers over more than 40 years. Their studies attempt to answer the question "How should goals be formulated to best serve client needs?" This research (Latham, Ganegoda, & Locke, 2011; Latham & Locke, 2002; Locke & Latham, 1985, 1990; Locke, Shaw, Saari, & Latham, 1981) has consistently shown that goal setting has a powerful effect on behavior. Some of the more germane

implications of Locke's research can be summarized as follows.

1. **Goals should be stated at moderate levels of difficulty.** We often talk about stretch goals (Hargrove, 2008) or ask clients to do more than they are initially willing to do. In line with this, clients may be eager to change and set overly ambitious target goals. Framing goals that are appropriately difficult rather than too easily attained or too difficult to reach can be a sticky matter because coaching is often about dreaming—it is about achieving the impossible. Though the idea of getting behind clients' intentions to dream outside the box and aim for the stars is laudable, goals need to be set with achievable targets. As people reach interim goals over time, they will build a certain measure of self-efficacy (Bandura, 1997a, 1997b) and may even attain the supposedly unreachable.

As a general principle, it is wise to frame short-term goals that clients work on during the coaching relationship so that they are challenging without setting the client up for failure. A corollary to this point is that setting goals that are too easy may reduce satisfaction and future motivation. Novice coaches may land on an action plan toward the end of a session where the person says, "Great. I can do that. In fact, I've already been doing something like that for months." If the client makes an agreement to do what she has already been doing, she will probably believe that coaching adds little value to her goal pursuit. In cases like this, the commitment must be framed so that it is more challenging.

2. **The more specific the goal statement, the better it is.** As much as goal specificity has been emphasized in the literature, a considerable gap continues to exist between what clients think are clearly stated goals for action and how detailed these goals actually need to be in order to make progress. Coaches may seem to be splitting hairs when they ask questions such as "When are you going to do that?" and "What will it look like?" and "How will you know that you have done what you said you were going to do?" These questions may seem superfluous, yet they are necessary. Indeed, this is one place where the magic of coaching can easily be demystified. Clients might be ready to end a session with what they think is a clear goal for the time between sessions. The coach then takes this one step further by asking them to imagine themselves engaging in their designed actions, almost like a behavioral rehearsal (Suinn, 1986). This allows clients to go through a trial run of their commitment to

further define its nature and possible impediments. They may come to realize that their action plan is missing a critical element for success.

3. **Goal setting includes the three types of goals—outcome, performance, and process.** Another way of thinking about the three goal types is that they represent facets of each objective addressed during coaching. Imagine someone who wants to develop a practice of daily meditation as a way of managing stress and feeling centered. An outcome of feeling centered can be assessed at the end of each meditation experience, the performance goal might be that the person sat on the cushion for 10 minutes with no allowance for distractions, and the process goal could be that throughout the 10 minutes she was able to stay in the present moment and come back to her breath without self-judgment. In other words, there is one action goal (meditating) with three faces.

4. **Feedback about progress is critical along the path to goal attainment.** Coaching involves an ongoing dialogue about clients' desires, the steps they will take to reach their goals, and assessment of progress along the way. As discussed, clients will likely be moving forward simultaneously on a number of action plans created at various points in the coaching relationship. Coaches help clients implement, monitor, and modify action plans to shape desired changes (Schwarzer, 2006). Feedback about progress is likely to be jointly designed so that clients take significant responsibility for evaluating their efforts and sharing their journey. This implies that objectively verifiable standards or assessments have been detailed. Benchmarks of progress may be identified to help motivate behavior and estimate time frames for completion.

Referring back to our discussion of outcome, performance, and process goals, specific standards might exist for each type. For instance, a client's report might sound like this: "Over the past two weeks, I lost 2½ pounds (outcome) by sticking to my eating plan at least six out of seven days each week (performance), and the interesting thing is that I actually enjoyed eating this way (process)."

5. **Imposed goals will not be as effective as client-generated goals.** The field of coaching stresses the centrality of goals that emerge from the client (Coach U, 2005; Skibbins, 2007; Steele, 2011). Though coaches might offer suggestions or advice at times, it is generally not their role to tell clients what to do. Still, coaching is about partnership; this implies that whatever objectives a client formulates derive

from a coaching dialogue. Some schools of coaching (Divine, 2009; Frost, 2009; Hunt, 2009) emphasize how coaches can add perspectives not yet appreciated by clients. Regardless, the overarching goal or meta-goal that represents a client's dream needs to derive entirely from the client. Although you may play a part in clarifying meta-goals, you will be more consistently engaged in dialogues that determine what clients might do from one session to the next as a means of reaching those goals. In other words, the steps toward the larger objective will be forged in the fire of dialogue between coach and client.

6. **Publicly acknowledged goals are more likely to be attained.** What constitutes *public acknowledgment* is key to understanding this point. People who self-direct their own change processes are more likely to succeed if they make their commitments known to others (Green, 2003; Kets de Vries, 2006). We see this in many self-help groups, where participants state openly to others what they are struggling with and what they intend to do to change (Etter, Bergman, & Perneger, 2000). Within the coaching sphere, clients inform their coaches of what they intend to do. This constitutes a public commitment, and it is enough to make a difference in behavior change. We all have ruminations about what we want, what we hope for, what we imagine, and so forth. Such wishes and hopes characterize our thought processes and sometimes have more potency than at other times. Nonetheless, so long as they remain inside our heads, they exist only as ideas or speculations. Saying them out loud to another person increases chances of action and consequently likelihood of success.

7. **The client's personality and motivation influence strategies for goal pursuit.** In coaching, the entire process of moving toward clients' dreams is coconstructed with intimate knowledge of clients' personal qualities, needs, style, motivations, and timing. Whatever action they undertake is unlikely to be an off-the-shelf solution. Even when generic guidelines are followed, such as those that might be part of a nutrition plan, personalized adaptations must be considered. The multiple dimensions of a client's patterns in approaching matters related to her coaching agenda must be appreciated. Coaching methods need to be closely aligned with what works for a particular person. Even when she reinitiates the pursuit of an agenda through coaching after a substantial lapse in time, this returning client must be viewed as an evolving being and therefore in a

different space than the being who was previously coached.

# SuPeRSMART Goal Structures

We have sufficiently emphasized the point that coaches focus on goals and goal setting not only in the beginning of coaching but systematically throughout the entire relationship. Moreover, goals are rarely static; they evolve with increasing levels of knowledge, self-understanding, and feedback from all the experimental initiatives that clients engage over time. As clients learn more about themselves and experience the products of their commitments, goals are likely to be further refined and shaped.

As a health, wellness, and fitness professional, you no doubt have been exposed to the principles of **SuPeRSMART goals** (Donatelle & Thompson, 2011; Powers, Dodd, Thompson, & Condon, 2005). Using this model for the three types of goals (outcome, performance, and process) is important to facilitate success. The following is a brief description of the elements of a SuPeRSMART goal-setting process (see table 11.1 for examples of each element).

## SuPeRSMART: Self-Controllable

Both short- and long-term goals need to be under the person's control. We cannot aim for something that is out of our control. For example, a client may wish to lose 10 pounds (4.5 kg) in the next month. That goal might be realistic for some, but it could prove beyond the reach of others even with their best efforts. People cannot fully manage all the factors (e.g., genetic, physiological, historical, environmental) that regulate the rate at which they lose weight. A self-controllable weight-loss goal for a client could be to consume a fixed amount of calories while expending a target amount of energy on a daily basis until he has lost the weight.

## SuPeRSMART: Public

Even before clients announce their goals to others, they need to make them public to themselves. That is, they need to vocalize to themselves that they are engaged in a specific process of goal pursuit. Because visions of a desired future propel us toward achievements (Senge, 2006), those who keep their attention on their goals are more likely to succeed. Reminders that focus the person's attention on her planned actions and on tracking progress can be most beneficial. For example, a client might need to put workout sessions in her agenda just as she would other appointments; moreover, she might

want to record the length and intensity of the sessions to keep track of her efforts.

## SuPeRSMART: Reward

As we have seen in earlier chapters, **intrinsic motivation** makes it more likely that a person will work to achieve his goal. Nonetheless, rewards for reaching short- and long-term goals can be effective forms of **extrinsic motivation**, especially when they are linked to the client's goals (e.g., buying a couple of scented candles after meditating regularly for three weeks, going on a weekend retreat at a meditation center when the practice has been fully adopted and maintained for six months). Remember that the reward must promote goal attainment rather than detract from it (e.g., a client would not reward himself with a giant brownie for losing a certain amount of weight).

## SuPeRSMART: Specific

The key here is in the details. Bearing in mind whether the goal type is outcome, performance, process, or a combination of the three, the specifics will vary. The details of outcome goals are stated in objective results, performance goals are stated in terms of standards of behavior, and process goals are stated in the framework of how actions would be engaged or experienced.

## SuPeRSMART: Measurable

This element of goals requires that clients be able to articulate their progression in a quantifiable fashion. When objective data are difficult to define or unavailable, subjective information such as self-ratings can be used. A client engaged in a meditation program could measure heart rate and blood pressure before and after each sitting, and he could subjectively assess his emotional tone and body tension.

## SuPeRSMART: Adjustable

Gollwitzer (1999) developed implementation intentions to help people engage in the behavior to which they commit. Implementation intentions are formulated as if-then statements: If situation $x$ happens, then I will do $y$. A practical illustration might be "When I get up in the morning, then I will meditate for 20 minutes." What is even more intriguing about Gollwitzer's theory is his addition of the even-if clause, such as "When I get up, then I will meditate, even if I feel rushed to get out of the house." According to Gollwitzer, the addition of an even-if condition solidifies the client's

**Table 11.1   Illustration of SuPeRSMART Goals**

| SuPeRSMART | Example |
|---|---|
| S = self-controllable | My goal is to lose weight. I am in control of the food I buy, prepare, and eat. I have a gym membership and I work from 8 to 5 on weekdays, leaving me time to exercise in the evenings and on weekends if I wish. |
| P = public | I will tell others around me that I plan to reduce my caloric intake and engage in regular physical activity with a goal of losing 20 pounds (9 kg). I will also write down my workout times in my agenda as a means of reminding myself; I will make weekly menus and grocery lists. |
| R = reward | For every 5 pounds (2.3 kg) I lose, I will buy myself a new article of workout clothing that I have wanted for quite some time. |
| S = specific | My goal is to lose 20 pounds (9 kg) in 20 weeks. In so doing, a related goal is to reduce my percentage of body fat from 27% to 22%. |
| M = measurable | I will measure my progress in the following ways:<br>I will record my weight each Monday morning starting January 5 and ending May 24.<br>I will have my percent body fat measured during the week of March 15 and again during the week of May 24.<br>I will keep a detailed record of my caloric intake each day, detailing the number of calories that I consume starting January 5 and ending May 24.<br>I will engage in cardiorespiratory exercise for the next 20 weeks 5 times a week for 45 minutes each time. Except for the 5-minute warm-up and cool-down, I will keep my heart rate between 60% and 75% of max. I will record each of my training sessions in terms of frequency, duration, and estimated caloric expenditure in a weekly training log beginning January 5 and ending May 24. |
| A = adjustable | My action plan is adjustable in the following four ways:<br>I have scheduled my training sessions for the next month without problem. If alterations occur in my work schedule that might affect my training, I will work with my coach to create alternative exercise strategies.<br>Though I plan to use the treadmill or step machine twice a week for 45 minutes and take an hour-long spinning class on the other 3 days, I will go for a run (same duration and intensity) if I cannot make it to the gym on a particular day.<br>I will plan in advance if I know that I will be eating out.<br>I will eat an occasional treat on special occasions if I so desire and I'll make sure to get back on track at the next meal. |
| R = realistic | My goal is realistic for the following four reasons:<br>A pound of fat (0.45 kg) contains 3,500 calories, and 20 pounds of fat (9 kg) represent approximately 70,000 calories. I currently eat approximately 2,000 calories per day. By decreasing my food intake by 300 calories a day and increasing my activity level, I will burn over 4,000 extra calories per week. Over the 20-week period, this will translate into a weight loss of at least 20 pounds (9 kg).<br>A trainer has confirmed that with the increased activity and estimated weight loss, the percentage of decrease in body fat is realistic.<br>I have the support of my partner and my coach.<br>In the past I have exercised regularly. Although the initial weeks may be challenging, I am committed to achieving this goal and know that I was able to train at similar levels in the past. |
| T = time-specific | I will begin my program on January 5 and continue until May 24. At that point I will reevaluate based on experiences and results. In the interim I will review progress biweekly with my coach. I will assess changes in my weight each week and changes in my percentage of body fat after 10 and 20 weeks. |

resolve to perform the intended behavior even if she is detracted from doing what she had originally planned to do. Coaches can use this implementation intention formula to promote client plans that are robust and actionable.

Of course, even with the most well-thought-out plan, the unexpected can happen. A child gets sick and the parent must stay home instead of going to work. The dog has to be taken to the vet, whose only available appointment is when one's scheduled yoga class is taking place. And so it goes. Life happens! To safeguard clients from an avoidable sense of failure or incompletion, goals need to be flexible—clients need a plan B. When something arises that alters plans, implementation intentions might unfold as follows: "If situation $x$ happens, then I will do $y$, even if $z$ occurs. If I am unable to do $y$ as planned, then I will do $y^1$." This could be translated into the following scenario: "When I get up ($x$), then I will meditate ($y$), even if I feel rushed to get out of the house. If I inadvertently get up too late, then I will meditate at night ($y^1$).

### SuPeRSMART: Realistic

This aspect of goals is often a prelude to a commitment check. Questions might be asked concerning any possible obstacles to engagement in the planned activities. Where there are challenges to implementation, similar to the emergent situations just addressed, strategies would be discussed for dealing with them. In coaching relationships, clients are likely to be working on a number of interconnected action plans at the same time. Sometimes a session will conclude with a client committed to two or more new action plans. You need to remain mindful of all the balls your clients are juggling at the same time, which will be part of the realistic assessment of goal setting.

### SuPeRSMART: Time-Specific

When is this going to happen? There may be a specific time frame in cases where an action is undertaken as an experiment. In a coaching relationship, normally there is at least an implicit notion that the actions will start shortly after the session and continue until the next one. At that point, progress is reviewed and action strategies revised as needed.

By persistently referencing all action plans to the SuPeRSMART template, clients quickly learn how to frame their proposals for commitments. They move away from loose formulations of action plans. "I'm going to get on this soon" morphs into phrases such as "Beginning tomorrow morning and for each morning thereafter until we meet again in two weeks, as soon as I wake up I will spend a minimum of 5 minutes (max 10) mentally focusing on my main priority for the day. I will sit quietly in my bedroom with no distractions and let come to mind the one thing I most want to achieve this day."

# INTERWEAVING GOALS

The final two core competencies within the ICF theme of facilitating learning and results are relevant not just in the end stages of coaching but in all sessions, beginning with the first. In the beginning, when initially hearing what clients truly want, coaches shape the conversation toward an action plan. At the next session, they explore how things went based on what was intended. So, if the process of each coaching session remains true to an action focus, what changes over time? The specific answer depends on the client and her topic. Generally speaking, the nature of actions designed and undertaken will be qualitatively different as the relationship progresses. These actions result not only from the ever-deepening base of information from which both coach and client operate but also from the accumulation of successes from previous efforts.

At first, clients' actions might serve to frame more clearly their intentions, capacities, resources, and desired outcomes (e.g., reduce caffeine intake, read about mindfulness, practice a five-minute breathing exercise daily as a way to manage stress). Then, clients might explore various avenues to achieve their dreams (e.g., move to the country or telecommute as ways to reduce stress). After a while, they would settle into actions that are more closely aligned with the specific results they are targeting (e.g., change career, reduce the amount of traveling they do for work). Toward the end, there might be a kind of shake-down process where actions and correlated engagements would be refined to ensure enduring results (e.g., consciously evaluate each component of the emerging changes against a template of the dream).

To examine this progression further, we will take you through a hypothetical coaching relationship that illustrates the kinds of action plans that must be considered in creating robust and enduring change. We begin our account with Norah, a fictional client, and examine how she and her coaching topic give rise to various action plans over the phases of the flow model of coaching. We will base our story first on an appreciation of what is important for Norah in the evolving relationship and second on the competency development model described in chapter 10.

## Goals in the Engagement Phase of the Flow Model of Coaching

The engagement phase of the flow model consists of three areas of focus that may be advancing at roughly the same time: insight, patterns, and resources. In this phase, the coach listens carefully to the client's agenda and begins to sort information into things she knows, things she doesn't yet understand, and perhaps things she needs to discover. She also is alert to gaps she perceives in the client's understanding of her topic. Furthermore, the coach seeks to discover patterns in the client's way of being and how she goes about goal pursuit. Finally, she helps her client discover resources, skills, and opportunities that could enable her to reach the desired goal. Within this straightforward coaching scenario, let's examine what actions the client might undertake in this first phase of a coaching relationship.

> The client, Norah, is a 48-year-old IT director in a large not-for-profit organization, where she has worked for the past 10 years. She has two children, aged 17 and 20. The older one is living in the student residence at a local university, and the younger one will be heading to college next year. Norah has been pursuing a master's degree in her field. Exhausted from the first year of her studies, she decided to take a solo vacation at an all-inclusive resort. Without her partner to accompany her, she ended up hanging around with the singles crowd on the first day. Rather than having fun, she found herself comparing her body unfavorably to those of the other women.
>
> After her shower the next morning, she took a good look at herself in a full-length mirror. She practically shrieked, "How awful! Ugh! How did I let myself become so fat?" In that moment, she made a commitment to do something immediately about her appearance. She had gained 15 pounds (7 kg) in grad school on top of the slow accumulation of weight over the past 20 years. According to her, she is about 35 pounds (16 kg) heavier than she was in her early 20s. Following her return home, she began jogging a mile (1.6 km) or so in the mornings. This was a few weeks before her first coaching session. Jogging had been okay for her, but there was no evident weight loss so she decided to hire you as her coach.
>
> When you first meet, she sketches her topic as follows: "I need to look better than I do.

> I have really let myself go. I want to lose all this excess weight. I need a plan that works." In your discussion, you discover that she is a caretaker at heart. She seems unaware of her own needs, generally putting others before herself. She describes her husband, Harry, as kind and accepting. He, too, is overweight and inactive, but it doesn't seem to bother him. When she came back from vacation and told him about her rude awakening, he said, "Oh, honey, don't be silly. You look great. Don't make more of it than what it is."
>
> Norah is very social and extroverted. She is a fabulous cook and frequently has friends and colleagues over for dinners. She knows how to do hard things, such as working a full-time job, completing a master's degree, and raising two kids, yet until her recent vacation she simply hadn't taken a close look at herself. So far, her self-examination has remained at the physical level. She tells you, "Maybe it's the nature of my work. I'm always analyzing things, except now I'm realizing there's one analysis I have conveniently avoided—me!"
>
> Norah acknowledges that the world of physical activity is foreign to her. Her parents didn't exercise, her kids are bookworms, and few of her friends are involved in sport. In her network, she's the answer lady when someone needs advice. She is knowledgeable and well informed about many things. She doesn't talk much about herself, but she's able to get information from just about anybody. She acknowledges that she's best with facts; she steers clear of emotional agendas. "That's just a big messy area for me," she says. "Personally, I don't trust emotions—they're always changing. Facts don't change."
>
> Toward the end of the first session, you ask Norah whether she has gained any clearer perspective about what she wants from coaching. She answers, "I want to make friends with my body. I want to treat it well, live in it well, and have it be a positive reflection of my inner self." You tell her that's a great reframing of her topic and ask her to detail what she just said a bit more. She replies, "I haven't had much of a relationship with my body—in fact, I've pretty much neglected it. I want to live in it better, and that means getting to know it better. I desperately want my body to look better. Generally, I feel pretty good on the inside, but my body doesn't reflect this. It looks totally neglected. I'm actually quite

**REFLECTION 11.1**

Take a moment and think about what you know so far. What are your overall impressions of Norah? Where is she strong? What does she need to develop? Where would you start? What other considerations might you have about the path ahead of her and the work she will need to undertake?

angry with myself for letting myself go so badly. So, this is a bit more than just getting fit, isn't it?" You agree.

Depending on the client's commitment to change and the coaching process, perspectives gained through the lens of the competency development model may come into play concerning what you and your client coconstruct. Bear in mind that sometimes our perceptions need to be kept private because the client has signed on for only a limited engagement and is not yet ready to expand her topic. Said differently, clients like Norah may have a mental map of the coaching relationship that restricts their thinking to simply getting involved in an appropriate and effective exercise program. Fortunately, Norah acknowledges that "… this is a bit more than just getting fit." The degree to which she is willing to engage in change processes that address the full spectrum of her needs is yet to be determined. Using the six areas of the competency development model, we can begin to look at this client.

### General Knowledge Competency

What does Norah know about issues related to her topic? Does she understand exercise? Does she know how to exercise correctly? Is she aware of the options and how each might address her needs? Does she know what needs to happen in order for her to reach her goals? Digging a bit deeper, what does she know about women and body image? Or perhaps given her age, does she have relevant knowledge about menopause and how that might play into her situation? As her coach, you may wonder how much she needs to understand. Part of the answer can be found in the contract you made with her. Are you simply going to help her find an exercise program? Or are you working with a multifaceted agenda?

If you were to judge Norah's competency in this area as low, we would agree with you. Maybe you would think that because she is so fact oriented, the evaluation here should be higher. Our perspective is that at this point in time, she doesn't possess the

relevant knowledge. This doesn't mean that it will be hard for her to master it. Given her orientation, we suspect that with a few leads, she will plow through as much data as she can to increase her general knowledge. Apart from what we proposed earlier, what else do you think Norah needs in this area of competency?

### Self-Knowledge Competency

How accurately does Norah know herself in regard to her relationship with her body and her weight? How aware is she of herself and what she needs? How does she deal with change? What is her mental map of how she goes about changing? Is she connected to her physical side? Does she live comfortably in her body and appreciate what she needs to do to keep her body functioning well?

Again, you would probably see her competency here as low and we would concur. Given that she has lived for so long in a state of denial or low awareness of her physical being, there is a chance that she will regress and fall back into old patterns. This issue speaks of her way of going about change. We would want to explore more fully her patterns of behavior in life transitions. What would you do to help her gain greater self-awareness and competency regarding her body, knowing its needs, nurturing it appropriately, and recognizing signals that things are not as they need to be?

### Emotional Competency

What are Norah's emotional capacities related to her topic? Even though she says that emotions are untrustworthy and she tends to avoid dealing with them, we don't yet know how much of an emotional component is relevant here. She did, however, express one clear emotion: anger toward herself for not attending to her body. We suspect that she may have some disquieting emotional moments in addressing her topic, but for now we might postpone examination of her emotional competencies until after she has begun to engage action. At this time, designing actions around emotional competency would not be a high priority.

### Somatic Competency

Because of the nature of Norah's topic, somatic competency bears some similarity to self-knowledge competency here. She doesn't know her body. She is largely disconnected from it. She probably has little sensitivity to her physical likes and dislikes or to somatic preferences.

Not having been involved in physical activities for most of her life, it's unlikely that she would have the physical skills necessary to perform various exercises or sports. We would guess her competency here would be low, though we would want to explore this in greater depth. For enduring change, increasing Norah's somatic competency would be pivotal. Where would you start in this regard?

## Interpersonal Competency

What are Norah's competencies in relationships with others that are relevant to her topic? There are two angles we can take here. The first speaks to her relationship competency. She likes people and seems to have a wide network. However, do you get the impression that something is a bit lopsided here? She is a caretaker. She is the answer lady. She attends to others, but who takes care of her? Does she even allow others to take care of her? The second angle is more closely related to her topic. Norah is probably capable of forming relationships quickly, but currently she doesn't have much of a support network related to physical activity. Her partner tells her not to be silly when she raises concerns about her physical state, and she hasn't confronted him about this.

We think there is work to be done in order for her to be more of a partner in dialogue rather than just a good listener. Also, she probably needs to build new social relationships related to an active lifestyle. Her competency in doing this is likely to be good, though the jury is out in terms of how able she is to bring herself, her needs, and her interests into social relationships that will support her new directions. Even though we would rate her somewhere between medium and high on this competency, we see some need for development and corresponding action planning in this area. What are your thoughts here?

## Moral Competency

What are Norah's judgments related to her topic? We noted in our discussion of emotional competency that she is angry with herself. We suspect she harbors negative judgments about how she has treated her body over her lifetime. She definitely had a strong reaction when she looked at herself in the mirror. Having such strong feelings of self-rejection will not make the change process easy. Does she have an ideal image of how her body must look for her to be accepting? To what degree will she live with a sense of "badness" for having been so inattentive to her appearance? Is there a chance that she will judge others for their complicity?

We can't be certain how much this competency will show up in her work, but we believe these questions have to be addressed if Norah is to move

> ### REFLECTION 11.2
>
> Now that we have looked at Norah's competencies related to her goal, what do you think she needs to do? For each of the competencies, try to identify at least one action or initiative that she might undertake to build her capacity in that area. Norah might have her own ideas, yet it is important for you as her coach to come prepared with thoughts to stimulate her exploration of necessary actions. Make sure that in designing these potential actions there is a sufficiently clear link between what you think might be useful and how she might see this as fostering her goal attainment.

toward her goal of making friends with her body. As a second area of focus, we wonder about the matter of fairness, which is a strong component of morality. Norah seems quite concerned about others, yet her self-focus seems lacking. Something is amiss here. Fairness is not only about how one treats others but also about self-regard. Will she experience difficulty in becoming what might seem to her to be self-centered as she undertakes the necessary work to pursue her goal?

From this assessment of Norah's competencies, you could explore possible actions she might pursue, particularly while in the engagement phase of the flow model. We have outlined some potential avenues for change initiatives for Norah (see table 11.2). As you read through these, some may make clearer sense than others. You might also realize that each of these action possibilities will take time in the coaching session to explore as well as time after the session to implement. Sometimes you might come across a great resource in the form of a book or film that speaks to a number of competency areas. These gems can help your clients increase their capacities more efficiently. It's a good idea to begin creating a file of resources of this nature, because your goal is not simply to get your clients involved in action plans directly tied to their goals but also to increase their capacity for self-directed action over their lifetimes. Coaching is about enduring change, not just a quick fix.

## Goals in the Goal-Pursuit Phase of the Flow Model

Before diving into this discussion, we offer you a reminder. The two phases of engagement and goal pursuit can be seen in any coaching session. This is because the flow model applies to the process

**Table 11.2　Potential Actions in the Engagement Phase of Coaching for Norah**

| Competencies | Potential directions and actions | |
|---|---|---|
| **General knowledge** | Reading about exercise—types, schedules, results<br>Reading about women—menopause, body image<br>Reading about bodily changes through the life span<br>Doing web searches concerning the latest findings of exercise science | |
| **Self-knowledge** | Journaling about her needs and wants each day<br>Reading appropriate self-help books—change processes, value clarification, and so on<br>Conversing with reliable friends about how they perceive her<br>Coaching dialogues about self-identity, values, needs, and so on | |
| **Emotional** | Coaching dialogues about emotions related to the topic<br>Reading about emotional intelligence<br>Examining emotional responses to her current physical being<br>Reflecting on emotional experiences throughout the day<br>Journaling about emotions | |
| **Somatic** | Performing sensory awareness exercises, such as body scans<br>Completing physical fitness testing<br>Having medical examinations<br>Exploring (sampling) physical activities and sports | |
| **Interpersonal** | Identifying active people in her network and scheduling lunches, coffees, and other meetings<br>Visiting local fitness centers to understand their interpersonal climates<br>Reading about the patterns of caretakers<br>Journaling about relationships and her patterns in relationships | |
| **Moral** | Reflecting on attitudes about her body<br>Practicing self-affirmations concerning body acceptance<br>Journaling about body judgments: self and others<br>Conducting a blame/shame inventory regarding her physical being both currently and throughout her life | |

of a single session as much as it maps the entire relationship. For the example with Norah, we are using the flow model as a map of her entire coaching experience. Of course, she will be involved in planning actions related to goal attainment in each of her coaching sessions, but as she progresses, the nature of her goals will evolve. This is what we want to examine in this case analysis.

Table 11.2 represents actions or goals intended to build a foundation; few of them directly target what Norah needs to be doing to achieve and maintain desired changes over the upcoming years. Most of them pertain to the areas of insight, patterns, and resources of the engagement phase.

As Norah moves into the goal-pursuit phase of the relationship, we assume that she has made progress or, in terms of the TTM, that she is in the action stage. We would predict that at this time some of her actions are directly targeting goals that will move her closer to her dream. Let's visit Norah at about month four of her coaching relationship.

Norah has lost 15 pounds (6.8 kg), but hers has not been an entirely linear journey. She continued her morning jogs until the weather got colder. She worked with a personal trainer at a gym and learned about proper form and program design. She devoured books and magazines on fitness and body image. She experimented with a variety of fitness classes and found some she loved. Her conversations with active people led to her joining a running club. She has been quite devoted and regular in exercising for the past eight weeks. Somewhere around the four-month mark of coaching, she said, "I'm getting closer to my goal. I don't have such a strong reaction when I look at myself in the mirror. . . ."

The quality of foods Norah consumed was never a problem; the issue was more about quantity and what she began to understand as her pattern of emotional eating. Things at work would get tense at unpredictable times of the year, and she would put in lots of uncompensated overtime. In those times, she would find herself snacking frequently. She is aware of this pattern now. Even so, she is in one of those stressful periods now, and her work has cut into her exercise time as well as halting her weight loss.

It came as a surprise to her that she suddenly began to experience more tension at home. Her partner subtly complained about the time she spent training or with her running group. On the other hand, her sister got excited by the changes she saw Norah making and asked if she could go to the gym with her. She is now Norah's most reliable exercise buddy.

It wasn't as if her personality changed, but Norah commented on some shifts she has noticed: "Maybe my patience is down. I seem less willing to take everyone else's problems on my shoulders, especially at work. I get irritated more easily—and here I thought exercise would make me calmer (*laughs*). I also have to say that at home I'm less willing to be the maid. When I was looking at myself over the past few months, I began to notice that I seem to be the only one in the household who takes responsibility for things. It's not that Harry doesn't help, but why should I have to ask him all the time? Doesn't he know what needs to be done?"

Regarding her intentions, Norah expresses greater commitment than ever. She subscribes to a number of fitness magazines. She talks more seriously about taking courses that might allow her to become a fitness instructor, "maybe as a hobby—but who knows," she adds.

Her old friendship network has fallen off a bit. She doesn't get as many calls from friends and when she has them over for a meal, she dominates the conversation with talk about her training. She notices that her friends' eyes seem to glaze over. After an evening of this sort, she finds herself judging her friends and thinking of them as a bit lazy and not very fit as a group.

> ### REFLECTION 11.3
>
> Once again, pause before continuing and reflect on what you have just read. What seems to be different in this portrait of Norah? What new agendas may be arising? Where, if anywhere, might you be developing new ideas about what would be helpful? What would your next steps be?

If you think this process of change is complicated, consider the fact that your client is a 48-year-old woman who has just awakened to the joys and power of movement and exercise. Like the ex-smoker who wants to preach on a soapbox about the benefits derived from his change, Norah seems to be in a kind of honeymoon phase with her new-found physicality. She has earned the results she achieved. She has been entirely committed to her training, except when work interferes, in which case she experiences an increasing and almost intolerable degree of resentment. The judgment that she previously directed toward herself now seems to be generalizing to all those people, including her partner and close friends, who are "too lazy" to do what their bodies need. As the pendulum swings, she has moved from one extreme almost to the other.

If Norah remains on this path without reflection and intervention, what do you imagine her life would look like? Can you predict that her increasing dissatisfaction with Harry might lead to separation? Would she jeopardize her job by devoting even more time to preparing for a career in the fitness industry? Would she begin losing old and valued friends because she is so self-absorbed in her personal pursuits? It is also reasonable to surmise that Norah might hit a plateau in her weight loss unless she addresses her emotionally driven eating patterns. What could happen then? With lots of ongoing interference with her training from incessant work demands, friction at home, and pesky emotions popping up everywhere, why not go back to the old Norah?

Let's examine Norah's evolving topic in light of the competency development model.

## General Knowledge Competency

What does Norah know about issues related to her evolving topic? The answer is a lot more than she did three months ago. Yet, her topic is not just about exercise; it's also about other ways of nurturing her physical wellness. It encompasses a more positive pattern of eating as well as a way of integrating exercise into her life. What does she need to learn that will give her perspective about where she is now and what she may want to do? Does she need to learn more about nutrition for healthy living? Does she need to appreciate the psychology of change more so that she can normalize some of what she is going through? Does she need to dig deeper into the sport sciences literature to understand plateaus in exercise-induced change? Would it be important to know about techniques for relapse prevention so that she can be self-sustaining once her coaching relationship has ended? Where would you go? What would you emphasize first?

## Self-Knowledge Competency

How accurately does Norah know herself in relation to her evolving topic? At this time, it appears that Norah has discovered what her preferences are within the world of physical activity. She probably also knows more about her patterns of excuses for not exercising—she's on to her own games. What shines through are the ways in which exercise may be enhancing her personal feeling of empowerment. She seems stronger in her self-expression and more likely to assert herself. There might be a learning edge for her related to changes in midlife. How does she see her life and her future? Before this awakening occurred, Norah expressed great tolerance for others and also allowed them to lean on her a lot. Why the change? How is it related to her physical program? Although she has gained self-knowledge regarding exercising, it appears that some of her deeper layers are also showing up. These will require better understanding so that she doesn't take a precipitous leap into actions such as quitting her job or divorcing her partner. What does she most need to learn about herself and her emerging way of being in the world?

## Emotional Competency

What are Norah's emotional capacities related to her evolving topic? Emotionality has clearly entered the picture. Initially, we weren't clear how her emotionality might be expressed over the course of the change process. Some of the emotional elements that have come up include pride in her improved physical appearance, excitement about her involvement in various exercise programs, emotionally driven eating, impatience with others, and perhaps resentment about being the maid. Her stated preference earlier was to avoid emotions because they are "messy" and "untrustworthy." A normal part of the change process, particularly as framed in Taylor's learning-through-change model (see chapter 3), is heightened emotionality. Norah seems to be reacting more emotionally to situations that she previously handled with great equanimity. This most likely signals a shift in her overall emotional state. Though her emotions may be founded on genuine frustrations and issues, they seem a bit intense. What's the learning edge for Norah? In your opinion, what competencies does she need to develop?

## Somatic Competency

What is Norah's body knowledge at this point? Though the core topic remains, it has also become more multidimensional. She is more aware of her emotionally driven eating patterns and may need to become more attuned to her somatic signals of hunger. There may also be physical components of her emotionality. How does tension show up? Regarding her exercise agenda, she has learned a great deal about her body. She has studied with a personal trainer and now appreciates how to treat her body well while she is exercising. Is this part of her learning over? We doubt it. In regard to her body image, is she more accepting of her body only because she has lost weight and improved her fitness level? How might she grow in the area of body love, for instance, being grateful for how her body serves her regardless of how it appears? How long does it take to move from a place of virtual disconnection of body and mind to a way of being that represents integrated functioning? What's the new agenda for Norah? How can she deepen her present level of somatic knowledge?

## Interpersonal Competency

What are Norah's competencies in relating to others with regard to her evolving topic? Norah's relationships have changed significantly over the past three months. While she continues to express a high degree of competence in meeting people, her capacity to manage herself in her long-term relationships seems a bit challenged. Most certainly, she's not likely to want to return to her maid or helper status with friends and family, yet she seems to lack understanding of how her change is affecting others. Her marital relationship feels strained, and although she is aware that she talks obsessively about her training when an audience appears, she does not want to be more inclusive, or perhaps she simply isn't capable of shifting gears to engage others in the conversation. What needs to happen? What development would help Norah navigate this passage?

## Moral Competency

What are Norah's judgments related to her evolving topic? We are not sure how much progress she has made here. The fact that her body no longer shocks her may represent movement. However, judgment has shifted from self to others. She has begun to judge others who don't exercise as lazy, and she seems to be more judgmental about how unfit her old friends are. What might happen if she relapses? Will even stronger feelings of body rejection arise? And what might these feelings provoke? In the final expression of her topic, what her body looked like did not seem to be the central concern. At this point in time, her absorption in the world of body shaping seems to prevent her from knowing her deep-seated prejudices and judgmental attitudes toward herself and others. Moreover, we continue to wonder about the theme of fairness. It seems to have arisen in her self-perception as the family maid—and a growing resentment toward her partner for not knowing what to do around the house. As noted, perhaps this is part of the pendulum swing and hopefully she will settle in a place where fairness includes herself as well as others. Overall, what work is needed now to move her toward healthy living with acceptance of self and others regardless of their physical manifestations?

We have examined Norah's current state again through the lens of the competency development model and you have reflected on her current needs for action. We now offer suggestions for action in table 11.3. Our goal is not to have Norah become the next fitness guru, but in her words, "I want to

**Table 11.3   Potential Actions in the Goal-Pursuit Phase of Coaching for Norah**

| Competencies | Potential directions and actions |
|---|---|
| **General knowledge** | Reading about nutrition and exercise<br>Reading about women in midlife<br>Reading about exercise adherence and relapse prevention<br>Reading about studies on exercise-induced body changes |
| **Self-knowledge** | Reading about the process of change and its unanticipated consequences<br>Coaching dialogues related to value clarification<br>Exploring career transition literature<br>Journaling about desires, satisfactions, and visions for the future |
| **Emotional** | Reading about emotionally driven eating<br>Practicing mindfulness and meditation<br>Self-reflecting to name her feelings and identify how her interpretation of specific events gives rise to particular feelings<br>Journaling about emotions |
| **Somatic** | Continuing development of body knowledge through personal training and exercise performance clinics<br>Focusing her supervision and practice in her running group to improve technique in one area (e.g., running)<br>Consulting sport science experts on training parameters for sustaining change<br>Identifying a clear pattern of physical activity that she can joyfully and reliably engage in over the foreseeable future |
| **Interpersonal** | Engaging in planned conversations with her partner regarding their experiences together over the past few months<br>Expressing feelings combined with requests for feedback from friends and colleagues<br>Holding family meetings about chores and responsibilities<br>Journaling about relationships and her new patterns |
| **Moral** | Reading about self-acceptance and empathy<br>Practicing self-affirmations concerning body acceptance<br>Continued journaling about body judgments of self and others<br>Practicing meditation exercises related to compassionate presence |

**REFLECTION 11.4**

In our review of the six competencies, we raised a number of questions regarding areas that Norah might address. Please take a few minutes now and write down your ideas for work that you might discuss with her so that she can further advance along this challenging path of change.

make friends with my body. I want to treat it well, live in it well, and have it be a positive reflection of my inner self." In this statement of her topic, we can say that her goal is still in the distance. She does not seem at peace with herself at this time. Her life is in flux and the risks of unproductive change or relapse seem moderately high.

For the purposes of this client presentation, we artificially divided the design and implementation of actions into the two phases of our coaching model, engagement and goal pursuit. As you can see in Norah's unfolding story, she is closer to her ultimate goal but continues to be in a transitional phase where emergent issues and unexpected shifts require attention and management. From the TTM perspective, we can say that she is in the action stage but has a way to go before she is in an easy flow of maintenance.

Four months into the coaching relationship seems to be a point when many clients contemplate ending the relationship. Hopefully, Norah will not quit at this time. Even if she doesn't, your reflections about potential steps may remain unrealized because she may choose other routes. Though we have invited you to think of potential steps that you might suggest in supporting your client's progress toward her overall goal, we offer a caveat concerning attachments you might develop to your plans. It is better to offer suggestions and ideas tentatively in dialogue with your clients. Ultimately, the choice belongs to them. It is quite possible that Norah may choose to devote her time and financial resources to working with personal trainers rather than remain in a coaching relationship. The honeymoon effect might have a strong hold on her right now.

Our hope is that Norah's final program—or at least the one she is engaged in when coaching concludes—incorporates heightened satisfaction with her body image, challenging and satisfying physical activities, healthy eating habits, mindfulness practices that keep her on top of her emotions, and nurturing relationships, including one with her partner, that provide mutual support and encouragement

for health and wellness. These elements seem well aligned with her stated purpose for coaching.

# TOWARD SELF-RELIANCE

The choice of coaching as a way of moving forward in life is not always an easy ride. Coaches encourage clients to push the envelope of change. They ask them to stretch into their futures by challenging themselves in new and exciting ways. Meanwhile, coaches are there to support, advise, and encourage. Then the relationship ends. The client has achieved his goals or is sufficiently on his way to make the remainder of the journey on his own. Will he continue or stop in midflight? The answer lies partly in the thoroughness of the process that client and coach have engaged in during their work together. The final two ICF core competencies, planning and goal setting and managing progress and accountability, reinforce clients' ways of thinking and acting regarding their commitments that will hopefully remain with them as templates for sustaining action.

In chapter 3, we presented nine intervention strategies associated with the TTM. Some were advocated as methods for getting people involved in change processes, while others were proposed as ways of helping them maintain their practices. These interventions are frequently employed in coaching relationships, so it is reasonable to expect that self-reliant clients will learn the strategies and incorporate them in their independent efforts in the future. To ensure that this happens, coaches need to be explicit about what they are doing. Because plans are codetermined, rationales for designing actions should be evident to the client. If necessary, and with their permission, there may be room for coaches to play an educator's role in instructing clients about maintaining these kinds of practices in their lives.

Of course, what happens after the end of coaching is not always predictable. A vast literature on relapse prevention is available with ideas about what people might do to ensure the continuity of desired behavior patterns. Clients will have done their utmost to adopt robust action strategies that will endure in the absence of the coaching relationship. In Norah's scenario, many of the suggested actions (see tables 11.2 and 11.3) might at first seem to be marginal to her path toward self-fulfillment. For instance, someone who decides to adopt a vegan diet is making a choice that will influence how and with whom his time is spent, his interior self-experience, his self-definition, his social image, and his moral perspective, among other perhaps unidentified effects. Coaches are exquisitely aware of these ramifications and help their clients construct processes that are built to last.

# ENDINGS AND NEW BEGINNINGS

As we conclude our coverage of the 11 ICF core competencies, it seems fitting that we address the critical passage clients and coaches experience in terminating their relationship. Endings are often referred to as *closure*, signifying a kind of relationship agenda rather than a static event. **Closure** implies that the client and coach engage in a process of reviewing experiences and extracting potential meanings for future relationships as the current work concludes.

With the growth of the coaching field in the 1990s, diverse opinions became evident concerning the temporal nature of the relationship. Some writers defined the ending according to the client's attainment of goals, whereas others imagined ongoing process-oriented relationships. Yet, with agendas of "action, action, action" (Martin, 2001), inevitably a moment will come when clients simply prefer a space of being rather than one of continually doing.

If we consider the likely agendas of clients in lifestyle wellness coaching, we can certainly imagine relationships lasting years. Similarly, it makes sense that some contractual coaching agreements would be shorter, that is, measured in months. A person who struggles with regularity in maintaining life–work balance and who wishes to pursue specific benefits obtained through engagement in leisure activities could reasonably maintain connections with a lifestyle wellness coach for at least a year, based on knowledge concerning the time that people need to solidify new habits (Buckworth & Dishman, 2002; Prochaska et al., 2002) and minimize the risk of relapse (Marlatt & Donovan, 2008). In short- or long-term relationships, the client and coach are likely to have established some rhythm and regularity of contact such that the ending will have significant meaning.

## Tasks and Meanings of Endings

The end of the coaching relationship offers opportunity for the completion of certain tasks and for various assessments. As Walsh (2007) implies, the closing of the relationship may allow the coach and client to achieve the following:

- Understand without ambiguity that the relationship is ending.

- Reflect on their work from all angles.
- Identify what was learned.
- Acknowledge feelings about the relationship.
- Consider the meaning of this relationship for potential future ones.

Beyond these general agendas, Walsh (2007) highlights specific tasks, reframed here according to how they might pertain to coaching roles:

1. Recognizing that ending the relationship is a process, coaches need to remain mindful of when and how to commence discussions of ending.

2. Each client will experience endings differently and a wide range of emotional reactions may be evidenced.

3. To ensure the maintenance and enhancement of client achievements, concrete actions that clients will undertake must be clearly defined.

4. Pertaining to the transfer of learning to new situations or to other agendas, coaches can facilitate discussions on how to link what occurred in the coaching process to what clients might be able to do independently in the future.

5. When issues not covered in the original contract emerge during the ending process, it may be appropriate to explore whether another cycle of working together would be of value.

6. Acknowledging other paths to personal growth and development suggests that coaches assist clients in identifying resources for these emerging directions. Referrals might be made to facilitate client engagement.

7. Closure needs to include a discussion of clear boundaries and guidelines for future contacts as well as for reinitiating the coaching relation.

8. Remaining aware of their own emotionality and unfinished business, coaches must be mindful of their potential projections onto clients' processes of completion.

Whenever coaching ends, there is a need to reflect on both outcomes and processes. Ideally, coach and client will be able to explore their experiences together, although this may not always be possible.

Certain questions can help inform future actions (Walsh, 2007):

- How has the client changed? What is different? What goals has the client reached? Which ones has he not achieved? What might have changed unexpectedly, for better or worse?

- How does the client feel about the work? Does he see the investment as worthwhile? Overall, was the experience one of satisfaction and accomplishment?

- What's next? What will the client do now? What plans or new goals would he like to consider? What is the logical next step in the process of personal development? How will the client engage in this work?

## Types of Endings

Knowing when to end a coaching relationship requires constant monitoring. Here are some guidelines to follow so that you are aware of the emerging need to end the relationship (Gabbard, 1995; Hepworth et al., 2010; Herlihy & Corey, 2006; Walsh, 2007):

- Having set clear objectives through explicit contracting, the degree of progress toward these goals will inform decisions about ending.

- Fostering awareness of your own needs as a coach will help you understand whether you are prolonging or hastening the ending for personal reasons.

- Keeping in mind that a meta-goal of coaching is to enhance the autonomous functioning of clients will enable you as a coach to pursue this objective in parallel with all of the other change agendas addressed in the coaching relationship.

- Whenever possible, inform yourself of clients' specific histories regarding endings and their culturally linked expectations of ending processes.

Of course, the end of the coaching relationship does not mean the end of learning. Learning is a lifelong process. You may facilitate the ending of coaching in a manner that engenders clients' skills for continuing their growth and development.

Walsh (2007) considers various types of endings in helping relationships. These are organized into three categories: unplanned endings initiated by the client, unplanned endings initiated by the coach, and planned endings.

### Unplanned Endings Initiated by the Client

In unplanned endings, the client terminates the relationship unexpectedly (Walsh, 2007). Such endings include some sense of surprise, and unfortunately the client may never share with the coach the reasons for ending. Clearly, the ambiguity surrounding these endings leaves matters open to interpretation. The following are possible scenarios occasioning abrupt endings:

1. **Clients' inability to discuss ending.** Here, the client perceives that he has made enough progress and he is unable or unwilling to talk with the coach about ending. Studies show that this scenario occurs in 20% to 50% of premature endings in various types of helping interventions (Sweet & Noones, 1989). An interesting dynamic explaining these results emerged from one study in which helpers anticipated that their clients would remain in the helping process two to three times longer than the clients themselves expected to do so (Pekarik & Finney-Owen, 1987). Just because a client ends the relationship without warning doesn't imply that the work was unsuccessful (Kazdin & Wassell, 1998).

Another finding was that when helpers were asked what they believed to be the most significant moments in the relationship, they often identified experiences different from those clients believed were most important (Stalikas & Fitzpatrick, 1995, 1996). One might say that the client is always right about his own experiences, but the reality is probably not that simple. Coaches may see things with greater objectivity, yet the client ultimately decides whether the process was of value. More to the point is the fact that no matter how insightful coaches are, they are not mind readers. A client may experience effects from a session that become evident only in the hours and days after the meeting. Coaches cannot know this, even though they may hope for such epiphanies. When clients receive what they came for, they may just presume the coach will understand without an explanation of why they are ending the relationship.

2. **Clients' dissatisfaction with progress.** Some clients expect immediate results. If they don't get them, they may quit and go shopping for another coach. Clients take varying amounts of time to reach the point of quitting because of disappointment with results. In some cases, they stay too long; in

others, not long enough. Strean (1986) offers several reasons why clients may end the relationship out of dissatisfaction:

- They think the helper isn't listening well.
- They experience the helper as being too directive.
- They believe the helper does not like them or is taking out her personal emotions on them.
- There may be sexual attraction between the helper and client.
- The helper may seem to identify too closely with the client's issues.
- The helper may seem uncomfortable with negative emotions such as anger or dissatisfaction.

To prevent this kind of ending, coaches need to request feedback from clients regularly, even as often as at the end of each meeting.

3. **Clients' discomfort with characteristics of the coach.** We might easily relate this to differences in cultural backgrounds, age, gender, or other obvious personal characteristics; however, discomfort can also result from something entirely peculiar to the client's personal history and experiences (Reis & Brown, 1999; Walsh, 2007). Clients can be highly skilled in face management, conveying positive impressions of their experiences while inwardly holding negative perceptions. Because the coaching relationship is a productive alliance to assist clients toward identified goals rather than to directly heal clients' histories, those who experience strong negative reactions to coaches based on their own idiosyncrasies should probably end the relationship rather than carry this extra issue into the sessions. There may also be cases where the lack of chemistry between coach and client was not identified at the beginning of the relationship. Although you may want to know which of your personal characteristics triggered the client's reactions, ultimately its significance is minor so long as you do your utmost to convey the core conditions of helping to clients. As a coach, you need to be aware of your own behaviors and seek regular feedback through discussions with colleagues and mentors.

4. **Clients' leaving during a hiatus in the coaching relationship.** Vacations, conferences, or unexpected life events may break the rhythm of a coaching relationship. During times like these, clients may consolidate lessons they have gained from the work, or they may come to realize that they are not as motivated to continue as they thought. At a deeper level, it is also possible that if a coach interrupts the regularity of meetings, regardless of the reason, the client may feel abandoned or frightened by the sense of dependency that she feels in the relationship. In most helping relations, vacations or lengthy breaks in contact increase the probability of clients' ending. Again, unless clients are open to a full discussion of their reasons, coaches may be left to wonder about the successes of their efforts.

5. **Clients' discomfort with the coach's approach.** No matter what your title, clients will have their own interpretations of what it is you do and how you should approach issues. Many clients expect helpers to tell them what to do (Shebib, 2010) or believe that they should be able to resolve issues in one or two meetings. Coaches may need to go to great lengths in describing their style and the processes of coaching. The more the client knows about the possible evolution of the work, the more positive the outcomes are likely to be (Frank & Frank, 1993). Clients in lifestyle wellness coaching *may perceive the process* in ways similar to expert-based prescriptive relationships like seeing a doctor to obtain medication. Engaging in dialogues about personal needs, styles, and histories related to their topic is a characteristic of coaching that some clients may not immediately appreciate. Asking for feedback and clarifying role expectations on a regular basis will improve the alignment between coaches' behaviors and clients' expectations.

## Unplanned Endings Initiated by the Coach

Coaches may decide to end their relationships with clients for a variety of reasons. These reasons may arise because of issues in the relationship or because of specific concerns or experiences of the coach. Walsh (2007) describes several possibilities, discussed here as they pertain to coaching relationships.

1. **Clients' lack of commitment.** A client may have begun with good intentions. Realizing that she has had difficulty sustaining desired changes on her own, she thought she would try working with a coach to give her that additional impetus to pursue her goals. Or, she may be strongly motivated by a sense of *should*, that is, she thinks she should work on self-improvement, become active, lose weight, become more assertive, make lifestyle changes, or do whatever else inspires her in the moment that she connects with her coach. Then

reality sets in. Changing is still hard. It does not automatically occur simply by hiring a coach. She has to do something, and that something requires effort that she is unwilling to commit. After weeks of hearing excuses for not following through on commitments, the coach may sensitively end the relationship. An important ethical issue can arise in this scenario. Some clients are willing to continue paying for coaching as long as they do not have to change and the coach is willing to go along with the charade. Coaching is based on clear agreements to pursue agreed-upon objectives, so coaches need to initiate discussions regarding closure when clients consistently fail to live up to their commitments. Not doing so means that the coach is behaving unethically.

2. **Clients overstep professional boundaries.** Boundaries have to do with limits. Bruhn, Levine, and Levine (1993) outlined five aspects of boundaries that are relevant to coaching: (1) contact time, which is the amount of time coaches and clients agree to spend working together, including time spent in phone and e-mail correspondence; (2) types of information shared, which includes the range of topics and discussions agreed to by coach and client; (3) physical closeness, which concerns issues of touch and physical closeness permitted in the relationship; (4) territory, which refers to the range of physical settings in which the client and coach will work together; and (5) emotional space, which deals with the level and range of emotions appropriate to the goals and purposes of the relationship. Some boundary violations may have to occur only once to justify a coach's decision to end the relationship. For example, a client may make an inappropriate sexual advance, and the coach may decide that the relationship is not viable.

3. **Clients engage in unacceptable behaviors.** Clients may behave in ways that are not acceptable to a coach. For instance, someone may use language that is racist, sexist, or foul. He may show up for appointments after drinking, or he may show indications of other substance abuse. Clients may repeatedly come unprepared or may multitask during sessions (e.g., answering phone calls, eating). You may decide that the client's behavior is unacceptable based on personal values or professional standards.

4. **Negative feelings toward clients.** As Walsh (2007) suggests, helpers do not like to admit that they may have strong negative feelings toward certain clients. Just as a client may discontinue the relationship based on the coach's personal charac-teristics, a coach may not want to work with certain people. When the coach identifies this attitude at the beginning of the relationship, he might easily resolve the situation by suggesting that the person work with another coach. More problematic is the case in which increasing dislike develops over time. The coach is then in a predicament of not want-ing to work with the client because of personality characteristics, the nature of the evolving topic, or the way the client behaves in sessions. This kind of situation would probably require that the coach review matters with a peer or mentor coach.

5. **Clients make poor progress.** Despite a client's best intentions and a coach's best efforts, the client simply may not be able to successfully engage the process of coaching or implement agreed-upon steps to reach her goals. This instance is different than the issue described earlier; here, the problem may be an underlying element of the client's capac-ity rather than his motivation. In these instances, the coach may reasonably wonder about her own capabilities, which may or may not be part of the problem. A more likely scenario is that the client has other hurdles to contend with before he is able to take on the challenges that he has set for himself in this coaching relationship. Referring back to the competency development model, the person may need significant development in a particular com-petency area before progress on the current goal can be realized. Although referring the client to another professional may be in order, the coaching relationship does not necessarily have to end. You could suggest a hiatus in coaching while the client works on an identified impediment to progress with someone else. Another example would be when a client wants help with a major lifestyle overhaul, but in the early stages of coaching a death occurs in her family and she is overcome by grief.

6. **The coach becomes overwhelmed.** Life hap-pens, and coaches like all humans are vulnerable to disease, disability, stress, and strain. Though they might be expected to manage their personal and work lives well enough that conditions such as burnout do not occur, they sometimes take on more than they can handle or the unexpected hap-pens. It makes sense to plan for contingencies and perhaps work in concert with other coaches who have compatible styles so that appropriate referrals can be made when situations of this nature occur.

## Planned Endings

A desirable progression in coaching may resemble the phases of the flow model of coaching in a relatively seamless manner. This does not always mean that the client has reached the fullness of his goals; rather, some other mutually determined criterion may become relevant to the decision. Here are some possible scenarios (Walsh, 2007).

1. **Desired goals have been achieved.** Clients may progress toward the attainment of mutually determined objectives until they feel they have achieved their purposes. Sometimes clients may set consecutive goals with the same coach and move through the phases of coaching until they feel satisfied. In these instances, the end may come after a number of successes.

2. **Agreed-upon time limit for the relationship has arrived.** Sometimes coaching is delineated according to a calendar of meetings. Clients agree to meet for a certain number of sessions to advance a particular agenda. They may not have concrete outcome goals as much as they have process goals of working in new ways or experiencing things differently with the assistance of a coach. For practical reasons, some clients may have budgeted a particular amount of money for coaching and scheduled a specific number of sessions to work on an agenda.

3. **Clients' topics suggest other avenues.** A coach and client may discover a host of other concerns that the client needs to address. For instance, someone may have serious health issues arising from overeating, smoking, or substance abuse that jeopardize their capacities. Through dialogue, the coach and client may create a plan of action for the client to address these matters with other processes or with other people. Contact with the coach could continue for an agreed-upon time during which strategies are planned for addressing the client's emergent issues.

## Potential Reactions to Endings

Feelings will vary when coaching relationships end. Ideally, clients feel a strong sense of achievement from the goals they have pursued and attained. Through coaching, clients may also have gained an enhanced sense of autonomy and personal efficacy. Beyond achieving specific goals, they may also have learned how to learn, how to plan, and how to strategize for success. Potentially, they will feel more accomplished and express greater confidence in themselves by virtue of having successfully committed to their goals.

At a process level, clients have reason to rejoice in their ability to work collaboratively with another person and to be open with that person without negative consequence. Transferring this learning to other relationships would provide them with yet another source of satisfaction. Although clients may experience such emotions as sadness regarding the ending of a significant coaching relationship, they may understand these experiences as normal and appropriate. If they allow these emotions to be legitimate and without judgment, this can also afford a meaningful benefit from the coaching process.

More problematically, clients may react with a sense of loss when the coaching relationship ends. This is more likely to occur when coaching has continued over a long time and when clients have been unsuccessful in achieving process goals of increased autonomy and self-efficacy. Another problematic reaction occurs when they deny that the ending has any meaning whatsoever or when they avoid discussing the matter. In these cases, they may be experiencing deeper reactions than they are consciously aware of or able to address. Eventually, their feelings may surface and color their perceptions of the effectiveness of their coaching experience.

Of course, some clients may react with anger at the ending of a coaching relationship. They may accuse the coach of not helping or not being sensitive to their needs. Clients who have not achieved their goals for whatever reason may react by expressing strong negative feelings toward the coach.

As a coach, you need to be aware of what might seem a reasonable request by clients for continuing contact through a new relationship, such as friendship or social connection. When clients are unwilling or unready to bring closure yet cannot justify the continuation of coaching, they may wish to transform the coaching relationship into a form of connection they can more easily justify.

Clients are not the only ones affected by endings. You may also experience enhanced feelings of self-efficacy through the work that you have done, and you may take appropriate satisfaction in clients' accomplishments. Just as clients who end long-term coaching relationships may understandably feel some sadness, coaches may experience similar emotions. Through those feelings, they will hopefully deepen their capacity for compassion.

What happens when clients do not achieve their goals, when they blame you for their failures, or when they terminate after a long period of unsuccessful effort? In these instances, you may experience guilt, a lessening of professional competency, or a tendency to blame the client for perceived failures. You may go so far as making inappropriate offers to continue working with clients who are ending the relationship because of their dissatisfaction with outcomes.

# COMMENTARY

Some theorists use deceptively simple terms to describe change processes. Bridges (2001), for instance, talks about the beginning, middle, and end. Although these concepts are commonly understood, they mask a myriad of dynamics when applied to personal change. In this chapter we have reflected on the final two ICF core competencies, which speak to the small goals, big goals, and dreams that people want to realize. We have also addressed maintenance of progress and completion. The final agenda of this chapter was the matter of endings. Clearly, the initial moments of a coaching relationship can be delicate and tricky to maneuver, and coaches must proceed with extreme sensitivity. The same is true of endings. As the client becomes a familiar face with predictable patterns and as interactions feel increasingly comfortable, coaches might think of endings as informal, almost matter-of-fact, "see you later" experiences. They are anything but that. Coaches may never truly know their effect on clients or grasp the full value, positive or negative, that they may have had. Consequently, they need to manage endings as carefully as they do beginnings.

In our next and final chapter, we address our own endings—yours in incorporating this material into your personal and professional life, and ours in presenting what remains to be said to usher you forward on your journey. We trust that this process will be one of your moving on to other learning and mastery encounters in the field of coaching. We hope that we have opened you further to these exciting explorations.

# 12

# COACHING AS A PATH OF CHANGE

## In this chapter, you will learn how...

- embracing a career in coaching places you on a profound path of personal change and development;

- changes generated in coaching—for both you and your clients—are likely to be transformational in nature;

- as a coach your basis of expertise will expand to include process as well as content components;

- your curriculum for lifelong learning as a coach requires focus on your personal evolution as well as professional skill development; and

- becoming a coach places you in the formative stages of this profession wherein you can help shape its future.

> To live is to change.
> To live well is to change often.
>
> —*John Henry Newman*

Coaching is challenging work for both client and coach—and it is exceptionally rewarding. It takes great courage to choose coaching as a path of change. For clients whose lives are often busy and complex, it means stepping away from old realities and consciously creating a dream future that often has little substance in their current lives. It abounds with transformations of comfortable habits into unfamiliar patterns. It requires sustained effort and doing things perhaps for the very first time. Though it is likely to be exhilarating, this work can also be fraught with doubts, anxieties, confusion, and even fear—more so for clients, and surprisingly often for coaches as well.

As someone who may be entering this profession with a solid belief in your personal wisdom and capacity to care for others, you will nonetheless encounter calls to action in virtually every corner of your existence as you deepen your involvement. The good news is that this doesn't all happen at once. At different moments, inner voices will gain volume as you discover yet another place where you are holding onto self-limiting beliefs or living in comfort zones that no longer serve you.

From a certain perspective, coaching can be thought of as a spiritual practice. You will continually confront questions about your higher purpose in the work you do. Coaching is a career that demands that you examine your deepest beliefs and values in order to know where you are positioned in judgment or habit. You may be inspirational and a great motivator in your current endeavors, yet these qualities could be insufficient for success in coaching. You will likely learn that no matter how quickly you get on top of your ingrained perspectives, you continue to find yourself listening with your own agendas in mind rather than those of your clients. You will notice how subtly you advance your own convictions because they have worked so well for you and others, though they may be a questionable fit for this particular client. You will trip over biases you never imagined you had.

None of this is meant to imply that there is something wrong with you. Human beings are hardwired for habit formation and conditioned from birth to prefer some things and reject others. We learn quickly and we develop our own success formulas, not fully realizing that there is an expiration date on most of the things to which we become attached. Our tried-and-true ways lose their potency, and old habits get us into increasing amounts of trouble. Beliefs that allowed us to have a sense of tribal belonging now run counter to ones in a wider multicultural society. Often, we feel the ground shifting beneath our feet.

Realities in the 21st century continually confront us with the need to adapt, change, adjust, shift, or move. Do you live in the same home where you grew up? The same town? The same country? Do you still speak your mother tongue at work and at home? Have you held the same job for more than five years? Has there been one and only one true love in your life with whom you continue to be in a relationship? Has your body changed in any significant ways? Do you think the same way that you did when you were a teenager? Change is the prevalent face of life, and it can feel relentless in its demands.

All of this has bearing because coaching is about change. More aptly, it is about transformational change. You buy a new shirt and wear it. That's probably a small change, but if you look at your wardrobe you might find that there is coherence and consistency in the style of clothing you wear. What if you switched your color scheme from soft, earthy tones to vibrant colors? Is that still a small change? Of course, it's unlikely you would make such a change without some significant provocation, and so we begin to drift closer to the concept of transformational change. A woman may treat herself to a total makeover due to some dissatisfaction with her old image and a need to do something new. A couple of things are likely here: First, there probably has been some internal shift that has given rise to this decision, and second, it's unlikely to last unless a host of other elements in her internal and external world support this change.

As we have seen repeatedly throughout this book, one thing affects another. No change occurs in isolation—the butterfly effect! Though some agendas for coaching will seem to be about making small life adjustments, the clients who bring you these supposedly small matters may show up in the first session with hope, doubt, unknown motivation, and a history of disappointment after having tried everything they possibly could to make this minor change. The agenda may seem small, but the process can be all encompassing. Yet, your rational mind says, "But it's just about cutting back on caffeine, or saying no to friends, or drinking eight glasses of water a day!"

Why do so many people choose coaching over other options? There is truth in the impression that modern-day coaching seems like the new panacea. Early books on coaching promoted its effectiveness with such glowing promise that success was all but guaranteed. Coaching clients were often portrayed as elite. They flourished on an ever-increasing spiral of success: The more they attained, the more they wanted, and coaching was their rocket to the stars. Many of the coaches who founded coaching schools were highly charismatic people who had profound effects on others. When you worked with them, you got results.

With exponential growth in the coaching field, at least two features of the coaching world are in greater focus at this time. The first is that clients who come to coaching are not always strongly motivated to change. They may want to adopt new behaviors, but when it comes down to the hard work of shifting patterns and habits, they may realize that coaching is not an easy fix. The second is that coaching involves hard work on both sides. For the coach it is anything but a sit-back-and-listen profession. We would describe it more as an edge-of-your-seat occupation, where the coach needs to be tuned in and turned on at every moment of the encounter.

For clients, it is not always a soft, embracing experience where empathic love and acceptance meet their every word. Coaching can be tough. Put another way, it is a highly assertive process where lengthy explanations are cut short and excuses are labeled as just that. This in no way implies that coaches lack compassion or that they are aggressive in demeanor. Rather, they are clear about their roles and the requirements for effective coaching to take place. When clients repeatedly show up with reasons why they didn't follow through, their coaches may respectfully challenge their explanations and even raise the question of ending the relationship.

In spite of the demands of this process, more and more clients are seeking out coaching relationships over other types of help, and as a result coaches need to be sharper about identifying the boundaries of their professional work. Coaching isn't for everyone. It would be accurate to say that a coaching approach to situations is becoming more prevalent in the Western world, but this doesn't mean that coaching relationships exist in all these cases. For instance, within the world of counseling and psychotherapy, one can easily find parallels between the ways therapists and coaches engage with their clients. They both may focus predominantly on the present and future, and they both facilitate clients toward action. Does this mean that these two professions are becoming more similar than different? We believe that the commonality in methodology adds credence and validity to the field of coaching, but the unwavering goal-driven pursuit of coaching sets it apart from helping professions that emphasize fundamental character change.

We have asserted throughout this book that the roots of coaching derive from many applied disciplines, including psychology, adult learning, social work, and psychiatry. Coaching is a highly specialized, bounded profession that intentionally sets limits on the kinds of clients for whom the process is appropriate. It assumes ways of collaborating that steadfastly respect and uphold contractual intentions for coach and client to work in partnership. As a profound change methodology, coaching can work with a wide range of client populations, including people who might not be so successful. In this respect, it is not an elitist approach. However, if a coach is to work with a specific population, she may need to have additional credentials that safeguard her work as an ethical practice. Think of this in all that we have been saying about the specialty or niche of lifestyle wellness coaching.

The question of motivation is key to coaching. Pioneering coaching references depict clients as having an abundance of motivation to change. As we have noted, this isn't always the case, and yet the methodology routinely yields robust outcomes. To illustrate, many coaches work in organizations where employees are told to submit to coaching sessions even though they might not want to change or they may perceive that they have been wrongly labeled. The power of coaching derives in part from the coach's ability to surface sources of motivation to change when clients show resistance at the outset. Through insight-producing dialogue, coaches generate a wider framework for the coaching process that embraces who the client is and how genuine benefit can be derived even under conditions that are less than auspicious.

## RECONFIGURING THE CONCEPT OF EXPERTISE

In the realm of health, wellness, and fitness, science continues to generate untold amounts of information about our biopsychosocial functioning as well as environmental influences on our state of being. In a certain light, our world seems to be drowning in information. One would think that with all we know, we should readily be able to live healthier lives. However, we know that this is not necessarily so. Information is often insufficient to motivate and sustain change. People know that smoking kills, that fast food is harmful, that condoms should be worn—and the list goes on. The simple fact is that changing long-standing beliefs, values, habits, and ultimately behaviors is extraordinarily challenging no matter what.

As a health, wellness, or fitness professional, you have foundational training in some specialty that provides you with expert knowledge. How do you integrate this knowledge into your work as a coach? Recognizing that a lack of information is rarely the most serious stumbling block to change, to what degree do you assert your expertise as a motivational source of change with your clients? In what ways does your expert knowledge become your clients' engine of change? Although information has a limited effect on motivation, when your coaching niche is based on your professional expertise in some content area (e.g., nutrition, exercise science, health promotion, nursing), clients may come to you for the final word about what they should do. Yet, effective coaching is substantially different from being an oracle of wisdom.

Let's look at this through a wider lens. People spend billions of dollars on advice they don't heed.

They go to seminars and workshops; they consult experts and gurus; they buy the latest books and videos. Then, they try to change, and soon afterward, they decide they need another expert, another book, another seminar, or whatever else appears to promise lasting change. This is not intended as criticism of the modern character but rather as a resounding acknowledgment of the challenge of change. It is not so much that we are gullible but more that, in this turbulent and uncharted world we live in, a survival mechanism may be to hope that just possibly someone has finally discovered the silver bullet.

Consider how expertise in lifestyle changes has helped you in your life. Think back to information you were offered about how you should live your life. Now, reflect on the innumerable times you were presented with this expert knowledge before it sank in. Of course, many messages from parents and experts may have been unhelpful, representing perhaps the limited scope of their visions or their own conditioning. But at least some of what they said constituted sound advice. Why didn't you listen then? What took you so long to get it? Well, you might say, it wasn't the right time to hear what was being offered. Or, perhaps you were determined to learn for yourself. Continuing with this reflection, might you acknowledge now that there's got to be something better than trial-and-error learning? The school of hard knocks is not the most efficient learning system in a rapidly changing world.

The advice givers in your world, including your parents, had intelligence and experience on their side. They had either lived long enough to know better or they had solid evidence behind their opinions. Yet, at times, you didn't listen, or perhaps didn't hear, just like the client who smokes a couple of packs a day and religiously schedules annual physicals only to be told once again, "Stop smoking." Prochaska and colleagues (2002) would remind us that some people simply aren't ready to change, and sometimes there's nothing we can ethically do to motivate them toward action.

This is truly a dilemma. You have so much information. You have spent years if not decades mastering a knowledge base with which to influence change. Yet, your expertise often has the same effect on your clients as others' expertise had on you at various moments in your life. How do we get out of this impasse? And why do we think coaching is a better way?

Let's come back to coaching and expertise. Your intelligence as a coach is not only about content knowledge regarding a particular subject matter. As reflected in the competency development model, your intelligence is represented in a multidimensional array of facts, skills, capacities, understandings, and accumulated wisdom. So, this is a far richer and more encompassing framing of expertise than would normally be understood. Your knowledge shows up in the myriad ways in which you understand your clients' patterns. It is represented in how you help them find the missing elements in their stories that will keep them from endlessly running in circles. It is found in how you surface resources that clients believed nonexistent. It manifests in your presence and how you hold the space for your clients. And it is represented by your offers of expert counsel at precisely the right moment and in a language that your clients can now hear. This kind of intelligence gives rise to clients' capacities to access that fourth dimension that we previously discussed.

As suggested, there is a strong component of social intelligence (Goleman, 2006) in the coach's expertise. This relates to the core fact that human beings are social creatures who benefit immensely from skillful, supportive help. Here it is important to ask once again the question we have examined throughout this book, "What constitutes support?" In everyday social relationships, support is often equated with a kind of collusion with others to think the same way they think. But we see support in coaching as far more than social friendliness. It is more appropriately understood as an elegant pattern of communication that shifts locked-in unproductive behaviors into more resourceful ways to propel constructive change. Support is also best appreciated as a process that occurs over time rather than as a one-time intervention. If clients have lived a certain way for two or three decades, how likely is it that sage and caring advice will instantaneously provoke permanent change? It can happen, but it is rare.

Likewise, it is a misconception to construe support as enthusiastic cheerleading; in fact, this form of support may backfire badly for both client and coach. Reality TV shows depict coaches working miracles with clients. You may ask, how wrong could this be? There is little doubt that someone inspirational enough to make it to stardom as a coach has some finely honed intervention skills. With the added motivations of tangible rewards and the accolades of an ever-curious TV audience, clients have ample external support for their change agendas. But the show ends. The coaches move on to their next challenges, and the clients are on their own. How well do they do? We suspect it varies greatly. The more coaches pour themselves into their clients to make them change, the more the process is about the coaches. Clients need to hear their own voices as they move toward autonomous action, not just the echoes of someone else's motivating words. Effective coaches encourage clients to find their own self-talk, their own way of being inspirational in their lives. This is an important component of the coach's social intelligence of change.

## COURAGE IN A SOCIAL PERSPECTIVE

People do amazing things. They overcome unimaginable limitations. They thrive in the harshest of circumstances. What one person is capable of, many more have the capacity to do. Yet, we seldom do it alone and rarely just for ourselves. Arctic explorers, transatlantic voyagers, and pioneers of all kinds may have been physically alone throughout their ordeals, but it is unlikely that they were alone in their thoughts. We are inspired by others, we strive so that others may feel proud, and we may even put ourselves in harm's way for the well-being of unknown others.

For better or worse, our lives are shaped by and directed toward inner and outer human connection. Our rich thought processes are replete with images and conversations, with feelings and the remembrances of touch. This is one of the deepest reasons why coaching is so effective. Coaching is about relationships; it is not about technically nailing a problem with precisely formulated solutions. Previously, clients may have bought books on their topic of concern. Perhaps they even looked online for potential solutions or bought special products. Whatever they came up with probably lacked the critical ingredients and resourcefulness to promote life-giving, sustainable progress. Ultimately, it is a human quality to want other people to hear our stories, to see us beyond the limited visions we hold of ourselves. We need someone who will open us to our full potential and lovingly hold us accountable because we have such difficulty being accountable to ourselves.

As long as we remain willing to understand the difficulties that people have in changing longstanding dysfunctional habits, we can keep our hearts open to helping them in processes of change. Doing so will not always be easy for us, and it will not be simple for them—though no doubt our efforts will smooth the path, lower the obstacles, and instill hope.

With our abundant knowledge about health, wellness, and fitness, we may sometimes focus too forcefully on the problem and not sufficiently on the beauty of the person sitting before us. What will inspire our capacity to be helpful is a determination to find the inner flame, the passion for life hidden in a corner of each client's existence. We need to seek the client's will to be more than her self-defined or externally defined limitations. Ultimately, we may not be able to change it all. Perfection is not a human reality. Striving is.

## YOUR LIFE AS A COACH

How you want your career to develop and how much emphasis you give to coaching will be informed partly by your desires and partly by your personal evolution. We cannot easily predict the future, although we may nonetheless plan for it. Once you embark on a course of learning and development associated with coaching, certain outcomes will become more likely. Understanding the skills and processes of coaching yields the power to change yourself for the better. As you learn to listen well to others, you will likely learn to listen to yourself better. As you express care and concern for the dilemmas that clients experience, you will most likely become more empathic to your own struggles and challenges. As you accompany them along the path of change, you will probably develop an intuitive understanding of how you can better manage your own passages and transitions.

Becoming an outstanding coach is about becoming the best of yourself. The course that you have chosen will nurture your growth and development as surely as it does that of your clients. Yet, this will not happen without clearly defined intentions and actions. Who are the clients you wish to serve? Where do you currently excel? What do you yet need to master?

## LIFELONG LEARNING

We have traveled with you through all these pages and wish to journey just a bit further. As we reflect on the field of coaching, we acknowledge that it is still in its formative years. Organizations such as the ICF have been highly successful in bringing a credible professional face to an industry that was virtually unheard of a few decades ago. Even so, it doesn't take much formal training to become certified as a coach. Is that reasonable? We believe that those who undertake basic training can be highly effective in many straightforward applications of a coaching methodology. As the complexity of client issues increases, however, coaches must have greater experience and training.

Coaching is not disconnected from other approaches to helping; in fact, as we have demonstrated, it depends on them for much of its skill base and understanding of human behavior. To be an effective coach with people who have challenging issues, you need to understand human behavior. Some of this information can be found in foundational psychology and human relations courses; other elements may be located in theories and practices related to communication, adult development, and behavior change. Beyond learning through formal studies, **reflective practice** is essential. This entails sincere self-reflection, engagement in peer supervision groups, and regular work with mentor coaches.

The learning process is ongoing in coaching; it is a gradual accumulation of understanding about the coaching field and about the intriguing and profound nature of human beings. Learning is never a search for the magic answer; rather, it is a gradual accumulation of understanding. In your personal learning journey, there may be times when you come across great teachers or inspired authors. You may be enthralled by their methodologies and become a true believer in a specific method of coaching. Or, you may sample a variety of coaching schools and find that each approach offers a new angle to apply to your work. Ultimately, you will discover your own approach to being the best coach you can be. It may not come easily or quickly, though hopefully you will be patient and not think that you have arrived long before you have. Each experience has something to offer, even when what you learn is something that you never plan to do again. Each course of study you undertake holds the capacity to stimulate understanding and deeper reflections about your clients. Your journey doesn't stop with the mastery of external sources of knowledge. Self-knowledge also needs to be embraced. The more you know about your own ways, the more readily you can step out of your clients' paths so they are able to follow their dreams rather than yours for them.

# SHORTCUTS

There are no shortcuts. Along the way, you may become intrigued with certain tools or techniques that seem to be essential to anyone who is a coach. You may, for instance, wonder about tests and questionnaires that would more rapidly reveal what you need to know about clients. As you develop your practice, you will come across many tools of this sort; we have even suggested a few earlier in the book. In the decades of our work in the helping professions and coaching in particular, we have used many tools and techniques. None has proven irreplaceable. As we review the great practitioners of the 20th and 21st centuries, we know that most of them had profoundly effective methods. Yet, in the cold light of research, what consistently shines through is not a particular technique but the human being who had the courage and humility to offer her services to another. The 11 ICF core competencies are about as encompassing a methodology as you will ever need in order to be an exceptional coach—and you will master them only with practice. When these are solidly in your grasp, it may be time to widen your horizons and expand your methods.

# CURRICULUM FOR COACHES

Returning to the theme of your development as a coach, we would now like to consider this from a more pragmatic perspective. Undoubtedly, waves of change are forthcoming for the coaching industry. We believe the ICF will incrementally raise the bar for certification as a professional coach in the years to come, and at the same time, society will hold coaches increasingly accountable through licensing requirements and professional reviews.

Currently, there are few academic programs in university settings for coach education. This will change. We believe that graduate diplomas, certificates, and degrees will become more the norm for coach education in the future, though it seems unlikely that professional coaching programs will be developed at an undergraduate level. Why do we envision this future?

Having carefully read the previous chapters, you will concur that coaching conversations can be complex, and coaches who are confronted with clients' normal challenges to change must have mastered concomitant levels of skill. If you take, by comparison, the preparatory training of other helpers, you will appreciate the discrepancies that currently exist between the training of a professional coach and that of other professionals.

In the field of social work, for example, people typically complete an undergraduate program leading to a BSW and then continue to pursue an MSW, which normally includes extensive practicum experiences under close supervision. In psychology, the requirements are steeper. For the most part, practicing psychologists throughout North America must hold a doctoral degree and undergo supervision both during and after graduation from their doctoral programs before they are allowed to practice on their own.

You might be thinking that these are more demanding professions, with clients who face more perplexing predicaments. However, you can never be certain who is requesting help on the phone or at your office door. More positively, we believe that you will want to be an exquisite coach who has the capacity to accompany your clients to their desired futures with grace and certainty. In service of this agenda, we have outlined an interrelated curriculum model for coach development (see Coach Development Curriculum). Some of this material was referenced earlier, but we want to take it to a more detailed level in this final section. Having trained professional coaches for years, we often recommend these pursuits for students as they are completing their intensive program with us. We invite you to think of the items in this curriculum within a time frame of 10 or more years rather than as objectives you need to accomplish right now.

## Coach Development Curriculum

### Professional education

Coursework and other learning experiences

- Eastern and Western philosophies
- General psychology
- Interpersonal dynamics
- Theories of personality
- Neuroscience
- Abnormal behavior
- Life-span development
- Helping skills
- Behavior change and management
- Health promotion
- Cultural studies
- Family relations
- Psychosocial assessment methods
- Transpersonal psychology
- Positive psychology
- Systems theory
- Theories of consciousness and evolution
- Communication theory and practice
- Professional ethics and morality
- Management theory
- Business development

### Personal development

Personal programs and learning

- Mindfulness practices
- Meditation
- Music and art appreciation
- Lifestyle management
- Stress management
- Spirituality
- Personal values
- Reading
- Personal and life coaching
- Psychological development including counseling or therapy
- Relationship work
- Journaling
- Purposeful physical training
- Bodywork of all kinds
- Travel

### Mentoring relations

Reflective or review experiences related to your coaching work

- Reflective practice
- Mentor coaching
- Peer coaching reviews
- Pursuit of additional and advanced certifications
- Professional seminars and workshops
- Presentations at peer-reviewed conferences
- Journaling and periodic reflective review

This curriculum model for coach development is fully in service of the experience of coaching itself. Here, you are on your own, doing what you have prepared yourself to do. What previous and concurrent work nourishes your capacities?

Personal development is the first sphere of influence. Who you are as a person, how you have developed, what you have done to create greater sensitivity and awareness, and the degree to which you are on top of your own game all strongly influence how you show up in coaching relationships. Think of this, in part, as your coaching presence. You cannot embody the way of a coach until you fully inhabit your own being—with comfort, acceptance, wisdom, power, and fullness.

Beyond self-knowledge and personal development is the sphere of mentoring. Here, we envision that all effective coaches have ongoing relationships where they review their coaching experiences with competent others. In your early practice, it would be wise for you to find a mentor coach to consult on a regular basis. As you advance in years of practice, you may find additional sources of support among peers. Though your need for mentoring may taper after a few years, it will never disappear completely. Having an experienced mentor who knows you well is a component of sound professional practice. As you become a senior coach, you may choose to become a mentor yourself. Such a shift in your practice base does not signal the end of the need for public review of your work, however. Surrounding yourself with other seasoned coaches in biweekly or monthly peer mentoring sessions would be of immense benefit to your evolutionary growth.

The final sphere that contributes to your coaching competency is that of professional education and development. In this regard, learning will be lifelong and extensive. Depending on your present professional and educational background, you may have more or less work in front of you. With the changing realities of today's world, all of us will remain on a steep learning curve to remain proficient in our work as coaches. Beyond courses and programs in coaching, you will want to enroll in many other forms of learning in the years to come. Given the multidisciplinary roots of coaching, continued learning may take many paths, though there are some fundamental areas that need to be integrated (see figure 12.1 for visual representation).

We have already indicated that your good intentions, capacity to listen, compassionate stance toward your clients, and knowledge gained through training will serve you well in the beginning. They will help you to know when you are in over

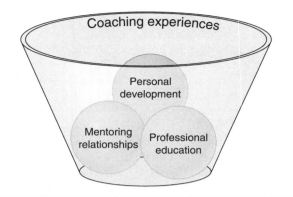

**Figure 12.1** The interrelationship of development agendas within the bowl of coaching experiences.

your head so that you can graciously bow out of coaching encounters that are beyond your current capacities. In time you will learn more, your practice will expand, and your reputation will grow. Your career needs to be understood in a scale of decades. Can you imagine doing this work for the next 40 years? We hope your answer is an enthusiastic and unequivocal *yes*. If you are less certain, then taking things one step at a time is sensible. Allow your learning and experiences to inform you about where you want to go and whether this work is deeply in your heart.

It may well be that your purpose in reading this book is to gain another set of tools for the profession you are passionately pursuing right now. You may not want to be a full-time coach but rather to incorporate some coaching methods in your current approach. This is entirely valid and of considerable merit. We simply want you to have an option along with a map of what another future might look like over time. Coaching as a profession is here to stay. It will continue to grow and its applications will spread. At the beginning of the 20th century there may have been 100 or so professional psychologists; currently, there are likely more than 100,000 psychologists in the United States alone. Think about becoming part of the coaching profession at this point in its history and evolving along with it for the duration of your career. What a thrilling journey that could be!

There is little doubt that mastering the challenges of a coaching career will be more than adequately compensated. The rewards of serving others on their paths to fulfillment are inestimable. We encourage you to embrace all the tasks and personal work that are necessary to bring you to the peak of your capacities and personal evolution as a coach—and as a human.

# COMMENTARY

No doubt you have worked hard to incorporate all the material presented throughout these pages. In doing so, you have learned some new things, reinforced others that were nascent within you, and perhaps talked to yourself about points of uncertainty. Whatever your path, the fact that you have completed this book will serve you well. You will have tackled practical skills. You will have ingested new models for understanding change and planning action. You will have gained perspective about the profession of coaching and how it applies to what you currently do. More centrally, we hope your efforts have opened your heart even wider to your clients and others. By realizing these results through your efforts with this book, you will have gained immeasurable potency for promoting health and wellness in this world. If you imagine your evolved capacities for personal and professional expression as having a kind of butterfly effect, what might be the ripples of your evolution throughout this planet Earth? What are the consequences of your growth on others' capacities to be their very best and to live in the fullness of their dreams?

# TTM DECISIONAL BALANCE

## Pros and Cons of Behavior Change

Use the decisional balance to help clients take action and bring about the change they want.

1. List the pros (left side) and cons (right side) of performing the behavior.
2. Establish the strength or importance of each entry on a scale of 1 to 10 (see the following example).
3. Add up the pros and cons separately. Subtract the cons from the pros.

If the behavior is something healthy clients want to adopt (e.g., start exercising, adopt a healthy diet, sleep seven hours a night), the pros should pro-gressively outweigh the cons as clients move from precontemplation to action. As a coach, you might help the clients identify new benefits of performing the behavior (pros) to strengthen their resolve to remain in action.

If the behavior is something unhealthy that clients want to stop (e.g., stop smoking, stop emotional eating, stop excessive drinking, refrain from expressing anger inappropriately), the cons should progressively outweigh the pros as the clients move from precontemplation to action. As a coach, you might help the clients identify negative effects of continuing to perform the unhealthy behavior (cons) to strengthen their resolve to remain in action.

Target behavior: _____

| Pros | Strength | Cons | Strength |
|------|----------|------|----------|
| 1. | | 1. | |
| 2. | | 2. | |
| 3. | | 3. | |
| 4. | | 4. | |
| 5. | | 5. | |
| Total pros | | Total cons | |
| Pros (_____) – cons (_____) = _____. | | | |

Example: Target behavior: Walking outside 30 minutes per day

| Pros | Strength | Cons | Strength |
|------|----------|------|----------|
| 1. Exercise burns calories. | 8 | 1. Takes time from other things. | 9 |
| 2. Clear my mind of the day's issues. | 6 | 2. Weather might not be good. | 7 |
| 3. Get some fresh air. | 5 | 3. Have to force myself out the door. | 8 |
| 4. Take time for myself. | 4 | 4. Not really exciting. | 7 |
| 5. Take the dog for a much-needed walk. | 6 | 5. | |
| Total pros | 29 | Total cons | 31 |

Pros (29) − cons (31) = −2.

The decisional balance is slightly negative (cons outweigh the pros), so this client needs to see further benefits of walking in order to adopt and maintain the new healthy behavior. As a coach, what could you do to help the client move forward?

Reproduced from J. Gavin and M. Mcbrearty, 2013, *Lifestyle wellness coaching*, 2nd ed. (Champaign, IL: Human Kinetics). Based on Prochaska, Norcross, and DiClemente 1994.

# SAMPLE LIFESTYLE WELLNESS COACHING AGREEMENT

## 1. Parties to the Agreement

Client's name: _____

Address:_____

Phone: _____ E-mail: _____

Coach's name:_____

Address:_____

Phone: _____ E-mail: _____

## 2. Agreement

| Coach | Client |
|---|---|
| As your coach, I agree to do the following:<br>1. Meet with you face to face for 10 consecutive weekly 60-minute sessions at a time that is mutually agreeable.<br>2. Be available by phone or e-mail for agreed-upon check-ins. You may call me twice between sessions if needed (short calls lasting no more than 10 minutes); I will respond to e-mails within 24 hours (except weekends and holidays).<br>3. Work with you through inquiry and dialogue to clarify your goals and design your action plan. I will also provide ongoing support for your goal-directed activities. | As your client, I agree to do the following:<br>1. Show up for scheduled meetings on time for 10 consecutive weekly 60-minute sessions, starting on January 25, 2013.<br>2. Commit myself to the coaching process and to the goals that we agree upon.<br>3. Call or e-mail you about my progress or issues that come up, within the limits that we have set. |

*(continued)*

Coach–client agreement    *(continued)*

| Coach | Client |
|---|---|
| 4. Give you feedback about issues that impede your progress.<br>5. Inform you about matters that I believe are affecting our working relationship.<br>6. Notify you at least 48 hours in advance if I need to cancel a meeting, except in case of dire emergency.<br>7. Respect the ICF code of ethics and keep all our sessions confidential. | 4. Be willing to talk to you about any issues that pertain to my progress or how we are working together. I will also let you know if anything you do or say does not feel right to me.<br>5. Pay for any sessions that I cancel less than 48 hours in advance, except in case of dire emergency. |

### 3. *Nature of the Coaching Relationship*

A coaching relationship is not psychological counseling or psychotherapy. The client is hiring the coach for a coaching relationship and not for any other type of professional work. The coach will partner with the client with the understanding that the client is responsible for creating his or her own results. Coach and client will work collaboratively, and the coach will provide support to the client in identifying and achieving goals.

### 4. *Logistics*

*Rates:* $___ per month payable by cash, check, or credit card at the beginning of each month. Additional phone calls (more than once between sessions) are $____ per 10 minutes. These are payable at the beginning of the next session.

*Place:* We will meet at my office at the sport center on Wednesdays from 5 to 6 p.m. for the next 10 weeks.

*Duration of this agreement*: From January 25, 2013, to March 29, 2013.

### 5. *Conditions or Actions That Would Make This Agreement Invalid*

| Coach | Client |
|---|---|
| 1. Client fails to attend two consecutive meetings without notice.<br>2. Client fails to live up to agreements on action plan for 2 weeks, unless extenuating circumstances exist.<br>3. Client fails to pay the agreed-upon fees at the agreed-upon times.<br>4. Client exhibits behavior that is inappropriate to the professional relationship. | 1. Coach fails to keep to scheduled meetings.<br>2. Coach fails to respond to e-mails or be available for agreed-upon phone calls.<br>3. Coach fails to be helpful in ways that have been agreed upon.<br>4. Coach gives advice or information that is wrong or jeopardizes me, the client, in some way. |

Signatures

_____

Coach

_____

Date

_____

Client

# ICF CODE OF ETHICS

## Part One: Definition of Coaching

### Section 1: Definitions

- **Coaching:** Coaching is partnering with clients in a thought-provoking and creative process that inspires them to maximize their personal and professional potential.

- **A professional coaching relationship:** A professional coaching relationship exists when coaching includes a business agreement or contract that defines the responsibilities of each party.

- **An ICF Professional Coach:** An ICF Professional Coach also agrees to practice the ICF Professional Core Competencies and pledges accountability to the ICF Code of Ethics.

In order to clarify roles in the coaching relationship, it is often necessary to distinguish between the client and the sponsor. In most cases, the client and sponsor are the same person and therefore jointly referred to as the client. For purposes of identification, however, the International Coach Federation defines these roles as follows:

- **Client:** The "client" is the person(s) being coached.

- **Sponsor:** The "sponsor" is the entity (including its representatives) paying for and/or arranging for coaching services to be provided.

In all cases, coaching engagement contracts or agreements should clearly establish the rights, roles, and responsibilities for both the client and sponsor if they are not the same persons.

## Part Two: The ICF Standards of Ethical Conduct

*Preamble: ICF Professional Coaches aspire to conduct themselves in a manner that reflects positively upon the coaching profession; are respectful of different approaches to coaching; and recognize that they are also bound by applicable laws and regulations.*

### Section 1: Professional Conduct at Large

As a coach:

1. I will not knowingly make any public statement that is untrue or misleading about what I offer as a coach, or make false claims in any written documents relating to the coaching profession or my credentials or the ICF.

2. I will accurately identify my coaching qualifications, expertise, experience, certifications, and ICF Credentials.

3. I will recognize and honor the efforts and contributions of others and not misrepresent them as my own. I understand that violating this standard may leave me subject to legal remedy by a third party.

4. I will, at all times, strive to recognize personal issues that may impair, conflict, or interfere with my coaching performance or my professional coaching relationships. Whenever the facts and circumstances necessitate, I will promptly seek professional assistance and determine the action to be taken, including whether it is appropriate to suspend or terminate my coaching relationship(s).

5. I will conduct myself in accordance with the ICF Code of Ethics in all coach training, coach mentoring, and coach supervisory activities.

6. I will conduct and report research with competence, honesty, and within recognized scientific standards and applicable subject guidelines. My research will be carried out with the necessary consent and approval of those involved, and with an approach that will protect participants from any potential harm. All research efforts will be performed in a manner that complies with all the applicable laws of the country in which the research is conducted.

7. I will maintain, store, and dispose of any records created during my coaching business in a manner that promotes confidentiality, security, and privacy and complies with any applicable laws and agreements.

8. I will use ICF member contact information (e-mail addresses, telephone numbers, etc.) only in the manner and to the extent authorized by the ICF.

## Section 2: Conflicts of Interest

As a coach:

1. I will seek to avoid conflicts of interest and potential conflicts of interest and openly disclose any such conflicts. I will offer to remove myself when such a conflict arises.

2. I will disclose to my client and his or her sponsor all anticipated compensation from third parties that I may pay or receive for referrals of that client.

3. I will only barter for services, goods, or other nonmonetary remuneration when it will not impair the coaching relationship.

4. I will not knowingly take any personal, professional, or monetary advantage or benefit of the coach–client relationship, except by a form of compensation as agreed in the agreement or contract.

## Section 3: Professional Conduct With Clients

As a coach:

1. I will not knowingly mislead or make false claims about what my client or sponsor will receive from the coaching process or from me as the coach.

2. I will not give my prospective clients or sponsors information or advice I know or believe to be misleading or false.

3. I will have clear agreements or contracts with my clients and sponsors. I will honor all agreements or contracts made in the context of professional coaching relationships.

4. I will carefully explain and strive to ensure that, prior to or at the initial meeting, my coaching client and sponsor(s) understand the nature of coaching, the nature and limits of confidentiality, financial arrangements, and any other terms of the coaching agreement or contract.

5. I will be responsible for setting clear, appropriate, and culturally sensitive boundaries that govern any physical contact I may have with my clients or sponsors.

6. I will not become sexually intimate with any of my current clients or sponsors.

7. I will respect the client's right to terminate the coaching relationship at any point during the process, subject to the provisions of the agreement or contract. I will be alert to indications that the client is no longer benefiting from our coaching relationship.

8. I will encourage the client or sponsor to make a change if I believe the client or sponsor would be better served by another coach or by another resource.

9. I will suggest my client seek the services of other professionals when deemed necessary or appropriate.

## Section 4: Confidentiality/Privacy

As a coach:

1. I will maintain the strictest levels of confidentiality with all client and sponsor information. I will have a clear agreement or contract before releasing information to another person, unless required by law.

2. I will have a clear agreement upon how coaching information will be exchanged among coach, client, and sponsor.

3. When acting as a trainer of student coaches, I will clarify confidentiality policies with the students.

4. I will have associated coaches and other persons whom I manage in service of my clients and their sponsors in a paid or volunteer capacity make clear agreements or

contracts to adhere to the ICF Code of Ethics Part 2, Section 4: Confidentiality/Privacy standards and the entire ICF Code of Ethics to the extent applicable.

## Part Three: The ICF Pledge of Ethics

As an ICF Professional Coach, I acknowledge and agree to honor my ethical and legal obligations to my coaching clients and sponsors, colleagues, and to the public at large. I pledge to comply with the ICF Code of Ethics, and to practice these standards with those whom I coach. If I breach this Pledge of Ethics or any part of the ICF Code of Ethics, I agree that the ICF in its sole discretion may hold me accountable for so doing. I further agree that my accountability to the ICF for any breach may include sanctions, such as loss of my ICF membership and/ or my ICF Credentials.

Approved by the Ethics and Standards Committee on October 30, 2008.

Approved by the ICF Board of Directors on December 18, 2008.

Reproduced from J. Gavin and M. Mcbrearty, 2013, *Lifestyle wellness coaching*, 2nd ed. (Champaign, IL: Human Kinetics). Reprinted, by permission, from International Coach Federation, 2011, *Code of ethics*. Available: http://www. coachfederation.org/about-icf/ethics/icf-code-of-ethics.

# GLOSSARY

**accountability**—A condition of the coaching relationship whereby clients are considered to be responsible for doing what they commit to do within their contracted coaching agreement and in service of their goal attainment.

**advice**—A suggested course of action directly communicated by a coach to a client typically in service of the client's goal attainment. Advice is usually based in the coach's area of expertise.

**andragogy**—Theory or model of adult learning; sometimes contrasted with pedagogy, which concerns the education of children and teens.

**boundary crossing**—An ethical matter in which a coach engages in a behavior with the client that holds the potential for jeopardizing the integrity of the relationship (e.g., attending a social event at the client's home).

**boundary violation**—An ethical matter in which a coach engages in a behavior with the client that jeopardizes the integrity of the relationship (e.g., going on a date with the client).

**closed question**—A type of question that limits the requested response from the client and thereby enables the coach to gather specific information and control the communication flow.

**closure**—In coaching, refers to the process of planned or unplanned ending or termination of the formal or contracted relationship with the client. Closure ideally involves a dialogue and may evolve over a number of sessions.

**coaching agenda**—Specific topics that clients bring to the coaching relationship. The client's coaching agenda forms the basis of the contractual agreement between coach and client.

**coaching approach**—Use of coaching skills and competencies in everyday interactions as contrasted with skill and methods of coaching applied in a formal contractual relationship between coach and client.

**coaching presence**—A coaching skill and manner of being that is represented by the coach's full availability to the client—in mind, body, and spirit—without attachment to the coach's own agenda.

**competency development model**—A coaching model that suggests a holistic approach whereby the multiple lenses of the client's strengths, lifestyle, habits, personality, thought patterns, feelings, and relationships are explored in relation to the client's agenda and goal pursuit.

**confrontation**—Coaching skill whereby the coach presents to the client evidence of his discrepant or inconsistent thoughts, feelings, or actions for consideration in service of the client's developmental goals.

**congruence**—Alignment between a person's values, beliefs, motivations, verbal and nonverbal messages, and actions.

**constructivist theory of knowing, or constructivism**—Knowledge generated by the learner's meaning-making process through her interactions with the world rather than by virtue of scientifically determined forms of objective data.

**containment**—The coach's ability to create psychological safety for the client as she expresses difficult personal issues or even intense emotions toward the coach.

**core coaching competencies**—Set of 11 coaching skills and approaches logically divided into four clusters as described by the International Coach Federation (ICF).

**core relationship conditions**—Qualities, often including trustworthiness, expertise, genuineness, and empathy, that coaches need to demonstrate in their relationship to clients so that clients can effectively engage the process of coaching.

**counterdependent**—A client behavior pattern indicating resistance to influence or direction from the coach or any other perceived authority related to the coaching agenda.

**countertransference**—Projection onto the client by the coach of feelings, attitudes, or behaviors originating in the coach's relationship with another significant individual in the coach's personal history. Also described as an unreal aspect of the relationship.

**decisional balance**—List of pros and cons for performing a desired behavior. The likelihood of adopting a new health-related behavior increases when the pros outweigh the cons.

**direct input**—Advice, suggestion, information, and instruction that a coach offers to clients in service of their goal attainment.

**emotional intelligence**—In contrast to the classic notion of IQ, this term encompasses a person's wisdom in emotional contexts related to self and others.

**empathy**—Ability to be aware of other people's feelings in a manner that mirrors the interior experience of the other without taking on the other's personal psychology or worldview regarding the issue at hand. Empathy differs from sympathy in that the former is akin to feeling with the other, whereas the latter is more about feeling for the other.

**espoused theories of action**—What people believe or say they do in certain situations as distinguished from what they actually do. Espoused theories may or may not be congruent with actual behaviors.

**ethics**—Moral principles adopted by an individual or a group to provide rules for conduct.

**experiential learning**—A concept most often associated with David A. Kolb, who proposed that learning from experience entails a cycle of experimenting, reflecting on our experience, reframing our theories of action, and finally applying our new learning or doing.

**extrinsic motivation**—A type of motivation occurring in situations where people pursue action in order to achieve some valued outcome or result (e.g., a prize, weight loss) rather than for the experience of the activity itself.

**feedback**—A coaching skill whereby the coach sensitively presents clients with information, observations, or results of their behaviors to support their development and reinforce effective patterns.

**flow model of coaching**—A model highlighting two phases within the coaching process: (1) engagement, which entails working with clients to create insight, identify patterns, and explore resources, and (2) goal pursuit, which includes a focus on action planning, committing to proceed, and staying the course until the goal is achieved.

**focusing**—A coaching skill whereby the coach directs the client's attention toward a specific theme, behavioral or communication pattern, or

experience. Might also apply to biases for types of information that a coach chooses to pay attention to.

**health**—Physical, mental, psychological, social, spiritual, environmental, and occupational well-being.

**holding environment**—Term borrowed from counseling and psychotherapy referring to the safety and trustworthiness of the relationship created by the coach for the client.

**identification**—A process whereby coaches experience clients' reality in such a manner that they take on the clients' issues as if they were their own.

**immediacy**—Combining such processes as confrontation and self-disclosure, this coaching skill focuses on the expression of what is happening precisely in the current moment of the coaching experience with the client, within the coach, or in their relationship.

**indirect question**—A coaching skill whereby the coach requests information from the client in a declarative sentence that implies to the client that certain information is needed in the dialogue (e.g., "I wonder what that might do for you").

**information**—Specific knowledge directly communicated by a coach in service of a client's goal attainment. May arise from the coach's area of expertise.

**instruction**—Specific directive communicated by a coach to a client with the purpose of helping the person acquire a technique, perform an activity, or engage in a behavior. Arises from the coach's knowledge or area of expertise.

**International Coach Federation (ICF)**—A not-for-profit organization formed in 1995 by individual coaches with a mission to advance the coaching profession worldwide. The ICF seeks to set high professional standards, provide independent certification, and build a network of credentialed coaches. More information can be found at www.coachfederation.org.

**interpretation**—A coaching skill whereby the coach provides new perspectives or ways in which the client can understand issues through a variety of techniques, including identifying unstated feelings, reframing issues, expressing ideas metaphorically, and storytelling.

**intervention**—In the context of coaches' engagements with clients, refers to any intentional action to address issues and influence client behavior in a desired direction.

**intrinsic motivation**—Motivation seen in situations where people pursue action for pleasure, learning, mastery, or aesthetic enjoyment. Motivation of this nature is associated with the activity itself rather than with outcomes derived from the activity.

**Johari window**—Model designed by Joseph Luft and Harry Ingham to demonstrate the relationships among self-disclosure, feedback, and self-awareness pertaining to a person's self-knowledge.

**kinesics**—The formal study of body motions, including all forms of nonverbal communication.

**learning style**—Personal preference for specific ways to process information and acquire knowledge.

**learning-through-change (LTC) model**—Model created by Marilyn Taylor suggesting that people involved in a change process will experience a cycle of learning where certain agendas must be addressed at certain times in order to successfully cope with and adapt to disconfirming events in life.

**leisure society**—Concept from the 20th century predicting a society where working hours would be reduced and free time would be more abundant, thus allowing a greater focus on leisure.

**lifestyle wellness coaching**—Coaching specialization, or niche, in areas related to health, wellness, and fitness.

**mindfulness**—Focused and nonjudgmental attention to the present moment.

**minimal encouragers**—An aspect of coaching communication whereby coaches acknowledge clients' verbalizations or behaviors with brief references or audible expressions such as "Mm-hmm" in order to reinforce client expression and openness.

**morality**—Determination of what is right or wrong on the basis of some broader cultural context or religious standard.

**morbid obesity**—Body mass index (BMI) of >35. BMI is a weight-to-height ratio calculated as weight (kg) / height (m)$^2$.

**motivation**—Factors, both intrinsic and extrinsic, that propel people to engage in goal pursuit.

**neurolinguistic programming (NLP)**—A multidisciplinary and eclectic methodology for understanding human behavior and interpersonal communications serving the purpose of identifying individual patterns in order to promote specific behavioral changes.

**obesity**—Excess weight in relation to a person's height or body weight beyond the socially accepted norms of attractiveness within a given group.

**open question**—A type of question in which the coach invites the client to expand on a theme or subject so that salient issues can be explored in depth.

**outcome goals**—Goals that typically focus on the result or end result of some activity such as physical training or specified nutrition regimens. Outcome goals may include weight loss or winning a contest.

**paradigm shift**—Refers to instances in which a significant and wholly new perspective arises in an area of knowledge, skill, or understanding and brings about questioning or reevaluation of old models or approaches.

**paralinguistics**—The study of nonverbal aspects of speech, including tone, volume, speed, and pauses.

**performance goals**—Goals of behavior or performance that are independent of others' actions. Examples include learning how to swim or running a distance in a specified time.

**personality**—The total of all the characteristics that make each person unique. Personality represents the habitual ways in which people behave, especially in relationships with other people. Personality also shows itself in a person's typical emotional responses to life events and circumstances.

**postmodern approaches**—Approaches to helping that include, among others, social constructionism, solution-focused brief therapy, and narrative therapy.

**process goals**—Goals that emphasize the qualities that one wishes to experience in carrying out certain behaviors or actions, such as enjoyment or pleasure.

**proxemics**—The study of physical distances of individuals in social settings and their effects on these individuals.

**psychological contract**—Set of assumptions about working together that coaches and clients independently bring to the relationship without verification from one another.

**psychosocial**—A characteristic of thoughts, feelings, or actions that represents both psychological and social dimensions. Psychosocial behaviors, for example, are thought to reflect intrapsychic or internal processes along with social ones.

**reflection of content**—A coaching skill involving the coach's sensitive mirroring of information provided in a client's communication to the coach; often referred to as *paraphrase*.

**reflection of feeling**—A coaching skill involving the coach's sensitive mirroring of the emotional or feeling elements of a client's communications to the coach.

**reflection of meaning**—A coaching skill that relies on such skills as questioning, reflection of content, and reflection of feeling to help the client uncover a deeper appreciation and awareness of issues.

**reflective practice**—Popularized by Donald Schön in the early 1980s, this term refers to one's ability and commitment to reflect on one's professional actions in order to engage in a continuous learning process.

**reframe**—A form of the coaching skill of interpretation whereby the coach reorganizes the client's messages and communicates them back in a way that offers more options and potential for change.

**regular physical activity**—Completing at least 150 minutes of moderate to vigorous physical activity each week.

**relapse**—Behavioral incidents in which a person reverts to a previous pattern of action that he had deliberately altered, usually in the pursuit of some health or wellness goal. For instance, relapse would be seen in a person smoking a cigarette after having stopped for a number of months.

**relapse prevention**—Strategies for identifying high-risk situations and preventing a return to behavior previously abandoned in the pursuit of some health and wellness goal.

**self-awareness**—Clear perception of the self, including one's personality traits; cognitive, emotional, and behavioral patterns; motivations; values; and beliefs.

**self-disclosure**—A coaching skill whereby the coach strategically reveals personal information or tells personal stories to support the client's progress and goal attainment.

**self-efficacy**—Most often associated with the psychologist Albert Bandura, this concept refers to confidence in one's abilities to engage in goal pursuit and achieve a desired objective regardless of obstacles that might stand in the way.

**self-fulfilling prophecy**—Based on a theory suggesting that when people expect themselves to behave in certain ways, typically reinforced by the feedback and opinions of others, their behavior conforms to these expectations—for better or worse.

**self-limiting beliefs**—Negative thought patterns that hold us back from pursuing desired goals. Example of self-limiting beliefs would be "I'm too old," "I'm not smart enough," "I'm not disciplined enough," or "I'm too fat."

**self-regulation**—The ability to control one's thoughts, emotions, urges, and actions in order to reach a desired goal.

**social support**—All those in clients' networks, including the coach, who can help them achieve their desired goal.

**summarizing**—A coaching skill whereby the coach mirrors back to the client key elements of a lengthy segment of communication or similar themes in client communication across a series of sessions.

**SuPeRSMART goals**—Goals that are **s**elf-controllable (under one's control), are **p**ublic to self and others, have a **r**eward attached to their achievement, and are **s**pecific, **m**easurable, **a**djustable, **r**ealistic, and **t**ime-specific.

**theory in use**—What people actually do in situations, as distinguished from what they believe or say they do.

**theory of action**—Set of values, beliefs, attitudes, norms, and so on that inform the way people plan to act and actually behave.

**transference**—Projection onto the coach by the client of feelings, attitudes, or behaviors originating in the client's relationship with other significant people in the client's history. Also described as an unreal aspect of the relationship.

**transformative learning**—Theory of education suggesting that adult learners play an active role in a learning process that ultimately alters their worldviews and belief systems.

**transtheoretical model (TTM)**—Model of individual behavior change composed of six phases: precontemplation, contemplation, preparation, action, maintenance, and termination.

**values**—Beliefs and attitudes that provide direction to everyday life.

**wellness**—Optimal state of health in seven dimensions: physical, social, emotional, mental, spiritual, occupational, and environmental.

**working alliance**—A phrase popular in counseling and psychotherapy referring to the agreement and collaboration of coach and client in engaging in necessary tasks and patterns of relationship toward the attainment of desired outcomes.

**worldview**—One's personal perspective incorporating beliefs about why things are the way they are, why people function as they do, how situations evolve, and what matters in life.

# REFERENCES

Abend, S.M. (1995). Discussion of Jay Greenberg's paper on self-disclosure. *Contemporary Psychoanalysis, 31,* 207-211.

Abernethy, B. (2001). Attention. In R. Singer, H. Hausenblas, & C. Janelle (Eds.), *Handbook of sport psychology* (2nd ed., pp. 53-85). New York: Wiley.

Ackerman, S.J., & Hilsenroth, M.J. (2003). A review of therapist characteristics and techniques positively impacting the therapeutic alliance. *Clinical Psychology Review, 23,* 1-33.

Adler, A. (1927). *Understanding human nature.* New York: Greenberg.

Adler, G., & Myerson, P.G. (Eds.). (1991). *Confrontation in psychotherapy.* Northvale, NJ: Aronson.

Adler, R.B., Rosenfeld, L.B., & Proctor, R.F., II. (2004). *Interplay: The process of interpersonal communication* (9th ed.). New York: Oxford University Press.

Ajzen. I., & Fishbein, M. (1980). *Understanding attitudes and predicting social behavior.* Englewood Cliffs, NJ: Prentice-Hall.

Ajzen, I., & Fishbein, M. (2004). Questions raised by a reasoned action approach: Comment on Ogden (2003). *Health Psychology, 23*(4), 431-434.

Allison, D.B., Fontaine, K.R., Manson, J.E., Stevens, J., & VanItallie, T.B. (1999). Annual deaths attributable to obesity in the United States. *Journal of the American Medical Association, 282*(16), 1530-1538.

Allison, M.J., & Keller, C. (2004). Self-efficacy intervention effect on physical activity in older adults. *Western Journal of Nursing Research, 26*(1), 31-46.

American Diabetes Association. (2011). *Data from the 2011 national diabetes fact sheet.* Retrieved from www.diabetes.org/diabetes-basics/diabetes-statistics/

American Psychiatric Association (APA). (2013). *Diagnostic and statistical manual of mental disorders* (5th ed.). Washington, DC: Author.

American Psychological Association (APA). (2012). Our health at risk. Retrieved from www.apa.org/news/press/releases/stress/2011/health-risk.aspx

Anderson, R., & Killenberg, G.M. (2009). *Interviewing: Speaking, listening, and learning for professional life* (2nd ed.). New York: Oxford University Press.

Andreas, S., & Faulkner, C. (Eds.). (1996). *NLP: The new technology of achievement: NLP comprehensive training team.* London: Brealey.

Argyris, C. (1970). *Intervention theory and method: A behavioral science view.* Reading, MA: Addison-Wesley.

Argyris, C., & Schön, D.A. (1974). *Theory in practice.* San Francisco: Jossey-Bass.

Armstrong, T. (2003). *You're smarter than you think: A kid's guide to multiple intelligences.* Minneapolis: Free Spirit.

Assagioli, R. (1965). *Psychosynthesis: A manual of principles and techniques.* New York: Hobbs, Dorman.

Auerbach, J.E. (2003). *Personal and executive coaching: The complete guide for mental health professionals.* Ventura, CA: Executive College Press.

Bachkirova, T., Cox, E., & Clutterbuck, D. (Eds.). (2010). *The complete handbook of coaching.* Los Angeles: Sage.

Baker Miller, J. (1991). The development of women's sense of self. In J. Jodan, A. Kaplan, J. Miller, I. Stiver, & J. Surrey (Eds.), *Women's growth in connection: Writings from the Stone Center* (pp. 11-34). New York: Guilford Press.

Baker Miller, J., & Stiver, I. (Eds.). (1997). *The healing connection: How women form relationships in therapy and in life.* Boston: Beacon Press.

Bandura, A. (1977). *Social learning theory.* Upper Saddle River, NJ: Prentice-Hall.

Bandura, A. (1986). *Social foundations of thought and action: A social cognitive theory.* Upper Saddle River, NJ: Prentice-Hall.

Bandura, A. (1992). Exercise of personal agency through the self-efficacy mechanism. In R. Schwarzer (Ed.), *Self-efficacy: Thought control of action* (pp. 3-38). Washington, DC: Hemisphere.

Bandura, A. (1995). *Self-efficacy in changing societies.* New York: Cambridge University Press.

Bandura, A. (1997a). Self-efficacy. *Harvard Mental Health Newsletter, 13*(9), 4-7.

Bandura, A. (1997b). *Self-efficacy: The exercise of control.* New York: W.H. Freeman/Times Books/ Henry Holt.

Bandura, A. (1998). Personal and collective efficacy in human adaptation and change. In J.G. Adair, D. Belanger, & K.L. Dion (Eds.), *Advances in psychological science: Personal, social and cultural aspects* (Vol. 1, pp. 51-71). Hove, UK: Psychology Press.

Bandura, A. (2000). Cultivate self-efficacy for personal and organizational effectiveness. In E.A. Locke (Ed.), *Handbook of principles of organization behavior* (pp. 120-136). Oxford, UK: Blackwell.

Bateson, G. (1979). *Mind and nature: A necessary unity.* New York: Dutton.

Baumeister, R.F., Heatherton, T.F., & Tice, D.M. (1994). *Losing control: How and why people fail at self-regulation.* San Diego, CA: Academic Press.

Beauchamp, T.L., & Childress, J.F. (2009). *Principles of biomedical ethics* (6th ed.). New York: Oxford University Press.

Beck, D.E., & Cowan, C. (1996). *Spiral dynamics: Mastering values, leadership, and change.* Malden, MA: Blackwell.

Bennis, W.G., & Shepard, H.A. (1956). A theory of group development. *Human Relations, 9,* 415-437.

Binswanger, L. (1963). *Being-in-the-world: Selected papers of Ludwig Binswanger.* New York: Basic Books.

Birdwhistell, R.L. (1970). *Kinetics and context: Essays on body motion communication.* Philadelphia: University of Pennsylvania Press.

Biswas-Diener, R. (2009). Personal coaching as a positive intervention. *Journal of Clinical Psychology: In Session, 65*(5), 544-553.

Bitter, J., & Byrd, R. (2011). Human conversations: Self-disclosure and storytelling in Adlerian Family Therapy. *Journal of Individual Psychology, 67*(3), 305-323.

Bize, R., Johnson, J.A., & Plotnikoff, R.C. (2007). Physical activity level and health-related quality of life in the general adult population: A systematic review. *Preventive Medicine, 45*(6), 401-415. doi:10.1016/j.ypmed.2007.07.017

Bloomgarden, A., & Mennuti, R.B. (Eds.). (2009). *Psychotherapist revealed: Therapists speak about self-disclosure in psychotherapy.* New York: Routledge.

Bordin, E.S. (1979). The generalizability of the psychoanalytic concept of the working alliance. *Psychotherapy: Theory, Research & Practice, 16*(3), 252-260.

Brammer, L.M., & MacDonald, G. (2003). *The helping relationship: Process and skills* (8th ed.). Boston: Allyn & Bacon.

Brems, C. (2001). *Basic skills in psychotherapy and counseling.* Belmont, CA: Brooks/Cole.

Brew, L., & Kottler, J.A. (2008). *Applied helping skills: Transforming lives.* Thousand Oaks, CA: Sage.

Bridges, W. (2001). *The way of transition: Embracing life's most difficult moments.* Cambridge, MA: Perseus.

Brinthaupt, T.M., Kang, M., & Anshel, M.H. (2010). A delivery model for overcoming psycho-behavioral barriers to exercise. *Psychology of Sport and Exercise, 11,* 259-266.

Brock, V.G. (2008). *Grounded theory of the roots and emergence of coaching.* Retrieved from http://libraryofprofessionalcoaching.com/wp-content/uploads/2011/10/dissertation.pdf

Brown, D., & Srebalus, D.J. (2003). *Introduction to the counseling profession* (3rd ed.). Boston: Allyn & Bacon.

Brown, L.S. (2007). Empathy, genuineness—and the dynamics of power: A feminist responds to Rogers. *Psychotherapy: Theory, Research, Practice, Training, 44*(3), 257-259.

Brownell, K.D. (1991). Dieting and the search for the perfect body: Where physiology and culture collide. *Behavior Therapy, 22*(1), 1-12.

Bruhn, J.G., & Levine, H.G., & Levine, P L. (1993). *Managing boundaries in the health professions.* Springfield, IL: C.C. Thomas.

Buckworth, J., & Dishman, R.K. (2002). *Exercise psychology.* Champaign, IL: Human Kinetics.

Bugental, J.F.T. (1965). *The search for authenticity.* New York: Holt, Rinehart & Winston.

Bureau of Labor Statistics. (2008). *Spotlight on statistics: Sports and exercise.* Retrieved from www.bls.gov/spotlight/2008/sports/

Burgess, A. (1962). *A clockwork orange.* London: Heinemann.

Cabana, S., Emery, F., & Emery, M., (1995). The search for effective strategic planning is over. *Journal for Quality and Participation, 18*(4), 10-19.

Capra, F. (1997). *The web of life: A new scientific understanding of living systems.* New York: Anchor Books.

Capuzzi, D., & Gross, D.R. (Eds.). (2009). *Introduction to the counseling profession* (5th ed.). Columbus, OH: Pearson/Merrill.

Carkhuff, R.R. (1969). *Helping & human relations: Vol I & II.* New York: Holt, Rinehart & Winston.

Carkhuff, R.R., & Berenson, B.G. (1977). *Beyond counseling and therapy.* New York: Holt, Rinehart & Winston.

Carron, A.V., Hausenblas, H.A., & Estabrooks, P.A. (2003). *The psychology of physical activity.* New York: McGraw-Hill.

Carver, C.S., & Scheier, M.F. (2010). Self-regulation of action and affect. In R.F. Baumeister & K.D. Vohs (Eds.), *Handbook of self-regulation: Research, theory and applications* (2nd ed., pp. 3-21). New York: Guilford.

Cashdan, S. (1988). *Object relations therapy: Using the relationship.* New York: Norton.

Centers for Disease Control and Prevention (CDC). (2009a). *Mortality: Multiple cause files* [Data file]. Retrieved from www.cdc.gov/nchs/data_access/Vitalstatsonline.htm#Mortality_Multiple

Centers for Disease Control and Prevention (CDC). (2009b). *Prevalence of overweight, obesity and extreme obesity among adults: United States, trends 1960-62 through 2005-2006.* Retrieved from www.cdc.gov/nchs/data/hestat/overweight/overweight_adult.htm

Centers for Disease Control and Prevention (CDC). (2009c). *Prevalence and trends data: Nationwide (States, DC, and Territories) 2009 physical activity.* Retrieved from http://apps.nccd.cdc.gov/BRFSS/display.asp?cat=PA&yr=2009&qkey=4418&state=US

Centers for Disease Control and Prevention (CDC). (2011a). *Facts about county-level estimates of leisure-time physical inactivity, 2008.* Retrieved from www.cdc.gov/diabetes/pubs/factsheets/county_inactivity_estimates.htm

Centers for Disease Control and Prevention (CDC). (2011b). *Obesity: Halting the epidemic by making health easier.* Retrieved from www.cdc.gov/chronicdisease/resources/publications/AAG/obesity.htm

Centers for Disease Control and Prevention (CDC). (2012a). *Childhood overweight and obesity.* Retrieved from www.cdc.gov/obesity/childhood

Centers for Disease Control and Prevention (CDC). (2012b). *Life expectancy.* Retrieved from www.cdc.gov/nchs/fastats/lifexpec.htm

Chang, V., Scott, S., & Decker, C. (2009). *Developing helping skills: A step-by-step approach.* Belmont, CA: Brooks/Cole.

Clark, D.M. (1995). Cognitive therapy in the treatment of anxiety disorders. *Clinical Neuropharmacology, 18,* 27-37.

Coach U. (2005). *The coach: Personal and corporate coaching training handbook.* Hoboken, NJ: Wiley.

Cohn, J.F., & Ekman, P. (2008). Measuring facial action. In J.A. Harrigan, R. Rosenthal, & K.R. Scherer (Eds.), *The new handbook of methods in nonverbal behavior research* (pp. 9-64). Oxford, UK: Oxford University Press.

Compton, B.R., Galaway, B., & Cournoyer, B. (2005). *Social work processes* (7th ed.). Pacific Grove, CA: Brooks/Cole.

Connor, M., & Norman, P. (2005). *Predicting health behavior: Search and practice with social cognition models* (2nd ed.). Maidenhead, Berkshire: Open University Press.

Cook-Greuter, S.R. (2000). Mature ego development: A gateway to ego transcendence? *Journal of Adult Development, 7,* 227-240. doi:10.1023/A:1009511411421.

Cook-Greuter, S.R. (2006a). Ego development: Nine levels of increasing embrace. Retrieved from www.stillpointintegral.com/docs/cookgreuter.pdf

Cook-Greuter, S.R. (2006b). 20th century background for integral psychology. *AQAL: Journal of Integral Theory and Practice, 1*(2), 144-184.

Cooper, C. (1998). *Fat and proud: The politics of size.* London: Women's Press Ltd.

Corey, G., Corey, M.S., & Callanan, P. (2011). *Issues and ethics in the helping professions* (8th ed.). Belmont, CA: Brooks/Cole.

Cormier, S., Nurius, P.S., & Osborn, C.J. (2009). *Interviewing and change strategies for helpers: Fundamental skills and cognitive behavioral interventions* (6th ed.). Pacific Grove, CA: Brooks/Cole.

Crespo, C.J., & Arbesman, J. (2003). Obesity in the United States. *Physician & Sportsmedicine, 31*(11), 23-28.

Crits-Christoph, P., Connolly Gibbons, M.B., & Hearon, B. (2006). Does the alliance cause good outcome? Recommendations for future research on the alliance. *Psychotherapy: Theory, Research, Practice, Training, 43*(3), 280-285.

Csikszentmihalyi, M. (2008). *Flow: The psychology of optimal experience.* New York: Harper Perennial Classics.

Culos-Reed, S.N., Brawley, L.R., Martin, K.A., & Leary, M.R. (2002). Self-presentation concerns and health behaviors among cosmetic surgery patients. *Journal of Applied Social Psychology, 32,* 560-569.

Cyr, A.V. (1999). *Overview of theories and principles relating to characteristics of adult learners: 1970s-1999.* Columbus, OH: ERIC Clearinghouse on Adult, Career, and Vocational Education.

Dallow, C.B., & Anderson, J. (2003). Using self-efficacy and a transtheoretical model to develop a physical activity intervention for obese women. *American Journal of Health Promotion, 17*(6), 373-381.

Davis, J. (2003). An overview of transpersonal psychology. *Humanistic Psychologist, 31*(2-3), 6-21. doi: 10.1080/08873267.2003.9986924

De Jong, P., & Berg, I K. (2008). *Interviewing for solutions* (3rd ed.). Belmont, CA: Thomson Higher Education.

De Shazer, S. (1988). *Clues: Investigating solutions in brief therapy.* New York: Norton.

DeForest, H., Largent, P., & Steinberg, M. (2005) *Mastering the art of feedback: Tips, tools and intelligence for trainers.* Alexandria, VA: ASTD Press.

Devaris, J. (1994). The dynamics of power in psychotherapy. *Psychotherapy, 31,* 588-593.

Dewey, J. (1916). *Democracy and education: An introduction to the philosophy of education.* New York: Macmillan.

Dilts, R., & DeLozier, J. (2000). *Encyclopedia of systemic NLP and NLP new coding.* Capitola, CA: Meta.

Dimeff, L., & Marlatt, G. (1998). Preventing relapse and maintaining change in addictive behaviors. *Clinical Psychology: Science and Practice, 5,* 513-525.

Divine, L. (2009). Looking at and looking as the client: The quadrants as a type structure lens. *Journal of Integral Theory and Practice, 4*(1), 21-40.

Donaldson, S.J., & Ronan, K.R. (2006). The effects of sports participation on young adolescents' emotional well-being. *Adolescence, 41*(162), 369-389.

Donatelle, R., & Thompson, A. (2011). *Health: The basics* (5th ed.). Toronto: Pearson Education Canada.

Donnelly, J.E., Blair, S.N., Jakicic, J.M., Manore, M.M., Rankin, J.W., & Smith, B.K. (2009). Appropriate physical activity intervention strategies for weight loss and prevention of weight regain for adults. *Medicine & Science in Sports & Exercise, 41*(2), 459-471.

Dychtwald, K. (1977). *Bodymind.* New York: Pantheon.

Egan, G. (2010). *The skilled helper: A problem-management and opportunity-development approach to helping* (9th ed.). Belmont, CA: Brooks Cole.

Ekman, P. (1993). Facial expression and emotion. *American Psychologist, 48,* 384-392.

Ekman, P. (2003). *Emotions revealed: Recognizing faces and feelings to improve communication and emotional life.* New York: Holt, Rinehart & Winston.

Ellison, L. (2001). *The personal intelligences.* Thousand Oaks, CA: Corwin.

Engel, G.L. (1977). The need for a new medical model: A challenge for biomedicine. *Science, 196,* 129-136.

Erikson, E.H. (1959). *Identity and the life cycle.* New York: International Universities Press.

Erikson, E.H. (1963). *Childhood and society* (2nd ed.). New York: Norton.

Erikson, E.H. (1968). *Identity, youth and crisis.* New York: Norton.

Etter, J.F., Bergman, M.M., & Perneger, T.V. (2000). On quitting smoking: Development of two scales measuring the use of self-change strategies in current and former smokers (scs-cs and scs-fs). *Addictive Behaviors, 25*(4), 523-538.

Evans, D.R., Hearn, M.T., Uhlemann, M.R., & Ivey, A.E. (2010). *Essential interviewing: A programmed approach to effective communication* (8th ed.). Belmont, CA: Brooks/Cole.

Farrell, P.A. (2001). Hear this: Sharpening your communication and listening skills. In S. Cullari (Ed.), *Counseling and psychotherapy: A practical guidebook for students, trainees, and new professionals* (pp. 59-91). Boston: Allyn & Bacon.

Fast, J. (2002). *Body language* (rev. ed.). New York: Evans.

Field, A.E., Barnoya, J., & Colditz, G.A. (2002). Epidemiology and health and economic consequences of obesity. In T.A. Wadden, & A.J. Stunkard (Eds.), *Handbook of obesity treatment* (pp. 3-18). New York/London: Guilford Press.

Fishbein, M., & Ajzen, I. (2005). Theory-based behavior change interventions: Comments on

Hobbis and Sutton. *Journal of Health Psychology,* 10(1), 27-31.

Fisher, C. (2012). *Decoding the ethics code: A practical guide for psychologists* (3rd ed.). Thousand Oaks, CA: Sage.

Fitzpatrick, K.K., Moye, A., Hoste, R., Lock, J., & Le Grang, D. (2010). Adolescent-focused psychotherapy for adolescents with anorexia nervosa. *Journal of Contemporary Psychology, 40,* 31-39.

Flaherty, J. (2010). *Coaching: Evoking excellence in others* (3rd ed.). Boston: Elsevier Butterworth-Heinemann.

Fradkov, A.L. (2007). *Cybernetical physics: From control of chaos to quantum control.* Berlin: Springer-Verlag.

Frank, J.D., & Frank, J.B. (1993). *Persuasion and healing: A comparative study of psychotherapy* (3rd ed.). Baltimore: Johns Hopkins University Press.

Frankl, V. (1969). *The will to meaning: Foundations and applications of logotherapy.* New York: New American Library.

Freire, P. (1970). *Pedagogy of the oppressed.* New York: Herder and Herder.

Freud, S. (1949). *An outline of psycho-analysis.* J. Strachey (Ed.). London: Hogarth Press.

Freud, S. (1953). The interpretation of dreams. In J. Strachey (Ed.), *The standard edition of the complete psychological works of Sigmund Freud* (Vols. 4 & 5). London: Hogarth. (Original work published 1900.)

Freud, S. (1964). *The standard edition of the complete psychological works of Sigmund Freud, Volume 23.* J. Strachey, F. Freud, & C.L. Rothgeb (Eds.). London: Hogarth Press.

Friedman, H.S., & Martin, L.R. (2011). *The longevity project: Surprising discoveries for health and long life from the landmark eight-decade study.* Carlton North, VIC: Scribe.

Fromm, E. (1962). *The art of loving.* London: Unwin Books.

Frost, L. (2009). Integral perspectives on coaching: An analysis of Integral Coaching Canada across eight zones and five methodologies. *Journal of Integral Theory and Practice, 4*(1), 93-120.

Gabbard, G.O. (1995). Countertransference: The emerging common ground. *International Journal of Psychoanalysis, 76,* 475-485.

Gardner, H. (1983). *Frames of mind: The theory of multiple intelligences.* New York: Basic Books.

Gardner, H. (2006). *Multiple intelligences: New horizons.* New York: Basic Books.

Gavin, J. (1992). *The exercise habit.* Champaign, IL: Human Kinetics.

Gazda, G.M., Asbury, F.S., Balzer, F., Childers, W.C., Phelps, R.E., & Walters, R.P. (1999). *Human relations development: A manual for educators* (6th ed.). Needham, MA: Allyn & Bacon.

Geldard, K., & Geldard, D. (2008). *Counselling children: A practical introduction* (3rd ed.). Los Angeles: Sage.

Gelso, C.J., & Fretz, B.R. (2001). *Counseling psychology* (2nd ed.). Belmont, CA: Thomson/Wadsworth.

Gelso, C.J., & Hayes, J.A. (2007). *Countertransference and the therapist's inner experience: Perils and possibilities.* Mahwah, NJ: Erlbaum.

Gendlin, E. (1981). *Focusing.* New York: Bantam Books.

Gibson, R.L., & Mitchell, M. (2008). *Introduction to counseling and guidance* (7th ed.). Upper Saddle River, NJ: Pearson/Merrill/Prentice Hall.

Gielen, U.P., Draguns, J G., & Fish, J.M. (Eds.). (2008). *Principles of multicultural counseling and therapy.* New York: Routledge.

Gladding, S.T. (2009). *Counseling: A comprehensive profession* (6th ed.). Upper Saddle River, NJ: Pearson.

Goldman, C. (2001). *Healing words for the body, mind and spirit: 101 words to inspire and affirm.* New York: Marlowe.

Goleman, D. (1995). *Emotional intelligence.* New York: Bantam Books.

Goleman, D. (2006). *Social intelligence: The new science of human relationships.* New York: Bantam.

Gollwitzer, P.M. (1999). Implementation intentions: Strong effects of simple plans. *American Psychologist, 54*(7), 493-503.

Gollwitzer, P.M., & Brandstätter, V. (1997). Implementation intentions and effective goal pursuit. *Journal of Personality and Social Psychology, 73,* 186-199

Grant, A.M. (2003). *Towards a psychology of coaching: The impact of coaching on metacognition, mental health and goal attainment.* Retrieved from www.eric.ed.gov/PDFS/ED478147.pdf.

Grant, A.M. (2006). An integrative goal-focused approach to executive coaching. In D.R. Stober & A.M. Grant (Eds.), *Evidence-based coaching* handbook: Putting best practices to work for your client (pp. 153-192). Hoboken, NJ: Wiley.

Grant, A.M. (2007). Past, present and future: The evolution of professional coaching and coaching psychology. In S. Palmer & A. Whybrow (Eds.), Handbook of coaching psychology: A guide for practitioners (pp. 23-39). London/New York: Routledge.

Green, E.C. (2003). Re-thinking AIDS prevention: Learning from successes in developing countries. Westport, CT: Praeger.

Grinder, J., & Bandler, J. (1976). The structure of magic: I & II. Oxford, UK: Science & Behavior.

Grof, S. (1988). The adventure of self-discovery: Dimensions of consciousness and new perspectives in psychotherapy. Albany, NY: State University of New York Press.

Groth-Marnat, G. (2009). Handbook of psychological assessment (5th ed.). Hoboken, NJ: John Wiley & Sons, Inc.

Gümüş, S., Öz, A., & Kırımoğlu, H. (2011). Sports and physical activity as a preventative social support approach to loneliness and hopelessness of adolescents. International Journal of Human Sciences, 8(2), 1-14.

Hackney, H.L. (2000). Practice issues for the beginning counsellor. Boston: Allyn & Bacon.

Hackney, H.L., & Cormier, LS. (2009). The professional counselor: A process guide to helping (6th ed.). Upper Saddle River, NJ: Pearson.

Hall, E.T. (1966). The hidden dimension. Garden City, NY: Doubleday.

Hall, E.T. (1976). Beyond culture. New York: Anchor Press.

Hall, E., & Hall, C. (1988). Human relations in education. New York: Routledge.

Hanh, T.N. (2007). The art of power. New York: HarperOne.

Hargrove, R. (2008). Masterful coaching (3rd ed.). San Francisco: Jossey-Bass.

Haslam, D. (2005). Gender-specific aspects of obesity. Journal of Men's Health & Gender, 2(2), 179-185.

Hayes, S.C. (2009). Acceptance and commitment therapy (ACT). Retrieved from http://contextualpsychology.org/act/

Hayes, S.C., Strosahl, K.D., & Wilson, K.G. (2011). Acceptance and commitment therapy (2nd ed.). New York: Guilford Press.

Health Canada. (2009). Canadian Alcohol and Drug Use Monitoring Survey: Alcohol. Retrieved from www.hc-sc.gc.ca/hc-ps/drugs-drogues/stat/_2009/summary-sommaire-eng.php#alc

Health Canada. (2010). Canadian Alcohol and Drug Use Monitoring Survey: Other illicit drug use. Retrieved from www.hc-sc.gc.ca/hc-ps/drugs-drogues/stat/_2010/summary-sommaire-eng.php#cannabis

Health Canada. (2011). Major findings from the Canadian Alcohol and Drug Use Monitoring Survey (CADUMS) 2011. Retrieved from www.hc-sc.gc.ca/hc-ps/drugs-drogues/stat/index-eng.php

Heart and Stroke Foundation. (2011). Denial putting Canadians at high risk of cutting their lives short: 2011 report. Retrieved from www.heartandstroke.com/site/c.ikIQLcMWJtE/b.6520045/k.BB7E/2011_Report__Denial_cutting_lives_short.htm

Heart and Stroke Foundation. (2012). Targeting obesity. Retrieved from www.heartandstroke.com/site/c.ikIQLcMWJtE/b.3479249/k.A5C3/Targeting_obesity.htm?gclid=CKrtxe3VtakCFUPf4AodPkb9MA

Helms, J., & Cook, D. (1999). Using race and culture in counseling and psychotherapy. Needham Heights, MA: Allyn & Bacon.

Henderson, K.A., & Ainsworth, B.E. (2002). Enjoyment: A link to physical activity, leisure, and health. Journal of Park & Recreation Administration, 20(4), 130-146.

Hendrix, H. (2008). Getting the love you want: A guide for couples (20th anniversary rev. ed.). New York: H. Holt.

Hepworth, D.H., Rooney, R.H., Rooney, G. D., Strom-Gottfried, K., & Larsen, J. (2010). Direct social work practice: Theory and skills (8th ed.). Belmont, CA: Brooks/Cole.

Herlihy, B., & Corey, G. (2006). Boundary issues in counseling: Multiple roles and responsibilities (2nd ed.). Alexandria, VA: American Counseling Association.

Hill, C.E., & Knox, S. (2002). Self-disclosure. In J.C. Norcross (Ed.), Psychotherapy relationships that work (pp. 255-265). New York: Oxford.

Hill, C.E., & O'Brien, K.M. (2003). Helping skills: Facilitating exploration, insight, and action. Washington, DC: APA Books.

Hill, G., & Hannon, J.C. (2008). An analysis of middle school students' physical education physical activity preferences. *Physical Educator, 65*(4), 180-194.

Hoeger, W.K., Turner, L.W., & Hafen, B.Q. (2007). *Wellness: Guidelines for a healthy lifestyle* (4th ed.). Belmont, CA: Thomson Wadsworth.

Holt, N.L., Black, D.E., Tamminen, K.A., Fox, K.R., & Mandigo, J.L. (2008). Levels of social complexity and dimensions of peer experiences in youth sport. *Journal of Sport & Exercise Psychology, 30*(4), 411-431.

Horney, K. (1939). *New ways in psychoanalysis.* New York: Norton.

Horton, I. (1996.) Towards the construction of a model of counseling: Some issues. In R. Bayne, I. Horton, & J. Bimrose (Eds.), *New directions in counselling* (pp. 281-296). London: Routledge.

Horvath, A., & Greenberg, L. (1994). Introduction. In A. Horvath & L. Greenberg (Eds.), *The working alliance: Theory, research, and practice* (pp. 1-9). New York: Wiley.

Hunt, J. (2009). Building Integral Coaching Canada: A practice journey. *Journal of Integral Theory and Practice, 4*(1), 121-149.

Hutchins, D.E., & Vaught, C.C. (1997). *Helping relationships and strategies* (3rd ed.). Pacific Grove, CA: Brooks/Cole.

Huxley, A. (1932). *Brave new world.* London: Chatto and Windus.

Ifedi, F. (2008). Sports participation in Canada, 2005. In Statistics Canada (Eds.), *Culture, tourism and the Centre for Education statistics research papers.* Ottawa: Statistics Canada. Retrieved from www.statcan.gc.ca/pub/81-595-m/81-595-m2008060-eng.pdf

Illich, I. (1972). *Deschooling society.* London: Calder and Boyars.

International Coach Federation (ICF). (2011a). *Benefits of Coaching.* Retrieved from www.coachfederation.org/find-a-coach/benefits-of-coaching/

International Coach Federation (ICF). (2011b). *Coaching FAQs.* Retrieved from www.coachfederation.org/clients/coaching-faqs/

International Coach Federation (ICF). (2011c). *ICF core competencies.* Retrieved from www.coachfederation.org/icfcredentials/core-competencies/

International Coach Federation (ICF). (2012). *2012 Global coaching study final report.* Lexington, KY: ICF.

Ivey, A.E., & Ivey, M.B., & Simek-Morgan, L. (1997). *Counseling and psychotherapy: A multicultural perspective* (4th ed.). Boston: Allyn & Bacon.

Ivey, A.E., Ivey, M.B., & Zalaquett, C.P. (2010). *Intentional interviewing and counseling: Facilitating client development in a multicultural society* (7th ed.). Belmont, CA: Brooks/Cole.

Jaafar, J., Kolodinsky, P., McCarthy, S., & Schroder, V. (2004). The impact of cultural norms and values on the moral judgment of Malay and American adolescents: A brief report. In B.N. Setiadi, A. Supratiknya, W.J. Lonner, & Y.H. Poortinga (Eds.), *Ongoing themes in psychology and culture* (online ed.). Melbourne, FL: International Association for Cross-Cultural Psychology. Retrieved from www.iaccp.org

Jakicic, J.M., Davis, K.K., Garcia, D.O., Verba, S., & Pellegrini, C. (2010). Objective monitoring of physical activity in overweight and obese populations. *Physical Therapy Reviews, 15*(3), 163-169. doi:10.1179/1743288X10Y.0000000003

James, R.K., & Gilliland, B.E. (2003). *Theories and strategies in counseling and psychotherapy* (5th ed.). Boston: Allyn & Bacon.

Joanisse, L., & Synnott, A. (1999). Fighting back: Reactions and resistance to the stigma of obesity. In J. Sobal & D. Maurer (Eds.), *Interpreting weight: The social management of fatness and thinness* (pp. 49-70). New York: Aldine de Gruyter.

Johnson, D.W. (2009). *Reaching out: Interpersonal effectiveness and self-actualization* (10th ed.). Upper Saddle River, NJ: Pearson Education.

Jung, C.G. (1969). *The psychology of the transference.* Princeton, NJ: Princeton University Press.

Kabat-Zinn, J. (2005). *Coming to our senses.* London, UK: Piatkus.

Kahn, W.A. (2005). *Holding fast: The struggle to create resilient caregiving organizations.* New York: Brunner-Routledge.

Katzmarzyk, P.T., & Ardern, C.I. (2004). Physical activity levels of Canadian children and youth: Current issues and recommendations. *Canadian Journal of Diabetes, 28*(1), 67-78.

Kazdin, A.E., & Wassell, G. (1998). Treatment completion and therapeutic change among children referred for outpatient therapy. *Professional Psychology: Research and Practice, 29*(4), 332-340.

Kegan, R. (1995). *In over our heads: Mental demands of modern life.* Cambridge, MA: Harvard University Press.

Kenny, M.C., Alvarez, K., Donohue, B.C., & Winick, C.B. (2008). Overview of behavioral assessment with adults. In M. Hersen & J. Rosqvist (Eds.), *Handbook of psychological assessment, case conceptualization, and treatment* (Vol. 1, pp. 3-25). Hoboken, NJ: Wiley.

Kernis, M.H., & Goldman, B.M. (2005). Authenticity, social motivation and psychological adjustment. In J.P. Forgas, K.D. Williams, & S.M. Laham (Eds.), *Social motivation: Conscious and unconscious processes* (pp. 210-227). New York: Cambridge University Press.

Kets de Vries, M.F.R. (2006). *The leader on the couch: A clinical approach to changing people and organizations.* San Francisco: Jossey-Bass.

Kimsey-House, H., Kimsey-House, K., & Sandahl, P. (2011). *Co-active coaching: Changing business, transforming lives* (3rd ed.). Boston: Brealey.

Kleinke, C.L. (1994). *Common principles of psychotherapy.* Pacific Grove, CA: Brooks/Cole.

Knapp, M.L., & Daly, J.A. (2002). (Eds.). *Handbook of interpersonal communication* (3rd ed.). Thousand Oaks, CA: Sage.

Knapp, M.L. & Hall, J.A. (2010). *Nonverbal communication in human interaction* (7th ed.). Boston: Wadsworth, Cengage Learning.

Knowles, M.S. (1980). *The modern practice of adult education: From pedagogy to andragogy.* Englewood Cliffs, NJ: Prentice Hall/Cambridge.

Kohlberg, L. (1981). *Essays on moral development.* San Francisco: HarperCollins

Kohut, H. (1984). *How does analysis cure?* Chicago: University of Chicago Press.

Kolb, D.A. (1984). *Experiential learning: Experience as the source of learning and development.* Upper Saddle River, NJ: Prentice Hall.

Kolb. D.A., & Fry, R. (1975). Toward an applied theory of experiential learning. In C. Cooper (Ed.), *Theories of group process* (pp. 33-58). London: Wiley.

Kornfield, J. (2008). *The wise heart: A guide to the universal teachings of Buddhist psychology.* New York: Bantam Books.

Kottler, J.A. (2008). *A brief primer of helping skills* (2nd ed.). Thousand Oaks, CA: Sage.

Kottler, J.A. (2010). *On being a therapist* (4th ed.). San Francisco: Jossey-Bass.

Kottler, J.A., & Shepard, D.S. (2011). *Introduction to counseling: Voices from the field.* Belmont, CA: Brooks/Cole.

Kratcoski, P.C. (2004). *Correctional counseling and treatment* (5th ed.). Long Grove, IL: Waveland Press.

Kurz, R., & Prestera, H. (1976). *The body reveals: An illustrated guide to the psychology of the body.* New York: Harper & Row.

Ladany, N., Walker, J.A., Pate-Carolan, L.M., & Evans, L.G. (2008). *Practicing counseling and psychotherapy: Insights from trainees, supervisors and clients.* New York: Routledge.

Lakoff, G., & Johnson, M. (1980). *Metaphors we live by.* Chicago: University of Chicago Press.

Lambert, M.J., & Barley, D.E. (2001). Research summary on the therapeutic relationship and psychotherapy outcome. *Psychotherapy: Theory, Research, Practice, Training, 38*(4), 357-361.

Larimer, M.E., Palmer, R.S., & Marlatt, G.A. (1999). Relapse prevention: An overview of Marlatt's cognitive-behavioral model. *Alcohol Research and Health, 23*(2), 151-160.

Latham, G.P., Ganegoda, D.B., & Locke, E.A. (2011). Goal setting: A state theory but related to traits. In T. Chamorro-Premuzic, S. von Strumm, & A. Furham (Eds.), *Wiley-Blackwell handbook of individual differences* (pp. 579-588). New York: Wiley-Blackwell.

Latham, G., & Locke, E.A. (2002). Building a practically useful theory of goal setting and task motivation. *American Psychologist, 57*(9), 707-709.

Lau, D.C.W., Douketis, J.D., Morrison, K.M., Hramiak, I.M., Sharma, A.M., & Ur, E., for members of the Obesity Canada Clinical Practice Guidelines Expert Panel. (2007). 2006 Canadian clinical practice guidelines on the management and prevention of obesity in adults and children [summary]. *Canadian Medical Association Journal, 176*(suppl. 8), s1-s13.

Lawley, J., & Tompkins, P. (2000). *Metaphors in mind: Transformation through symbolic modeling.* London, UK: The Developing Company Press.

Lazarus, A.A., & Zur, O. (Eds.). (2002). *Dual relationships and psychotherapy.* New York: Springer.

Lazarus, R.S., & Lazarus, B.N. (1994). *Passion and reason: Making sense of our emotions.* New York: Oxford University Press.

Levinson, H. (1976). *Psychological man.* Oxford, UK: Levinson Institute.

Lewin, K. (1935). *A dynamic theory of personality.* New York: McGraw-Hill.

Lippke, S., Ziegelmann, J.P., & Schwarzer, R. (2005). Stage-specific adoption and maintenance of physical activity: Testing a three-stage model. *Psychology of Sport and Exercise, 6*(5), 585-603.

Locke, E.A., & Latham, G.P. (1985). The application of goal setting to sports. *Journal of Sport Psychology, 7*, 205-222.

Locke, E.A., & Latham, G.P. (1990). Work motivation and satisfaction: Light at the end of the tunnel. *Psychological Science, 1*(4), 240-246.

Locke, E.A., Shaw, K.N., Saari, L.M., & Latham, G.P. (1981). Goal setting and task performance: 1969-1980. *Psychological Bulletin, 90*, 125-152.

Lofgren, I., Herron, K., Zern, T., West, K., Patalay, M., Shachter, N.S., et al. (2004). Waist circumference is a better predictor than body mass index of coronary heart disease risk in overweight premenopausal women. *Journal of Nutrition, 134*(5), 1071-1076.

Lorenz, E.N. (1972, December). *Predictability: Does the flap of a butterfly's wings in Brazil set off a tornado in Texas?* Paper presented at the American Association for the Advancement of Science, 139th Meeting, Boston. Retrieved from http://eapsweb.mit.edu/research/Lorenz/Butterfly_1972.pdf

Luborsky, L., & Barrett, M.S. (2006). The history and empirical status of key psychoanalytic concepts. *Annual Review of Clinical Psychology, 2*, 1-19.

Luft, J. (1969). *Of human interaction*. Palo Alto, CA: National Press.

Luszczynska, A., Gutiérrez-Doña, B., & Schwarzer, R. (2005). General self-efficacy in various domains of human functioning: Evidence from five countries. *International Journal of Psychology, 40*(2), 80-89.

Lynch, A., Elmore, B. & Morgan, T. (2012). *Choosing health*. San Francisco: Pearson Education.

Marlatt, G.A., & Donovan, D.M. (2008). *Relapse prevention: Maintenance strategies in the treatment of addictive behaviors* (2nd ed.). New York: Guilford Press.

Marlatt, G.A., & Gordon, J.R. (1985). *Relapse prevention: Maintenance strategies in the treatment of addictive behaviors*. New York: Guilford Press.

Marquez, D.X., & McAuley, E. (2001). Physique anxiety and self-efficacy influences on perceptions of physical evaluation. *Social Behavior & Personality, 29*(7), 649-660.

Marshall, S., & Biddle, S. (2001). The transtheoretical model of behavior change: A meta-analysis of applications to physical activity and exercise. *Annals of Behavioral Medicine, 23*, 229-246.

Martin, C. (2001). *The life coaching handbook: Everything you need to be an effective life coach*. Carmarthen, Wales: Crown House.

Maslow, A.H. (1962). *Toward a psychology of being*. Princeton, NJ: Van Nostrand.

Mathews, B. (1988). The role of therapist self-disclosure in psychotherapy: A survey of therapists. *American Journal of Psychotherapy, 42*, 521-53.

May, R. (1996). *The meaning of anxiety* (rev. ed.). New York: Norton.

Mcbrearty, M. (2010). *Women, obesity, and weight loss: Bridging the intention-behaviour gap*. Dissertation Abstracts International (Section A, 71).

Mearns, D., & Thorne, B. (2007). *Person-centred counselling in action* (3rd ed). London: Sage.

Mehr, J.J., & Kanwischer, R. (2011). *Human services: Concepts and intervention strategies* (11th ed.). Boston: Allyn & Bacon.

Mehrabian, A. (1981). *Silent messages: Implicit communication of emotions and attitudes* (2nd ed.). Belmont, CA: Wadsworth.

Mental Health America. (2012). *Mind your stress—on the job*. Retrieved from www.mentalhealthamerica.net/go/mind-your-stress-on-the-job

Merriam, S.B. (2004). The role of cognitive development in Mezirow's transformational learning theory. *Adult Education Quarterly, 55*(1), 60-68.

Mezirow, J. (1994). Understanding transformation theory. *Adult Education Quarterly, 44*(4), 222-232.

Mezirow, J. (2000). Learning to think like an adult: Core concepts of transformation theory. In J. Mezirow (Ed.), *Learning as transformation: Critical perspectives on a theory in progress* (pp. 3-34). San Francisco: Jossey-Bass.

Miles, L.L. (2007). Physical activity and health. *Nutrition Bulletin, 32*(4), 314-363. doi:10.1111/j.1467-3010.2007.00668.x

Muennig, P., Lubetkin, E., Jia, H., & Franks, P. (2006). Gender and the burden of disease attributable to obesity. *American Journal of Public Health, 96*(9), 1662-1668.

Murphy, S., Xu, J., & Kochanek, K. (2012). Deaths: Preliminary data for 2010. *National Vital Statistics Report, 4*(60).

Myers, D., & Hayes, J.A. (2006). Effects of therapist general self-disclosure and countertransference disclosure on ratings of the therapist and session. *Psychotherapy: Theory, Research, Practice, Training, 43*(2), 173-185.

Nagy, T.F. (2011). *Essential ethics for psychologists: A primer for understanding and mastering core issues*. Washington, DC: American Psychological Association.

National Center for Health Statistics (NCHS). (2011). *Health, United States, 2010: With special feature on death and dying*. Retrieved from www.cdc.gov/nchs/data/hus/hus10.pdf#066

National Institute of Mental Health (NIMH). (2005). *Any disorder among adults*. Retrieved from www.nimh.nih.gov/statistics/1ANYDIS_ADULT.shtml

Neenan, M., & Dryden, W. (2002). *Life coaching: A cognitive-behavioural approach*. East Sussex, UK: Brunner-Routledge.

Norcross, J. (2002). *Psychotherapy relationships that work: Therapist relational contributions to effective psychotherapy*. London: Oxford University Press.

Ogden, C.L., Carroll, M.D., Kit, B.K., & Flegal, K.M. (2012). *Prevalence of obesity in the United States, 2009-2010*. Centers for Disease Control and Prevention. Retrieved from www.cdc.gov/nchs/data/databriefs/db82.pdf

Ogden, J., & Hills, L. (2008). Understanding sustained changes in behaviour: The role of life events and the process of reinvention. *Health: An International Journal, 12*, 419-437.

Paffenbarger, R.S., & Lee, I. (1998). A natural history of athleticism, health and longevity. *Journal of Sports Sciences*, 1631-1645. doi:10.1080/026404198366957

Palmer, P.J. (2000). *Let your life speak: Listening for the voice of vocation*. San Francisco: Jossey-Bass.

Palmer, S. & Whybrow, A. (Eds.). (2007). *Handbook of coaching psychology: A guide for practitioners*. London/New York: Routledge.

Parrott, L. (2003). *Counseling and psychotherapy* (2nd ed.). Pacific Grove, CA: Thomson/Brooks/Cole.

Patterson, C.H. (2000). *Understanding psychotherapy: Fifty years of client-centred theory and practice*. Ross-on-Wye: PCCS Books.

Pedersen, P., Crethar, H.C., & Carlson, J. (2008). *Inclusive cultural empathy: Making relationships central in counseling and psychotherapy*. Washington, DC: American Psychological Association.

Pekarik, G., & Finney-Owen, K. (1987). Outpatient clinic therapist attitudes and beliefs relevant to client dropout. *Community Mental Health Journal, 23*(2), 120-130.

Peterson, C., & Seligman, M. (2004). *Character strengths and virtues: A handbook and classification*. Washington, DC: Oxford University Press.

Piaget, J. (1952). *The origins of intelligence in children*. New York: International University Press.

Pi-Sunyer, X.F. (2002). The obesity epidemic: Pathophysiology and consequences of obesity. *Obesity Research, 10*(2), 97S-104S.

Pi-Sunyer, X.F. (2004). The epidemiology of central fat distribution in relation to disease. *Nutrition Reviews, 62*(7 suppl.), S120-S126.

Powers, S.K., Dodd, S.L., Thompson, A.M., & Condon, C.C. (2005). *Total fitness and wellness* (Canadian ed.). Toronto: Pearson Education Canada.

Prochaska, J.O., & Norcross, J.C. (2010). *Systems of psychotherapy: A transtheoretical analysis* (7th ed.). Belmont, CA: Brooks/Cole.

Prochaska, J.O., Norcross, J.C., & DiClemente, C.C. (1994). *Changing for good*. New York: Avon Books.

Prochaska, J.O., Norcross, J.C., & DiClemente, C.C. (2002). *Changing for good: The revolutionary program that explains the six stages of change and teaches you how to free yourself from bad habits*. New York: Quill.

Puhl, R., & Heuer, C.A. (2009). The stigma of obesity: A review and update. *Obesity, 17*(5), 941-964.

Quenck, N.L. (2009). *Essentials of Myers-Briggs type indicator assessment* (2nd ed.). Hoboken, NJ: Wiley.

Raines, J.C. (1996). Self-disclosure in clinical social work. *Clinical Social Work Journal, 24*(4), 357-375.

Ratcliff-Daffron, S. (2003). *Andragogy: Malcom S. Knowles*. Retrieved from www.trainandeducate.com/docs/ipte_te2.pdf

Rehab International. (2012). *Statistics: What is gambling addiction*. Retrieved from http://rehab-international.org/gambling-addiction/gambling-addiction-statistics

Reis, B., & Brown, L. (1999). Reducing psychotherapy dropouts: Maximizing perspective convergence in psychotherapy dyad. *Psychotherapy, 36*, 123-136.

Rogers, C.R. (1951). *Client-centered therapy: Its current practice, implications and theory*. Boston: Houghton Mifflin.

Rogers, C.R. (1957). The necessary and sufficient conditions of therapeutic personality change. *Journal of Consulting Psychology, 21*(2), 95-103.

Rogers, C.R. (1961). *On becoming a person.* Boston: Houghton Mifflin.

Rogers, C.R. (1980). *A way of being.* Boston: Houghton Mifflin.

Rogers, C.R., & Farson, R.E. (1995). Active listening. In D.A. Kolb, J.S. Osland, & I.M. Rubin (Eds.), *The organizational behavior reader* (6th ed., pp. 203-214). New York: Wiley.

Rogers, C.R., & Sanford, R. (1984). Client-centered psychotherapy. In H.I. Kaplan & B.J. Sadock (Eds.), *Comprehensive textbook of psychiatry IV* (pp. 1374-1388). Baltimore: Williams & Wilkins.

Rorive, M., Letiexhe, M.R., Scheen, A.J., & Ziegler, O. (2005). Obesity and type 2 diabetes. *Revue de medicine de Liège, 60*(5-6), 374-382.

Rosenstock, I.M., Strecher, V.J., & Becker, M.H. (1988). Social learning theory and the health belief model. *Health education quarterly, 15*(2), 175-183.

Ruby, M.B., Dunn, E.W., Perrino, A., Gillis, R., & Viel, S. (2011). The invisible benefits of exercise. *Health Psychology, 30*(1), 67-74. doi:10.1037/a0021859

Ruiz, M.A. (2001). *The four agreements: A practical guide to personal freedom* (special ed.). San Rafael, CA: Amber-Allen.

Saint-Exupéry, A. de (1958). *Le petit prince* (2nd ed.). London: Heinemann.

Scharmer, C.O. (2007). *Theory U: Leading from the future as it emerges.* San Francisco: Berrett-Kohler.

Schneider, K.J. (2008). (Ed.). *Existential-integrative psychotherapy: Guideposts to the core of practice.* New York: Taylor & Francis Group.

Schön, D.A. (2003). *The reflective practitioner: How professionals think in action.* Aldershot, UK: Ashgate.

Schwarzer, R. (1992). Self-efficacy in the adoption and maintenance of health behaviors: Theoretical approaches and a new model. In R. Schwarzer (Ed.), *Self-efficacy: Thought control of action* (pp. 217-243). Washington, DC: Hemisphere.

Schwarzer, R. (2001). Social-cognitive factors in changing health-related behaviors. *Current Directions in Psychological Science, 10*(2), 47-51.

Schwarzer, R. (2006). *Health action process approach.* Retrieved from http://userpage.fu-berlin.de/~health/hapa.htm

Segal, D.L., June, A., & Marty, M.A. (2010). Basic issues in interviewing and the interview process. In D.H. Segal & M. Hersen (Eds.), *Diagnostic interviewing* (4th ed., pp. 1-22). New York, NY: Springer.

Seligman, M.E.P. (1975). *Helplessness: On depression, development, and death.* New York: Freeman.

Seligman, M.E.P. (2006). *Learned optimism: How to change your mind and your life.* New York: Vintage Press.

Seligman, M.E.P., & Csikszentmihalyi, M. (2000). Positive psychology: An introduction. *American Psychologist, 55*, 5-14.

Selye, H. (1956). *The stress of life.* New York: McGraw-Hill.

Senge, P.M. (1990). *The fifth discipline: The art and practice of the learning organization.* New York: Currency Doubleday.

Senge, P.M. (2006). *The fifth discipline: The art and practice of the learning organization* (rev. ed.). New York: Doubleday/Currency.

Senge, P., Scharmer, C.O., Jaworski, J., & Flowers, B.S. (2004). *Presence: Human purpose and the field of the future.* New York: Doubleday.

Sexton, T.L., Whiston, S.G., Bleuer, J.C., & Walz, G.R. (1997). *Integrating outcome research into counseling practice and training.* Alexandria, VA: American Counseling Association.

Sharpley, C.F., Fairnie, E., Tabary-Collins, E., Bates, R., & Lee, P. (2000). The use of counselor verbal response modes and client-perceived rapport. *Counselling Psychology Quarterly, 13*(1), 99-116.

Shebib, B. (2010). *Choices: Interviewing and counselling skills for Canadians* (4th ed.). Toronto: Pearson Education Canada.

Sheehy, G. (1976). *Passages: Predictable crises of adult life.* New York: Dutton.

Sheldon, K.M., Cummins, R., & Kamble, S. (2010). Life balance and well-being: Testing a novel conceptual and measurement approach. *Journal of Personality, 78*(4), 1093-1134.

Sheldon, K.M., & Kasser, T. (1995). Coherence and congruence: Two aspects of personality and integration. *Journal of Personality and Social Psychology, 68*, 531-543.

Silsbee, D.K. (2010). *The mindful coach: Seven roles for facilitating leader development* (rev. ed.). San Francisco: Jossey-Bass.

Simone, D. H., McCarthy, P., & Skay, C. L. (1998). An investigation of client and counselor variables that influence likelihood of counselor self-disclosure. *Journal of Counseling and Devlopment, 76*, 174-182.

Skibbins, D. (2007). *Becoming a life coach: A complete workbook for therapists.* Oakland, CA: New Harbinger.

Skinner, B.F. (1938). *The behavior of organisms: An experimental analysis.* New York: Appleton-Century-Crofts.

Skinner, B.F. (1953). *Science and human behavior.* New York: McMillan.

Smith, D., & Fitzpatick, M. (1995). Patient-therapist boundary issues: An integrative review of theory and research. *Professional Psychology: Research and Practice, 26*(5), 499-506.

Smith, J.V. (2007). *Therapist into coach.* New York: Open University Press.

Smits, J.A.J., Tart, C.D., Presnell, K., Rosenfield, D., & Otto, M.W. (2010). Identifying potential barriers to physical activity adherence: Anxiety sensitivity and body mass as predictors of fear during exercise. *Cognitive Behaviour Therapy, 39,* 28-36.

Sommer, R. (2007). *Personal space: The behavioral basis of design* (updated ed.). Bristol, UK: Bosko Books.

Sommers-Flanagan, J., & Sommers-Flanagan, R. (2009). *Clinical interviewing* (4th ed.). Hoboken, NJ: Wiley.

Stalikas, A., & Fitzpatrick, M. (1995). Client good moments: An intensive analysis of a single session. *Canadian Journal of Counseling, 29*(2), 160-175.

Stalikas, A., & Fitzpatrick, M. (1996). Relationships between counselor interventions, client experiencing, and emotional expressiveness: An exploratory study. *Canadian Journal of Counselling, 30*(4), 262-271.

Statistics Canada. (2008). *Leading causes of death, by sex.* Retrieved from www.statcan.gc.ca/tables-tableaux/sum-som/l01/cst01/hlth36a-eng.htm

Statistics Canada. (2009). *Who participates in active leisure?* Retrieved from www.statcan.gc.ca/pub/11-008-x/2009001/article/10690-eng.pdf

Statistics Canada. (2010). *Physical activity during leisure time, 2010.* Retrieved from www.statcan.gc.ca/pub/82-625-x/2011001/article/11467-eng.htm

Statistics Canada. (2012a). *High blood pressure, by age group and sex.* Retrieved from www.statcan.gc.ca/tables-tableaux/sum-som/l01/cst01/health03a-eng.htm

Statistics Canada. (2012b). *Life expectancy at birth, by sex, by province.* Retrieved from www.statcan.gc.ca/tables-tableaux/sum-som/l01/cst01/health26-eng.htm

Statistics Canada. (2012c). *Body mass index, overweight or obese, self-reported, adult, by age group and sex.* Retrieved from www.statcan.gc.ca/tables-tableaux/sum-som/l01/cst01/health81a-eng.htm

Statistics Canada. (2012d). *Health trends: Age-standardized rates, both sexes, Canada (Catalogue No. 82-213-XWE).* Retrieved from www12.statcan.gc.ca/health-sante/82-213/

Statistics Canada. (2012e). *Diabetes, by sex, provinces and territories.* Retrieved from www.statcan.gc.ca/tables-tableaux/sum-som/l01/cst01/health54a-eng.htm

Steele, D. (2011). *From therapist to coach: How to leverage your clinical expertise to build a thriving coaching practice.* Hoboken, NJ: Wiley.

Stober, D.R. (2006). Coaching from the humanistic perspective. In D.R. Stober, & A.M. Grant (Eds.), *Evidence-based coaching handbook: Putting best practices to work for your client* (pp. 17-50). Hoboken, NJ: Wiley.

Stober, D. R. & Grant, A. M. (2006). *Evidence-based coaching handbook: Putting best practices to work for your client.* Hoboken, NJ: John Wiley & Sons, Inc..

Stoltzfus, T. (2008). *Coaching questions: A coach's guide to powerful asking skills.* Virginia Beach, VA: Pegasus Creative Arts.

Strachan, D. (2001). *Questions that work: A resource for facilitators.* Ottawa, ON: ST Press.

Strean, H. (1986). *Countertransference.* Philadelphia: Haworth Press.

Stringer, E.T. (2007). *Action research* (3rd ed.). Thousand Oaks, CA: Sage.

Sue, D.W., & Sue, D. (2008). *Counseling the culturally diverse: Theory and practice* (5th ed.). Hoboken, NJ: Wiley.

Suinn, R.M. (1986). *Seven steps to peak performance: The mental training manual for athletes.* Lewiston, NY: Huber.

Surya Das, L. (1997). *Awakening the Buddha within: Tibetan wisdom for the Western world.* New York: Broadway Books.

Sweet, C., & Noones, J. (1989). Factors associated with premature termination from outpatient treatments. *Hospital and Community Psychiatry, 40*(9), 947-951.

Tamminen, A.W., & Smaby, M.H. (1981). Helping counselors learn to confront. *Personnel and Guidance Journal, 60,* 41-45.

Taylor, M. (1986). Learning for self-direction in the classroom: The pattern of a transition process. *Studies in Higher Education, 11*(1), 55-72.

Tenenbaum, G., & Eklund, R.C. (Eds.). (2007). *Handbook of sport psychology* (3rd ed.). Hoboken, NJ: Wiley.

Tennant, M. (2006). *Psychology and adult learning.* New York: Routledge.

Teyber, E., & McClure, F.H. (2011). *Interpersonal process in therapy: An integrative model* (6th ed.). Belmont, CA: Brooks/Cole.

Tjepkema, M. (2004). Measured obesity—adult obesity in Canada: Measured height and weight. In Statistics Canada (Ed.), *Nutrition: Findings from the Canadian community health survey,* pp. 1-32. Ottawa: Statistics Canada.

Tolle, E. (2004). *The power of now: A guide to spiritual enlightenment.* Novato, CA: New World Library.

Trenholm, S., Jensen, A., & Hambly, H. (2010). *Interpersonal communication: A guided tour for Canadians.* Toronto: Oxford University Press.

Trotzer, J.P. (2006). *The counselor and the group: Integrating theory, training, and practice* (4th ed.). New York: Routledge.

Truax, C.B., & Carkhuff, R.R. (1967). *Toward effective counseling and psychotherapy: Training and practice.* Chicago: Aldine.

Turock, A. (1980). Immediacy in counseling: Recognizing clients' unspoken messages. *Personnel and Guidance Journal, 59,* 168-172.

U.S. Department of Health and Human Services (HHS). (2008). *Physical activity guidelines for Americans.* Retrieved from www.health.gov/PAGuidelines/factsheetprof.aspx

Vallerand, R.J. (1997). Toward a hierarchical model of intrinsic and extrinsic motivation. In M.P. Zanna (Ed.), *Advances in experimental social psychology* (pp. 271-360). New York: Academic Press.

Vallerand, R.J., & Rousseau, F.L. (2001). Intrinsic and extrinsic motivation in sport and exercise: A review using the hierarchical model of intrinsic and extrinsic motivation. In R. Singer, H. Hausenblas, and C. Janelle (Eds.), *Handbook of sport psychology* (2nd ed., pp. 389-416). New York: Wiley.

Varela, F.J., Thompson, E., & Rosch, E. (1992). *The embodied mind: Cognitive science and human experience.* Cambridge, MA: MIT Press.

Vohs, K.D., & Baumeister, R.F. (2010). *Handbook of self-regulation: Research, theory and applications* (2nd ed.). New York: Guilford.

Von Bertalanffy, L. (1968). *General system theory: Foundations, development, applications* (rev. ed.). New York: Braziller.

Vygotsky, L.S. (1978). *Mind in society: The development of higher psychological processes.* Cambridge, MA: President and Fellows of Harvard College.

Walker, A.P., Walker, B.F., & Adam, F. (2003). Nutrition, diet, physical activity, smoking, and longevity: From primitive hunter-gatherer to present passive consumer—How far can we go? *Nutrition, 19*(2), 169. doi:10.1016/S0899-9007(02)00948-6

Walsh, J.F. (2007). *Endings in clinical practice: Effective closure in diverse settings* (2nd ed.). Chicago: Lyceum Books.

Watkins, C.E., Jr. (1986). Transference phenomena in the counseling situation. *The Personnel and Guidance Journal, 62*(4), 206-210.

Watkins, C.E., Jr. (1990). The effects of counselor self-disclosure: A research review. *Counseling Psychologist, 18*(3), 477-500.

Weger, H., Jr., Castle, G.R., & Emmett, M.C. (2010). Active listening in peer interviews: The influence of message paraphrasing on perceptions of listening skill. *International Journal of Listening, 24*(1), 34-49.

Weinberg, R.S., & Gould, D. (2011). *Foundations of sport and exercise psychology* (5th ed.). Champaign, IL: Human Kinetics.

Weiner, I.B., & Bornstein, R.F. (2009). *Principles of psychotherapy: Promoting evidence-based psychodynamic practice* (3rd ed.). Hoboken, NJ: Wiley.

Welfel, E.R. (2010). *Ethics in counseling and psychotherapy: Standards, research, and emerging issues* (4th ed.). Belmont, CA: Wadsworth/Cengage.

Wells, T.L. (1994). Therapist self-disclosure: Its effects on clients and the treatment relationship. *Smith College Studies in Social Work, 65,* 23-41.

Whitmore, J. (1992). *Coaching for performance: A practical guide to growing your own skills.* Boston: Brealey.

Whitworth, L., Kimsey-House, H., Kimsey-House, K., & Sandahl, P. (2007). *Co-active coaching* (2nd ed.). Mountain View, CA: Davies-Black.

Widiger, T.A., & Trull, T.J. (1997). Assessment of the five-factor model of personality. *Journal of Personality Assessment, 68*(2), 228-250.

Wilber, K. (2000a). *A brief history of everything* (2nd ed.). Boston: Shambhala.

Wilber, K. (2000b). *A brief theory of everything: An integral vision for business, politics, science and spirituality.* Boston: Shambhala.

Wilber, K. (2000c). Integral psychology: Consciousness, spirit, psychology, therapy. Boston: Shambhala.

Wilber, K., Patten, T., Leonard, A., & Morelli, M. (2008). Integral life practice: A 21st-century blueprint for physical health, emotional balance, mental clarity, and spiritual awakening. Boston: Integral Books.

Williams, P. (2008). The life coach operating system: Its foundations in psychology. In D.B. Drake, D. Brennan, & K. Gortz (Eds.), *The philosophy and practice of coaching: Insights and issues for a new era* (pp. 3-26). West Sussex, England: Wiley.

Williams, P.A., & Cash, T.F. (2001). Effects of a circuit weight training program on the body images of college students. *International Journal of Eating Disorders, 30*(1), 75-82.

Williams, P., & Davis, D.C. (2007). *Therapist as life coach: An introduction for counselors and other helping professionals* (rev. ed.). New York: Norton.

Winnicott, D.W. (1958). The capacity to be alone. *International Journal of Psycho-Analysis, 39,* 416-420.

World Health Organization (WHO). (1946). Constitution of the World Health Organization. *American Journal of Public Health Nations Health, 36*(11), 1315-1323.

World Health Organization (WHO). (1998). *Obesity: Preventing and managing the global epidemic. Report of a WHO consultation on obesity. WHO/NUT/NCD/98.1.* Retrieved from http://whqlibdoc.who.int/hq/1998/WHO_NUT_NCD_98.1_(p1-158).pdf

World Health Organization (WHO). (2012). *Obesity and overweight fact sheet no. 311.* Retrieved from www.who.int/mediacentre/factsheets/fs311/en/index.html

Yalom, I.D. (1980). *Existential psychotherapy.* New York: Basic Books.

Young, D.R., Jerome, G.J., Chen, C., Laferriere, D., & Vollmer, W.M. (2009). Patterns of physical activity among overweight and obese adults. *Preventing Chronic Disease, 6*(3). Retrieved from www.ncbi.nlm.nih.gov/pmc/articles/PMC2722396/

Young, J.E., Klosko, J.S., & Weishaar, M.E. (2003). *Schema therapy: A practitioner's guide.* New York: Guilford Press.

Young, M.E. (2009). *Learning the art of helping: Building blocks and techniques* (4th ed.). Upper Saddle River, NJ: Prentice Hall.

Zunker, C., Cox, T.L., Ard, J.D., Ivankova, N.V., Rutt, C.D., & Baskin, M.L. (2011). Maintaining healthy behaviors following weight loss: A grounded theory approach. *Journal of Ethnographic & Qualitative Research, 5*(3), 186-204.

Zur, O. (2004). To cross or not to cross: Do boundaries in therapy protect or harm? *Psychotherapy Bulletin, 39*(3), 27-32.

Zur, O. (2009). Therapeutic boundaries and effective therapy: Exploring the relationships. In W. O'Donahue & S.R. Graybar (Eds.), *Handbook of contemporary psychotherapy: Towards an improved understanding of effective psychotherapy* (pp. 341-355). Thousand Oaks, CA: Sage.

# INDEX

*Note:* The italicized *f* and *t* following page numbers refer to figures and tables, respectively.

# ABOUT THE AUTHORS

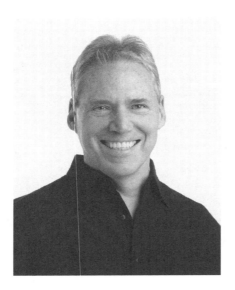

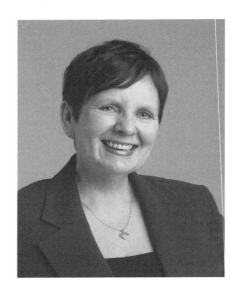

**James Gavin, PhD,** has been designing and delivering coach training programs to health, wellness, and fitness professionals since 1998. He is the director of the Centre for Human Relations and Community Studies and a full professor in the department of applied human sciences at Concordia University in Montreal, Canada. He has consulted with health, wellness, and fitness centers for 25 years and has been a practitioner of counseling psychology for more than 35 years. Gavin was awarded a Diplomate in Counseling Psychology by the American Board of Professional Psychology, the highest award recognizing achievement and excellence in the practice of counseling psychology. He has written and researched extensively concerning personality matching related to active living since the early 1980s and has presented around the world at health fitness conferences since 1985. Gavin is also the author of *Psychology for Health/Fitness Professionals.* He is a long-time practitioner of aikido, iaido, and yoga and has pursued other passions such as triathlon training, kayaking, and tai chi.

**Madeleine Mcbrearty, PhD**, is codirector and faculty member for the Professional and Personal Coaching Certification (PPCC) program offered through the Centre for Human Relations and Community Studies at Concordia University in Montreal, Canada. As an organizational change agent and executive coach, she works with people in community and not-for-profit organizations. She conducts workshops to promote wellness in the workplace and is currently involved in a number of projects concerned with physical fitness and psychological well-being. As a personal coach, her passion is to walk alongside those who want to achieve their personal life vision. The focus of Mcbrearty's academic research is personal change. She works with women in weight management as a means of understanding intrapersonal change processes.